Peter Machamer

pay what

HISTORY
OF MEDICAL
ILLUSTRATION

"I DO NOT WISH
THE PUBLIC TO READ
ENTIRELY WITHOUT
EFFORT WHAT I HAVE
WRITTEN NOT ENTIRELY
WITHOUT EFFORT"

Petrarch

ROBERT HERRLINGER †

HISTORY OF MEDICAL ILLUSTRATION

FROM ANTIQUITY TO A.D. 1600

Preface by F. N. L. Poynter Ph.D. D. Litt. Hon. M.D. (Kiel),
Director of the Wellcome Institute of the History of Medicine, London
President of the International Academy of the History of Medicine

PITMAN MEDICAL & SCIENTIFIC PUBLISHING CO. LTD.

Published and distributed by Pitman Medical and Scientific Publishing Co. Ltd.

Printed and bound in the Netherlands by C. C. and G. F. Callenbach N.V. – Nijkerk.

Translated from the German edition – published by Heinz Moos Verlagsgesellschaft mbH & Co KG, München – by Graham Fulton-Smith.

ROBERT HERRLINGER †

HISTORY OF MEDICAL ILLUSTRATION

FROM ANTIQUITY TO A.D. 1600

Preface by F. N. L. Poynter Ph.D. D. Litt. Hon. M.D. (Kiel),
Director of the Wellcome Institute of the History of Medicine, London
President of the International Academy of the History of Medicine

PITMAN MEDICAL & SCIENTIFIC PUBLISHING CO. LTD.

Published and distributed by Pitman Medical and Scientific Publishing Co. Ltd.

Printed and bound in the Netherlands by C. C. and G. F. Callenbach N.V. – Nijkerk.

Translated from the German edition – published by Heinz Moos Verlagsgesellschaft mbH & Co KG, München – by Graham Fulton-Smith.

IN MEMORIAM: ROBERT HERRLINGER

A number of books on "Medicine in Art" have been published in recent years, but the book which is here presented to English-speaking readers for the first time is not another addition to that list. It is not concerned with medical aspects of the works of the old masters, but with the illustrations of down-to-earth medical texts executed by mainly unknown artists with the sole aim of conveying practical instruction. It is only incidentally that many of these illustrations, especially those from the earlier Middle Ages, are now found to provide unexpected treasure for the historian of art. They are primarily pictorial records illustrating medical thought and practice over two thousand years, and are of great concern to the historian of medicine.

In the course of time we might have expected an accumulation of separate studies by experts in these disciplines to provide some kind of general view of the place of these illustrations in the history of European art and of their value as medical documents. What is completely unexpected – and what makes the publication of this volume a unique and exciting event – is that it is the work of a single individual who combined in himself all the necessary qualifications and skills. For Robert Herrlinger was a highly qualified art historian and a medical historian, as well as a practising physician. His sudden death at the age of fifty-three robbed his special type of scholarship of its leading exponent only a few months after the original German edition of this work came from the press.

To claim this book as the most important which Herrlinger produced may seem exaggerated in that he was also the author of one of the most popular current German textbooks of anatomy, which reached its fourteenth edition in 1968, and of another on anatomical nomenclature which has gone into twenty-seven editions. Although these have the individual stamp of his personal scholarship, they might well have been written by another anatomist as expert as himself: but only he could have provided us with this masterly historical survey of medical illustration.

Robert Herrlinger, who came of an old and cultured German family, was born in Antwerp on April 24, 1914. After completing his studies at Heidelberg, where he was awarded an M.D. as well as a Ph.D. in the History of Art, he came to London for a year to work as a physician in the German Hospital at Dalston. On this visit, as on his later visits to England, art galleries and medical centers were rival attractions. Both of his interests grew side by side, the one as truly professional as the other. For ten years after the Second World War he worked as a practising physician, but he also began to teach in the neighboring university town of Würzburg and proved to be a born teacher, his broad sympathies and humanistic interests being readily appreciated by young students. At this time he was not only constantly working on new editions of his anatomical textbook but also publishing original papers on the history of anatomical illustration and especially on Leonardo and other Renaissance figures. In 1960 he gave up his medical practice when he was appointed professor of the history of medicine in Würzburg; two years later he was appointed to a similar chair in the Christian-Albert University in Kiel. Here too he rapidly won over medical students to an interest in his own subjects and during the long vacation would lead groups of them on expeditions to the ancient medical shrines of Cos, the birthplace of Hippocrates; and Epidaurus, with its ruined temple of Aesculapius. By this time his scholarly work had won him international as well as national recognition.

He was Assistant Secretary of the International Academy of the History of Medicine, in which professors of over thirty countries are represented, and during the last few years of his life he was President of the German Society for Hospital History. He had just begun a term of office as President of the German Society for the History of Science when, on February 8, 1968, he died suddenly from coronary heart disease.

A singularly happy family life – with a wife, also a doctor, who shared his interests; two sons who followed him into medicine; and two daughters – reinforced the energy which he always put into his career as a teacher and historian.
Of his many publications, this work on medical illustration is the one which is most peculiarly his own. It was intended to be a comprehensive history up to the present time, and the fact that the second volume – which was planned – was never completed is our loss. Nevertheless, this single volume is complete in itself; and the period which it covers, from antiquity to the beginning of the seventeenth century, is the one which is the least known and is the most rewarding field for research.

Our present interest in visual aids and their role in education gives us a special reason to turn back to the past to see how other ages and other cultures have attempted to solve the communication problem. Before the days of photography, motion pictures, and television, and still more before the days of printing and mechanized transport, the only way to convey to more than a few immediate observers the necessary instruction in certain practical techniques was to get an artist to make a drawing of the procedure. Such a drawing was more than an illustration of the accompanying text – in many cases it was the essence of the instruction.

One of the oldest medical manuscripts left to us is the early sixth-century Vienna codex of the Roman physician Dioscorides on *materia medica.* In the days when nearly all medical prescriptions were made up of tinctures, extracts, and infusions

of particular parts of plants, it was most important that the plants should be accurately identified. The name alone would be quite insufficient, and so the work of Dioscorides is set out as a picturebook of medicinal plants, with a few paragraphs of text attached to each illustration indicating the conditions for which the plant should be used and the method of administration. The text would certainly be essential to the physician, but for the pharmacist and the herb gatherer the picture would be of primary importance. What set out to be a practical manual becomes for us one of the earliest collections of botanical illustrations, from which we can judge not only what were considered the essential points of recognition but also the extent to which the artists were observers of nature and the accuracy and skill with which they represented what they saw.
Similarly, the only work on surgery from the great Islamic culture of the Middle Ages is that of Abulcasis, who wrote his book in Cordova in the tenth century. This contains the earliest illustrations of a whole range of surgical instruments, with explanations of the operations for which they should be used. This work was translated into Latin and copied from manuscript to manuscript until it was eventually printed, with woodcuts of the figures. Imagine the simple surgeon, as he was in those days, trying to convey to a cutler or blacksmith how a certain instrument should be fashioned with only a verbal description to help him! But show the cutler or smith the figure, and the design is taken in at a glance. So too with many of the surgical procedures which are depicted in medieval miniatures. These miniatures are at the same time fine examples of early primitive art and clear guides to the surgeon as to where to apply the cautery, where to let blood, or how to deal with a depressed fracture of the skull.

With the advent of printing, woodcuts take the place of painted miniatures; and in the German books of the late fifteenth and early sixteenth centuries are to be found a great variety of illustrations, of great simplicity and charm, which are most informative to the medical historian. They bring home to us, for example, far more than any study of texts could do, the ignorance of anatomy that prevailed at that time. There was little or no firsthand study of human anatomy by actual dissection until the early sixteenth century: before then, the descriptive texts of Galen had been taken as an adequate guide. Beginning with the artists of the Italian Renaissance and their study of human proportions, of surface anatomy, and of the muscles and their movements, genuine anatomical study spread to the medical schools, and eventually reached its finest achievement in the work of Vesalius with its great series of full-page illustrations. As is well known, it was at the special command of King Henry VIII that an English edition of Vesalius's work was published in 1545, with illustrations copied by Thomas Geminus that were the first copperplate engravings of any consequence produced in England.

Robert Herrlinger does full justice to this classic period of anatomical illustration, giving special attention not only to Vesalius but also to Leonardo da Vinci. Basing his work on his own dissection of more than a score of bodies, Leonardo left us a wealth of anatomical drawings, many of which are now preserved in the Royal Library at Windsor. Because these were not published for nearly four hundred years, it has usually been thought that they could have had little influence on the development of anatomy in Leonardo's own time. Some experts on Leonardo, however, have reminded us that it was customary for manuscripts and drawings to be passed around a small circle of interested scholars, and it seems probable that this was so with at least some of these drawings. Herrlinger, with his special insight as an art historian, argues that their influence can be traced in the best pre-Vesalian anatomical work, that of Berengario da Capri, published in 1521.

Other branches of medicine besides anatomy also provide fascinating illustrations from this period. The beautiful illustrations in the great herbal of Leonhart Fuchs are an outstanding contribution to botany, while the pictures of orthopedic operations echo in a remarkable way the earliest classical illustrations of similar procedures.

The technical quality of the reproductions in this volume, and especially of the superb color plates, testifies to the success with which the publisher matched the exacting standards of his author. The text is a mine of detailed information, and rarely can instruction have been so delightfully presented to the public.

F. N. L. Poynter

Contents

Foreword

> A history of anatomical illustrations seen from the point of view not of the history of medicine but of the history of art would be an extremely worthwhile undertaking that would place the whole problem in an entirely new light.
>
> Henry E. Sigerist

A good illustration is often better than a thousand words. Often the written word fails completely to communicate certain information, where a picture easily succeeds.

Originally, of course, writing itself derived from pictures: Egyptian hieroglyphs, for instance, were stylized drawings of objects. Likewise, Japanese and Chinese characters were drawings before they were simplified to their present forms.

When we take into account the important part that illustration plays in communication and when we then look back over the entire history of thought, the whole picture of man's cultural development comes into focus. For example, since thought often cannot be easily transmitted without drawings or diagrams, art plainly has an important role in the history of thought. Moreover, medicine and anatomy – forms of self-knowledge – are important aspects of man's cultural development. And it is medical illustration which unites art and medicine in this complicated scheme. Medical illustration is, therefore, part of the history of art, which is in turn part of the history of thought.

Just as the history of art is not concerned solely with general aspects of artistic form, but also with the history of individual works of art, likewise medical illustration also has its significant individual works. We need only reflect upon the singular achievements of Leonardo da Vinci in the field of anatomical illustration. But in this book we will view not only the singular achievements in medical illustration, but also the step-by-step development of the art. And we will see that as painting and drawing progressed, so medical illustration advanced and was refined. Moreover, it is the aim of this book to demonstrate close parallels between the development of fine art and the development of medical illustration.

In this book, antiquity has been treated in greater detail than later periods in order to show that the most important possibilities of didactic medical illustration had already been discovered in the classical era. Then, as medical illustration developed, emphases were modified and forms were varied as artists followed the prevailing trends in graphic arts.

The techniques by which illustrations were reproduced is another subject altogether. The reproduction of graphic art can be traced from the linear and graphic illumination of manuscripts through wood and copperplate engraving to the complex technological processes that have come into use during the last two centuries. In subsequent treatment of practical graphic art, we shall observe that while the technical aspects of its development limit the artist, they also open up new possibilities.

There are certain kinds of abstract illustrations – diagrams, charts, statistical tables – which may seem at first glance to have no relation to art. But if the graph is classified as a medical illustration, we touch upon the introduction of quantitative thinking into medicine, which in turn is related to the history of thought. Convincing arguments have been offered for regarding quantitative thinking as the beginning of modern medicine (SHRYOCK). Therefore, this history of medical illustration will also refer to such developments.

Thus, what at first glance seems to be a simple theme is in reality rather complex. Since space does not permit truly comprehensive treatment of our topic, we can only hope to bring the main lines of development into focus. Nevertheless, we hope that nothing has been omitted which might have revealed totally new aspects of the subject.

The foreword is also the place for thanking those who made this book possible. Throughout many years of work I have received support in a great many quarters, whether during my visits to libraries and museums, in correspondence with librarians and custodians, or in my discussions with academic colleagues. It is impossible to list all of them, but I should like to mention a few by name.

My publisher, HEINZ MOOS, is to be specially thanked for supplying the original idea for such an unconventional book, and for encouraging me in my inclinations. He showed, moreover, generous understanding in view of the various obstacles which stood in the way of an earlier completion of the manuscript: not only my re-appointment from Würzburg to the University of Kiel, which brought new commitments, but also the need to examine and assess a number of manuscripts in the original. I received various help for this purpose, particularly in the form of travel allowances from the German Research Association. The libraries where I have regularly worked over the years deserve particular mention: the University Libraries in Erlangen, Würzburg and Kiel, the Wellcome Historical Medical Library in London, and the various departments of the British Museum. I am also grateful for the hospitality given by many others. These source studies would have remained monologues had I not received inspiration and advice from academic colleagues. For this first volume I am greatly obliged to my colleagues L. BELLONI, F. GUERRA, E. HINTZSCHE, C. E. KELLERT, L. MÜNSTER, H. MUSPER, C. NISSEN, F. N. L. POYNTER, D. H. TURNER, E. WICKERSHEIMER and W. WIEGAND. No book can be produced without technical assistance, and this is especially true for such an unusual work. I should therefore like to thank our photographer at the Kiel Institute for the History of Medicine and Pharmacy, Miss D. SCHERR, my secretaries in Würzburg and Kiel, Mrs. G. JÜRGEN and Miss A. PHILIPP, who were supported by Mrs. W. SCHRÖDER; and, finally, my colleagues Dr. E. FEINER and Prof. F. KÜDLEIN for their unselfish assistance in looking through the typescript and suggesting corrections. I am grateful for all their cooperation: without it this book would never have been printed.

Kiel, August 5, 1967 ROBERT HERRLINGER

Antiquity

When did medicine begin to use scientific illustration? This question cannot be fully answered merely by quoting the oldest literary references to particular illustrations or by naming an original which happens to have survived. Our answer must also entail speculation about a stage in the history of medicine at which medical illustration becomes conceivable, or where it must have become necessary in order to make clear a lecturer's or writer's points.

This stage was reached in Hellenic Alexandria, where the intellectual milieu of the *Museion* was also the focal point of medicine in the Greek and Roman worlds until their final eclipse by the Arabs in 643 A.D. The end of the 4th or beginning of the 3rd century B.C. can be identified as the threshold of that era which also produced the first medical illustrations. For there are sufficient reasons for assuming that the two eminent anatomists HEROPHILUS and ERASISTRATUS, who taught in Alexandria at that time and probably put the systematic study of anatomy on a scientific basis, also employed illustrations in their lectures. These illustrations were used by the anatomists to demonstrate what could not be conveniently shown on the object or to represent subject matter in a few lines so that their pupils could more easily memorize the data.

We shall not discuss whether it is accurate to attribute botanical and zoological illustrations to DIOCLES of CARYSTUS, a contemporary of PLATO (4th century), or to ARISTOTLE (384-322). There is a herbal manuscript written by DIOCLES which one would like to think was illustrated, and ARISTOTLE'S *Historia animalium* contains descriptions which refer to illustrations.[1]

There is no doubt that the idea of scientific illustration originated in classical Greek thought. On the other hand, the Corpus hippocraticum, which is the largest collection of classical medical manuscripts, contains nothing even to suggest the existence of explanatory illustrations.[2] (The origin of geographical cartography, which probably was parallel to that of medical illustration, is even less clear, but it also appears to have originated in Alexandria.)

The history of botanical illustration ultimately suggests the inclusion of all plant illustrations irrespective of their artistic form within the early history of scientific illustration. If we restrict ourselves to this theme we also arrive chronologically in the Hellenic period[3] and geographically in Alexandria. The earliest botanical illustrations can be assigned with confidence to this place and period.

Hieroglyphic literature contained neither geographical nor medical illustrations. In

[1] WELLMANN, MAX: Das älteste Kräuterbuch der Griechen, in: Festgabe für Franz Susemihl, Leipzig 1898, pp. 1-31. – JÄGER, WERNER: Diokles von Karystos, Berlin 1938. – AUBERT, H. and WIMMER, FR.: Die Tierkunde des Aristoteles, Leipzig 1868.

[2] EDELSTEIN, LUDWIG: Die Geschichte der Sektion in der Antike. Quellen u. Studien z. Gesch. d. Naturwiss. u.d. Medizin *3*/2 (1932), pp. 50-106.

[3] NISSEN, CLAUS: Die botanische Buchillustration, Stuttgart, 1951.

ancient Egypt, illustration was evidently not employed to clarify texts of this type.[4]

Numerous imitations of Hellenic graphic art have been handed down which, although preserved only as copies, are still quite revealing. They cover the whole variety of medical subjects to which illustration proves useful: anatomy, surgery, obstetrics, and medicinal plants. We shall examine them in this order as our earliest evidence of genuine medical illustration.

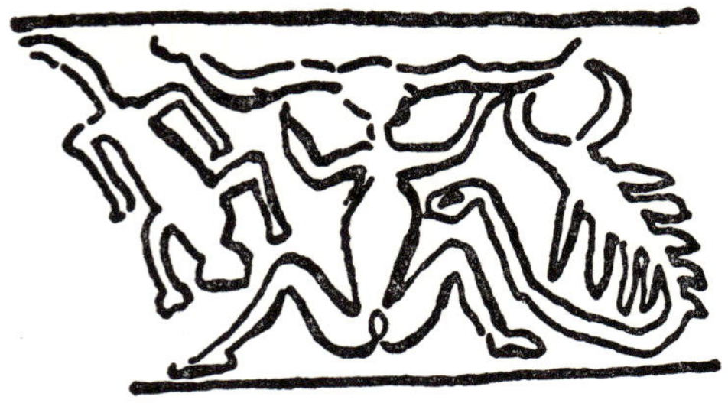

Fig. 1 Fertility goddess from Ur. Mesopotamian scroll seal.

Anatomy was first taught from the human cadaver about 300 B.C. in Alexandria, where the intellectual prerequisites already existed for the illustration of details observed directly on the object.

KARL SUDHOFF began the laborious work of collecting, organizing, and establishing the origins of the illustrations contained in the profusion of medieval manuscripts.[5] He discovered a series of characteristically related pictures which he initially termed the "five-figure series" and later renamed "squatting figures." Their origin, and this has never been seriously questioned, was assigned to Alexandria. In this context, "Alexandria" refers to an epoch extending over many centuries, during which graphic art was undergoing a process of formal transition and appears to be only vaguely definable. The origins of anatomical illustrations per se are less easily ascertained than those of surgical and botanical illustrations.

As a general and somewhat hypothetical rule, the Alexandrian *five-figure series* consists of five full-figures, each representing one system of organs:

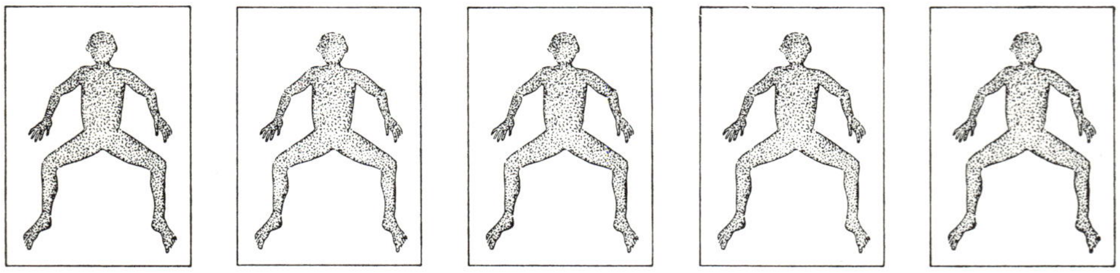

arteriae venae ossa nervi lacerti (= musculi)

Fig. 2a

A sixth figure, illustrating pregnancy, might have initially belonged to this series before subsequently achieving independent status. It is also possible that there were originally nine pictures, as accompanying texts indicate (fig. 2b).

The first five figures are characterized by the curious "squatting posture" – a position

[4] BETHE, ERICH: Buch und Bild im Altertum. Edited from papers left by ERNST KIRSTEN. Leipzig and Vienna, 1945. (This small, compactly written work provides the best introduction to the problem of scientific illustration in antiquity.) For a recent treatment, see WEITZMANN, KURT: Ancient Book Illumination (eq. Martin Classical Lectures, Vol. XVI), Harvard Univ. Press, Cambridge, Mass., 1959. Contains recent literature and hypotheses which go further than BETHE. We exclude Egyptian tomb reliefs, which do not belong to medical illustration in our use of the term.

[5] SUDHOFF, KARL: Kurzes Handbuch der Geschichte der Medizin. Berlin, 1922. Sudhoff includes on p. 129 a bibliography of what he considers to be the most important monographs.

which still requires a satisfactory explanation. GARRISON employs the expression "frog posture." On the other hand, it might be more apt to speak of "mensa figures";

Fig. 2b

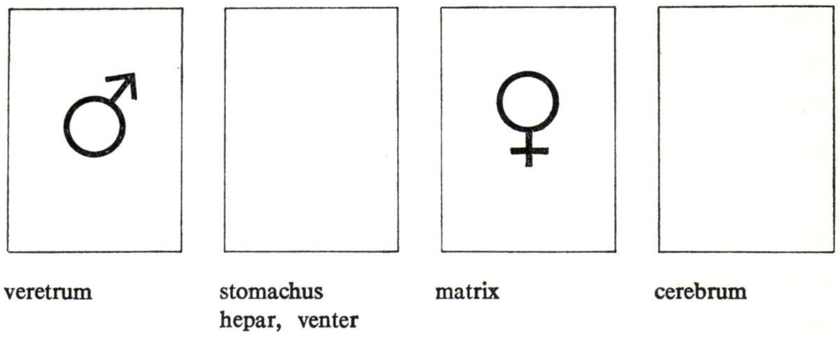

Figures 2a/b From the reconstructed Latin text in Arch. Gesch. Med. 3 (1910), 361.

for, of all the possible explanations for the posture of the oldest figure reproduced in medical illustration, the most probably is the position of a corpse laid upon a table (*mensa*) for dissection. For this purpose the legs are spread apart in order to make the inside of the thighs and genitals accessible. In any case, "squatting" is a posture which can only be adopted by a living person and is therefore a misleading conception. Later, the artist occasionally provided the figure with a convenient stool. The expression "squatting figure" thus becomes even more persuasive, but it is false in the original developmental context. It is possible that the historical roots of our phenomenon are deeper, extending perhaps into prehistoric times. L. H. WELLS and other historians have recently connected the matrix-figure with a primitive fertility goddess common to many early cultures, and subsequently with pre-classical illustrations of male gods (for instance the Egyptian god Bes, fig. 3), which were depicted in a similar manner. This hypothesis does not invalidate SUDHOFF'S theory, for the adoption of fertility gods as models for anatomical figures may well have occurred in Alexandria.[6]

SUDHOFF conceived his idea of a "squatting figure" series while examining two manuscripts in the Munich State Library. The first (Codex latinus 13002) originates from the monastery at Prüfening near Regensburg and was written and illustrated in 1158. The second (Codex latinus 17403) comes from the monastery at Scheyern in Upper Bavaria and dates from the first half of the 13th century.[7] Both monasteries were Benedictine abbeys and centers of Romanesque book illustration, and both manuscripts were based upon the same unknown prototype. The Prüfening series still remains the oldest of its type, although SUDHOFF himself discovered other

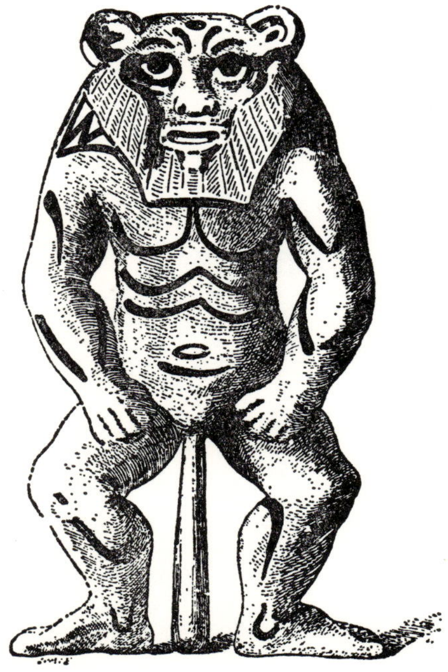

Fig. 3 The Ancient Egyptian god Bes, from a copy in Wells.

[6] WELLS, L. H.: J. Hist. Med. Allied Sci. (Baltimore) *XV* (1960) pp. 59-63 and *XVII* (1962) pp. 385-387. – MACKINNEY, LOREN and THOMAS HERNDON: ibid. *XVIII* (1962), p. 295, footnote 17.

[7] SUDHOFF, KARL: Tradition und Naturbeobachtung in den Illustrationen medizinischer Handschriften und Frühdrucke vornehmlich des 15. Jahrhunderts (Studien z. Gesch. d. Med. I), Leipzig 1907, pp. 49-65. – Sudhoff's monochrome phototype plates give an imperfect impression of the orginal. The Prüfening Codex is a pen-and-ink drawing in brown and red ink; the Scheyern Codex also has a colored frame. See also: SUDHOFF, KARL: Ein Beitrag z. Gesch. d. Anatomie im Mittelalter (Studien z. Gesch. d. Med. 4), Leipzig, 1908, pp. 1-10.

examples in Dresden,[7] Oxford,[8, 11] Basel[9] (plate II), Raudnitz Castle in Bohemia,[10] and Stockholm.[12] In 1950, BELLONI found a further example (fig. 4) in the Biblioteca Trivulziana in Milan.[13]

The assumption that these are examples of Alexandrian anatomy would be somewhat rash had not similar "squatting figures" been discovered in Persian manuscripts[7, 8] dating from different centuries. These discoveries strengthen the hypothesis that medieval Constantinople was the common source of such illustrations. First, it was here that literary fragments were washed ashore from the ruins of Alexandria. Then, there is a botanical manuscript originating directly from Constantinople which actually arrived there by the same route postulated for the anatomical illustrations (see p. 19). Moreover, the accompanying text of all the

Fig. 4 From the Codex 836 in the Biblioteca Trivulziana, Milan, 14th century.

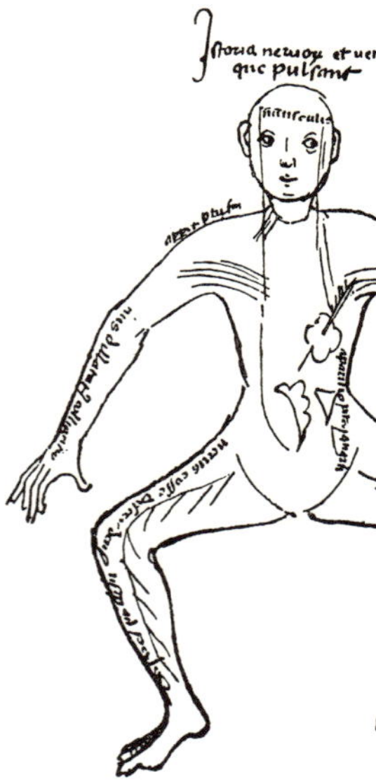

[8] SEIDEL, ERNST and SUDHOFF, KARL: Drei weitere anatomische Fünfbilderserien aus Abendland und Morgenland. Archiv. Gesch. Med. *3* (1910), pp. 165-187.

[9] SUDHOFF, KARL: Ein Beitrag z. Gesch. d. Anatomie im Mittelalter (Studien z. Gesch. d. Med. *4*), Leipzig 1908, pp. 11-51.

[10] SUDHOFF, KARL: Abermals eine neue Handschrift der anatomischen Fünfbildserie. Archiv. Gesch. Med. *3* (1910), pp. 353-368.

[11] SUDHOFF, KARL: Die Oxforder anatomische Fünfbildserie des Cod. Ashmol. 399. Archiv. Gesch. Med. *7* (1914), pp. 363-366.

[12] SUDHOFF, KARL: Die graphische Weiterbildung der anatomischen Fünfbilderserie aus der Alexandrinerzeit und eine anatomische Serie aus Stockholm. Arch. Gesch. Med. *8* (1915), pp. 129-139.

[13] BELLONI, LUIGI: Gli schemi anatomici trecenteschi del Codice Trivulziano 836. Riv. Storia Scn. Med. Nat. *41* (1950), pp. 193-207.

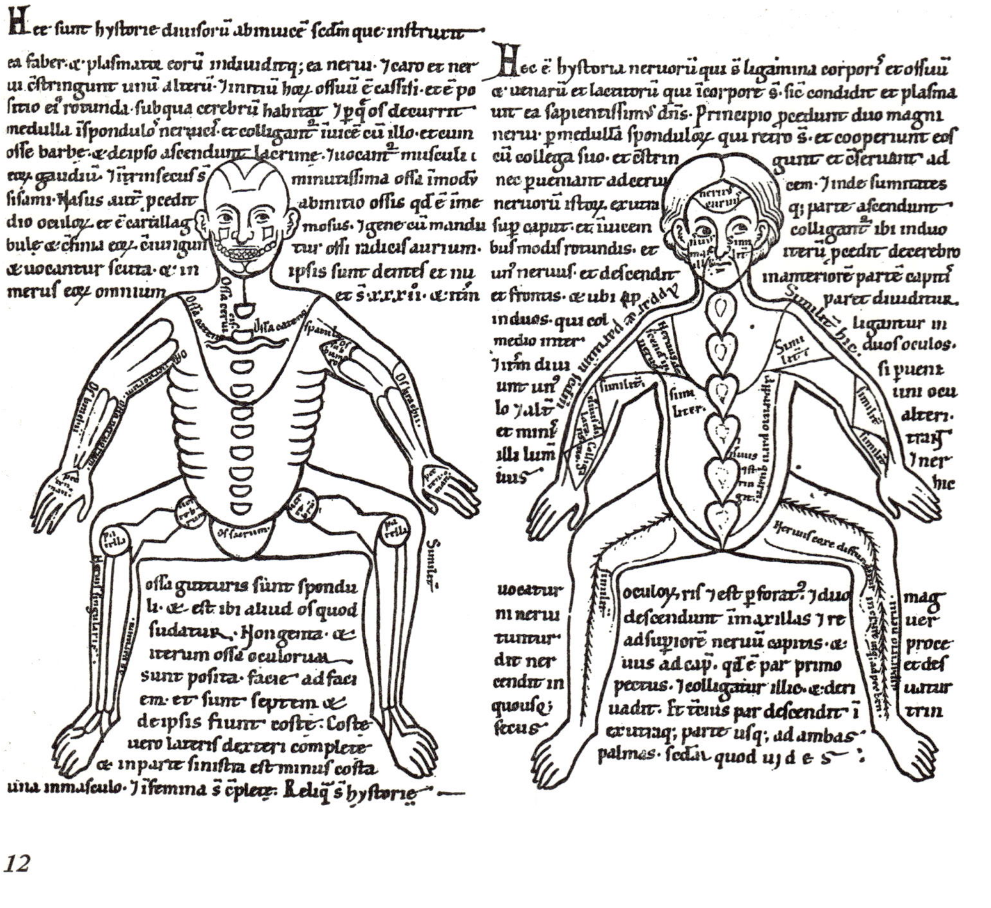

Fig. 5 From the Prüfening Codex, Bayer. Staatsbibliothek, Munich, Cod. lat. 13002. Written and illuminated in 1158.

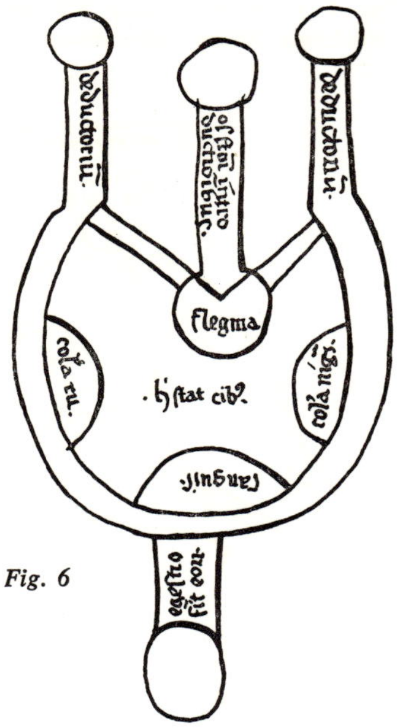

Fig. 6

Figures 6 to 10 Diagrams of organs from the Codex Roncioni 99, University Library, Pisa.

Figures 7 to 9

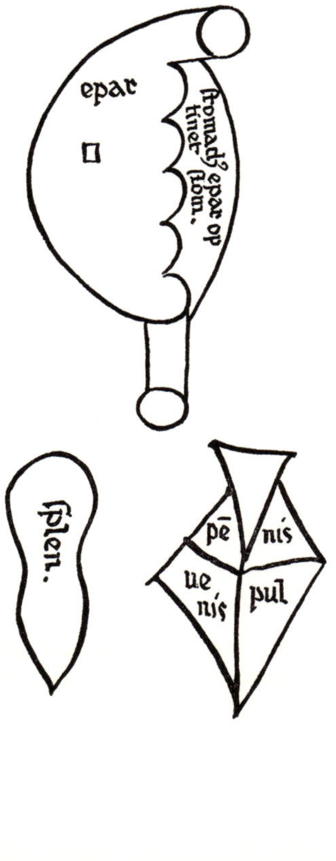

illustrations, with the exception of the Basel manuscript, refers to GALEN, who gained his knowledge of anatomy principally in Alexandria. As GALEN himself testifies, even by the 2nd century A.D. Alexandria was the only place where anatomy was being taught directly from the human skeleton.[14]

We see then that medieval illustrations known to modern scholarship all indicate that anatomical graphic art originated in the period of Alexandrian Hellenism. Although these copies are quite faded, we can still detect the rudiments of semi-schematic illustrations which, drawn in typically bold outline, were perhaps developed from a naturalistic model for the purpose of demonstrating exenteration and dissection of the displayed cadaver. The complete outline of the human figure was also employed for demonstrating the abdominal situs or genital organs. The majority of these typical figures demonstrate the great organ systems, the *partes similares* of the ancients: skeleton, musculature, blood vessels, and nerves. In these late copies it is impossible to determine the extent to which details were given. In part they contain absolute nonsense which was created by successive generations of copyists who, mostly through lack of understanding, made more and more technical errors.

Apart from the representations of systems, there are smaller pictures of the organs which exhibit the form characteristic of very old, probably late Grecian, originals. They have been discovered in numerous manuscripts and still appear in 15th-century incunabula. Typically, they appear as schematic representations involving a maximum simplification of form and are frequently only rendered comprehensible by their accompanying text. They are so simplistic they almost look like symbols. The figures reproduced in the margins on this and the next page are from the Codex Roncioni 99 in Pisa and are intended to represent the stomach, the liver, spleen and lungs, eyes and nose. The stomach is shown in figure 6 (central inscription: *hic stat cibus*, "here lies the chyme") as a sack suspended on both sides by a *ductorium* which flanks the stomach orifice (*os stomachi introductionibus*). Situated on the stomach wall are the four humors: the *flegma* on the cardia, the *cholera nigra* and the *cholera rubra* on each side corresponding to the topographical position of the spleen and gallbladder, and the *sanguinis* at the stomach outlet which leads into the intestine (*egestio fit eorum*). Figure 7, for the liver, shows the five lobes of this organ in position on top of the stomach. The stomach outlet conforms to the intestinal connection in the stomach scheme, but the artist has erroneously connected the top tube into the liver, whereas it should actually lead into the stomach as the os stomachi. This is quite obvious because the same figure occurs in another manuscript (Ashmol. 399, Oxford) where the os stomachi is correctly represented. This comparison also shows that the small quadrangle on the liver is meant to symbolize the gallbladder. Figure 8, representing the spleen, is

[14] SUDHOFF, KARL (see footnote 5); EDELSTEIN, LUDWIG (see footnote 2); SINGER, CHARLES: Galen, On Anatomical Procedures. Translation etc. London, 1956.

Fig. 10

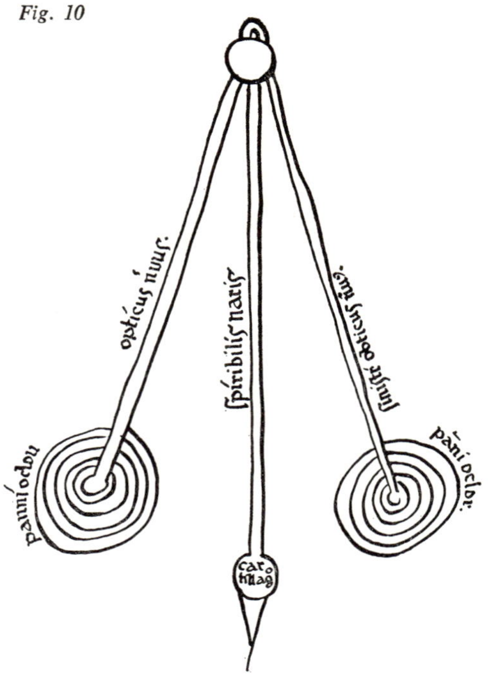

easily comprehended, but figure 9, for the lungs, is quite abstract. Figure 10 symbolizes the eyes with their respective nerves (*opticus nervus*) and shows the nose (*cartillago*) connected to a *spiribilis naris* which is also conceived as a hollow "nerve." All three canals emerge from an unspecified center which "is probably meant to depict the brain or a brain cell."[15] Similar but less abstract organ schematics are still encountered in the first printed medical works of the 15th century (see p. 62). In our opinion the individual drawings of the "five-figure series" are also abstractions and should not be interpreted as mutilated naturalism.

The earliest illustrations from the field of surgery present us with other problems, for historically their form has an entirely distinct origin. Instead of demonstrating morphological features which can be reduced to symbols, they illustrate methods of practical medical treatment which, for didactic purposes, were depicted as actual events. It is also noteworthy how the graphic treatment reveals essential information about art history: in fact, in this case the illustration is as important to art history as it is to medical history.

The most important and earliest piece of evidence is the illustration of a parchment codex with a commentary by Apollonius of Kition to the treatise *Peri arthron* ("Concerning the Joints") of the Corpus hippocraticum. This priceless manuscript, which was written and illustrated for the Byzantine physician Nicetas as part of a collection of several surgical treatises, was possibly commissioned by Emperor Constantine vii Porphyrogenitus (905-959), who authorized the systematic copying of Greek manuscripts. In 1492, it was acquired in Crete by a Florentine bibliophile and incorporated into the treasures of the Medici court. It now belongs to the Biblioteca Laurenziana in Florence (Ms. LXXIV, 7).

The original text of the Hippocratic manuscript on the structure of the joints dates from the 4th century B.C. The present form of the text derives from a copy produced in Alexandria where, about 70 B.C., Apollonius of Kition wrote and authorized the illustration of his commentary *Peri arthron* for a King Ptolemy. As far as the medical illustration is concerned,[16] the 10th-century version appears to conform closely to the Alexandrian original, including a scene of the naked figures of both patient and strangely enough his physicians (see plate I). The framework, painted in blue, red, and gold, displays ornamental motifs characteristic of Syrian book illustration during the early Christian era. The form of the original framing structure for the surgical scenes remains unknown. It is possible, however, that semicircular arches similar to those of Alexandrian calendar tables were employed to ornament the original. The frame-like position of the columns and the sham architecture of late classical mural decoration are typically Alexandrian. Alter-

[15] Sudhoff, Karl: Graphische Darstellungen innerer Körperorgane. Arch. Gesch. Med. 7 (1914), pp. 367-372.

[16] Kudlien, Fridolf: Die handschriftliche Überlieferung des Galenkommentars zu Hippokrates De articulis. Berlin 1960.

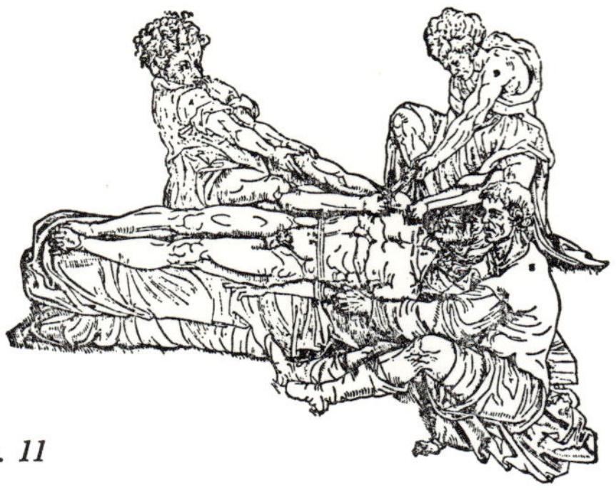

Fig. 11

natively, unless the frame structure was omitted, there could have been a rectangular decorated frame surrounding each picture in the manner which we shall see to be characteristic of other Alexandrian book illustrations.[17]

The Florentine manuscript contains thirty full-page illustrations which are fundamentally similar to the reproduction shown on plate I. The influence of these superb miniatures on European book illustrations following the sudden appearance of the codex in Florence was considerable. If we accept what has long been regarded as expert opinion, the Nicetas Codex was copied and partially redrawn by FRANCESCO PRIMATICCIO (1504-1570) who, born in Bologna, later became court artist at Fontainebleau and helped to introduce Italian Mannerism to France. These sepia watercolors – now in the Bibliothèque Nationale in Paris – are attractive proof of how an antique motif can be transformed by a great artist into a totally different design, when the essential content of the original is preserved and a different formal idiom employed.[18] It is also fascinating that the artist has not pushed modernization to extremes but has preferred to retain the character of the original Greek design by clothing his figures in classical rather than contemporary dress. Modernization does not appear until several decades later, when a more liberal treatment of part of the design was undertaken. This treatment transcended copying and served as a basis for the illustration (fig. 12) by AMBROISE PARÉ (Paris, 1564). Moreover, PRIMATICCIO'S drawings were only the early sketches for woodcuts intended for the illustration of the *Chirurgia* of GUIDO GUIDI (VIDUS VIDIUS), a topographically exquisite specimen of Parisian printing craft from 1544 (fig. 11). Finally, it is noteworthy that the amazing history of this series of thirty Hellenic surgical illustrations not only reveals the durability of these pictures, but also serves as evidence that a medical text from the 4th century B.C. still retained its authority and educational value twenty centuries later. Even today, the manual reduction of dislocations conforms to procedures first described in the Hellenic era. There are ample reasons for supposing that in addition to the Hellenic science of dislocations and bone fractures, other sectors of surgery also made use of illustrations. Unfortunately, the greater part of these most likely have been permanently lost. What remains is merely a small series of three operation scenes – the couching of a cataract and the excision of hermorrhoids and nasal polyps – which, from abundant medieval surgical illustration, can be identified with some certainty as copies of late classical graphic art. Three variations have been preserved, all of which are in British libraries. The manuscript Sloane 1975 in the British Museum (plate III) dates from the 12th century and displays the three scenes together on

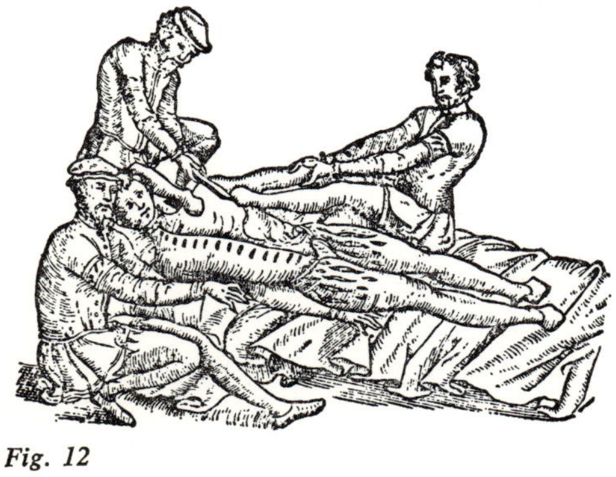

Fig. 12

17 WEITZMANN (footnote 4), p. 21.

18 This hypothesis which derives from H. OMONT has recently been disputed by C. E. KELLETT, who attributes the Paris drawings to the Italian artist SALVIATI (1510-1563). Cf. OMONT, H.: Foreword to "Collections de Chirurgiens grècs avec dessins attribués au Primatrice," Paris (Imprimerie Berthaud Frères) n.d. – KELLETT, C. E.: The Chirurgia of Vidus Vidius, 1544. An occasional lecture May, 1959, in: Mannerism and Medical Illustration. Lectures . . . given at the University of California, Los Angeles, 1961 (private printing).

one page: the hemorrhoidal excision is at the top left and above the excision of the nasal polyps; to the right and in somewhat larger detail is the couching of cataract. All three pictures have one feature in common which is not so typically found in any other of the numerous medieval illustrations of surgical scenes: in each case, there is a vessel, either a basin or a box. In two of the scenes the vessel appears as a basin for catching the blood; during the nasal operation, the basin is held by the patient himself. In the couching scene, where there is no blood emission, the patient holds an ointment box.

This is a familiar scene in manuscripts from the classical era. SUDHOFF reminds us, for example, that there is a pronounced developmental link between the representation of the washing of Odysseus's feet on Grecian urns and the same act depicted in connection with the apostles in medieval miniatures, and that our example is clearly a parallel case.[19]

It is probable that, as we have already observed in anatomy, Alexandrian surgery worked less with naturalistic instructional illustrations than with semi-schematic or schematic figures. This is especially indicated by the subject matter of the highly canonized doctrine relating to cauterization. From the time of Hippocrates on,[20] searing with a hot iron not only was held to divert pain or, in the sense of modern neural therapy, to intercept the course of pain sensation, but was also employed for the treatment of numerous complaints of a general and surgical nature. The texts preserved from the Corpus hippocraticum are so fragmentary that is impossible to form a reasonable conception of the extent and topographical application of cauterization. It is probable, however, that illustrations of cauterization points soon became part of this category of literature or were even introduced at the very beginning. Such illustrations appear to reveal more of the first thousand years of our chronological reckoning than the purely descriptive texts. Cauterization was also practiced by the Arabs as an important part of therapy. The number of medieval Latin manuscripts containing illustrations of cauterization points is considerable.[21] They first appear in an 11th-century Codex Laurentianus[22] and continue to appear in the incunabula. In addition there are numerous copies written in the major European languages.

The oldest of these manuscripts conform most closely to the missing classical prototypes: they contain reference illustrations with short texts that specify only the place and nature of the particular malady. In the artistically less engaging series of pictures reproduced in the aforementioned codex at the Biblioteca Laurenziana in Florence, the patients – most of whom are naked – lie on a sack-like couch

[19] SUDHOFF, KARL: Beiträge zur Geschichte der Chirurgie im Mittelalter I (Studien z. Gesch. d. Med. 10), Leipzig, 1914, pp. 11-16.

[20] Ancient Egyptian medicine was familiar with the cautery but only as a "caustic knife" for purely surgical symptoms (JONCKHEERE).

[21] SUDHOFF: Studien 10 (see footnote 19), p. 81. – MACKINNEY, LOREN: Medical Illustrations in Medieval Manuscripts. London 1965, pp. 48-54. – HUARD, PIERRE and MIRKO DRAZEN GRMEK: Mille ans de Chirurgie en Occident: V^{e}-XVe siècles. Paris (Les Editions Roger Dacosta), 1966.

[22] Florence, Biblioteca Laurenziana, Cod. LXXIII, 41.

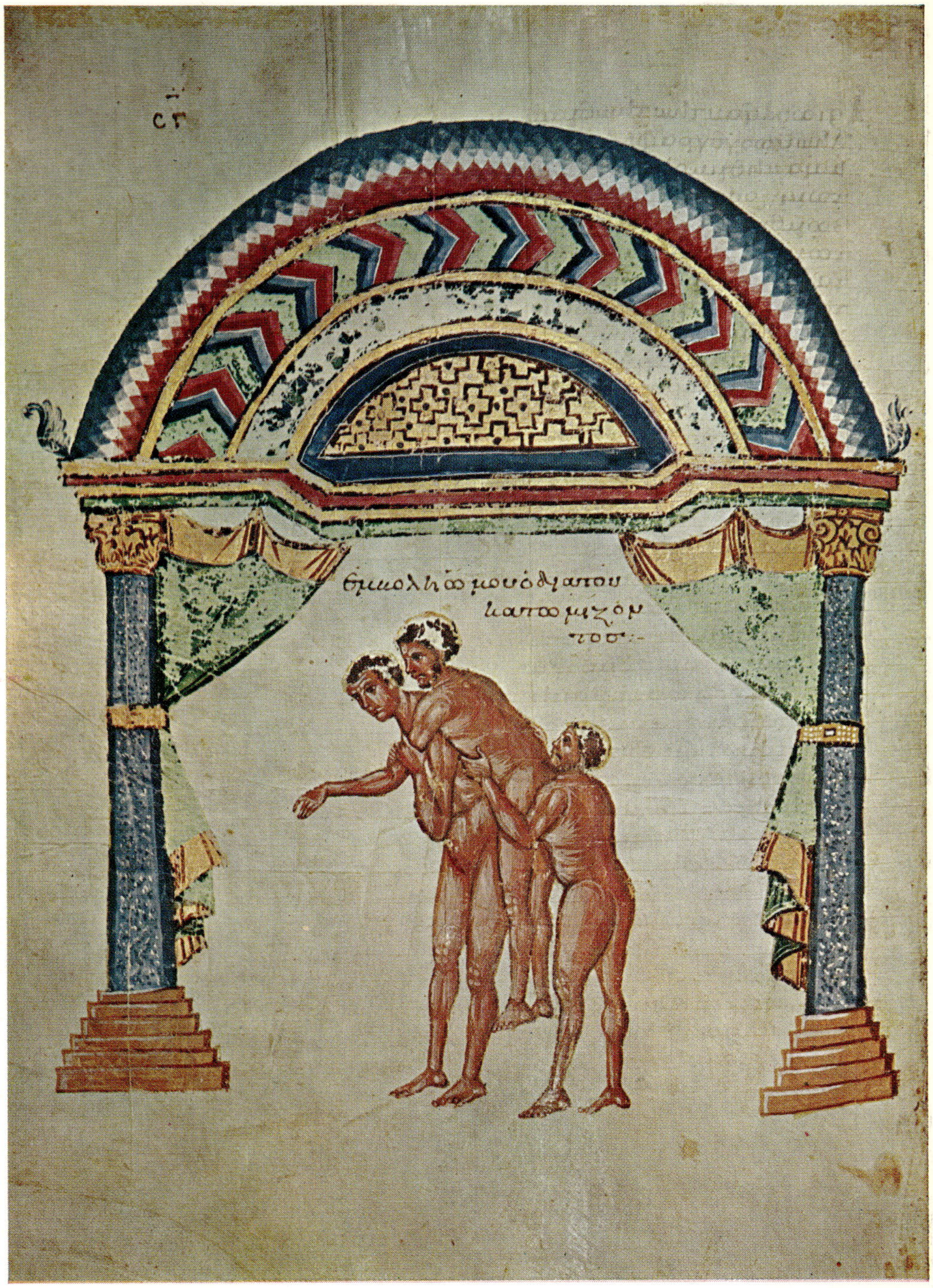

Plate I Resetting a dislocated shoulder according to Peri arthron, *Corpus hippocraticum, 4th century B.C. Byzantine miniature from the Commentary of Apollonios of Kition, 1st century B.C., a copy of which was painted in the 10th century A.D., MS. LXXIV, 7, Bibl. Laurenziana, Florence.*

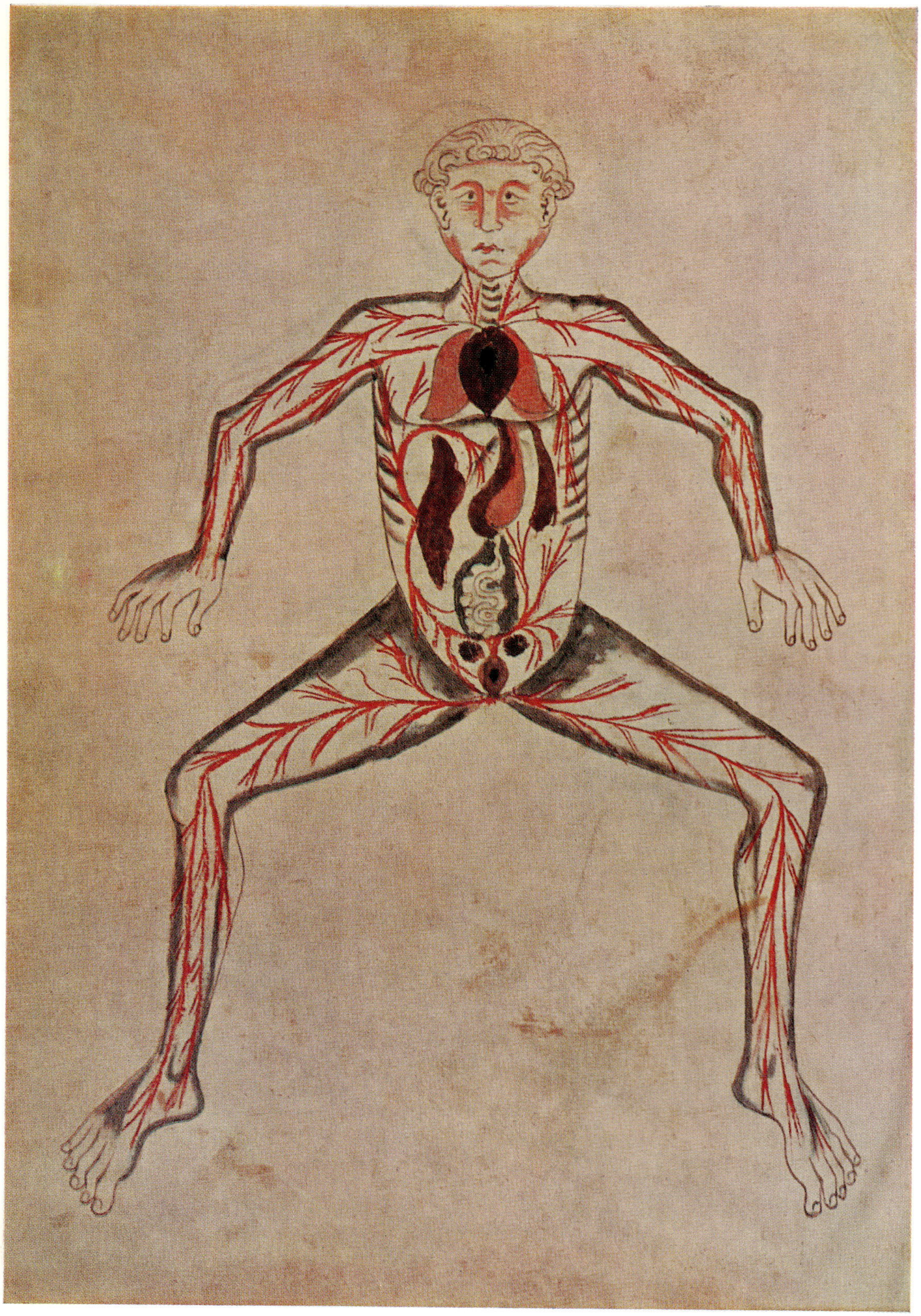

Plate II Last figure of a five-figure series of illustrations, Provence, 13th century. MS. D II. 11, fol. 171v, Universitätsbibliothek, Basel.

of Byzantine origin. In several manuscripts the medical scenes are framed by Roman arches, as in the famous Codex Casanatensis[23] and the vividly colored series of illustrations in the mid-14th-century manuscript Rawlinson C 328 in Oxford (plate IV). In the Rawlinson manuscript, the physician wears the clothing of the period. The illustration on the lower left demonstrates, however, that the design must be consideraby older. Note, for example, that the patient, described in the text as suffering from elephantiasis, reclines on an oval couch similar to the couch that can be identified as Byzantine in the illustrations of the Codex Laurentianus. In the top left-hand illustration of plate IV, the physician is using a bellows to kindle the fire for the cautery. The right-hand pictures show the patients sitting on low benches. In the first of these, the physician is applying his cautery to the forehead of a patient with "dolor capitis." In the other, the mode of demonstration undergoes a remarkable transformation: in a pose reminiscent of St. Sebastian, a youth is leaning against a stake and the cautery is being applied to his breast for the treatment for asthma. Instead of the whole figure of the physician, only the right hand appears from behind the column armed with a cautery.

Is it in fact a cautery? The question is clearly justified, for the second patient, with the scrotal hernia or hydrocele – described on the picture as 'ernia' – is to all appearances prepared for cauterization, but the cautery itself is of unusual length, if the line is indeed intended to represent a cautery. Actually we are inclined to think of this rather as a didactic device for aiding demonstration. If so, it is one of the early uses of *indication lines*, which will appear more prominently in later illustrations. The iconographic development of the indication line in medical illustration appears to start with this example, and we are tempted to believe that we can observe the process virtually unfolding before us (see pages 54-60).

If we are right in thinking that these illustrations show that a realistic element can become a purely symbolic or diagrammatic element, we can regard these cauterization pictures as early examples of a phenomenon which will receive more of our attention in the last phase of its development during the 16th and 17th centuries. A modern graphic artist would never draw the whole human figure merely to demonstrate cauterization points on the head or scrotum. This is, moreover, didactically impractical because these features would be so small on a full-figure drawing as to render the necessary topography obscure. In all didactic graphic art of this category – for example, the illustrations to *Peri arthron* – on no occasion is only one part of the body represented. Even where this would have facilitated demonstration, we are inevitably presented with the whole human figure. This is a typical example of those rules which have long-term effects.

We believe then, that the cautery in the Oxford Rawlinson Codex (and in all comparable manuscripts) is intended not as an objective instrument, but rather as

[23] Ms. 1382 in Biblioteca Casanatense, Rome. Reproduced in SUDHOFF, Studien z. Gesch. d. Med. 10 (1914), Plate XXV, with references to the uncopied parts.

an indication line. Similarly, the oval couch supporting the patient in the lower left-hand scene of plate IV is no longer meant as a real couch – it only signifies "a bedridden patient." This becomes clear when we consider the famous mosaic on the high ceiling of the Santa Maria Nuova in Ravenna, showing the cripple of Capernaum being lowered down through the roof of a house to Jesus Christ (fig. 13) as described in the New Testament (Luke 5 : 19). The representation is both naturalistic. and symbolic: the house is not a "real" house and Jesus stands (apparently) outside because the figure is reproduced in exaggerated proportion to emphasize his importance. Furthermore, the oval bed of the invalid serves merely to make the essential point that he is truly sick and recumbent. The two scenes we have just compared, contained respectively in the 6th-century Ravenna mosaic and the 14th-century Oxford Codex, share the same formal idiom.[24] It is the idiom of the late classical, early Byzantine era.

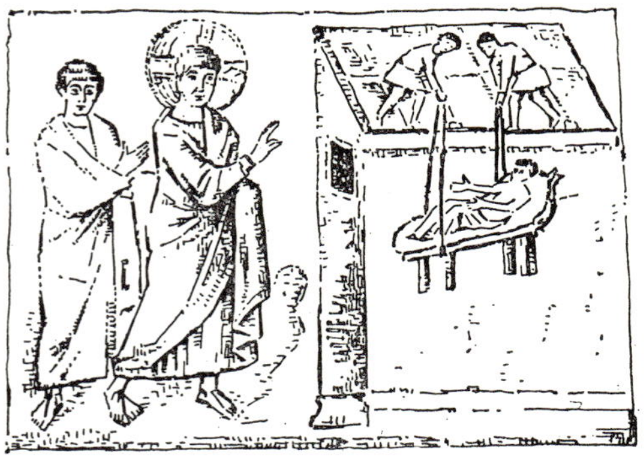

Fig. 13

A special group of late classical clinical illustrations can be recognized in medieval pictures which, even after the invention of printing, survived longer than those so far considered. We are referring to illustrations of the uterus, with and without the fetus. The Bibliothèque Royale in Brussels has preserved under No. 3714, a 9th-century manuscript containing an obstetrical catechism by Soranus of Ephesus (2nd century A.D.) in the revised version of Moschion (6th century). The Brussels illustrations actually belong to the original text of Moschion, but it seems certain that they derive from Soranus, who was a pupil at the Alexandrian academy and practiced in Rome under Trajan and Hadrian.

The illustrations are schematic in the manner of mnemonic pictures. The form of each uterus is the same and all contain small puppet-like fetuses which are drawn in different positions and described in the text. There is no strict proportional relationship between fetus and uterus, and even the positions are unrealistic. Their didactic value as mnemonic devices is nevertheless evident (plate V). The depiction of the uterus without the fetus, that is, in a purely anatomical form, belongs to the category of schematic organ-illustration. One figure with a two-horned uterus contained in the 13th-century Codex Roncioni (fig. 14) corresponds approximately to a description by Aristotle in the *Historia animalium* which, according to the text, had an accompanying illustration.[25] This may well have been similar. More problematical is the interpretation of a group of three schematic uterus figures reproduced in a Vicentine manuscript dating from the first half of the 13th century.[26] The cupping-glass form of the uterus is certainly from the same source

Fig. 14

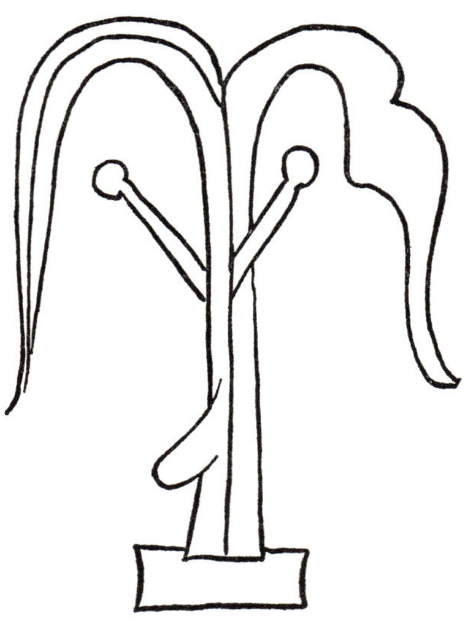

[24] Sudhoff has published the respective illustrations (surgical practice scenes), in the Arch., 10 (1917): from the Florentine Pseudo-Apuleius-Manuscript, Plut. LXXIII, 16 = XII century.

[25] Ferckel, Christoph: Diagramme der Sexualorgane in mittelalterlichen Handschriften. Arch. Gesch. Med. *10* (1917), pp. 255-263.

[26] Sudhoff, Karl: Uteruszeichnung in einer bisher unbekannt gebliebenen Mus(t)io-Handschrift zu Vicenza. Arch. Gesch. Med. *17* (1925), pp. 1-11.

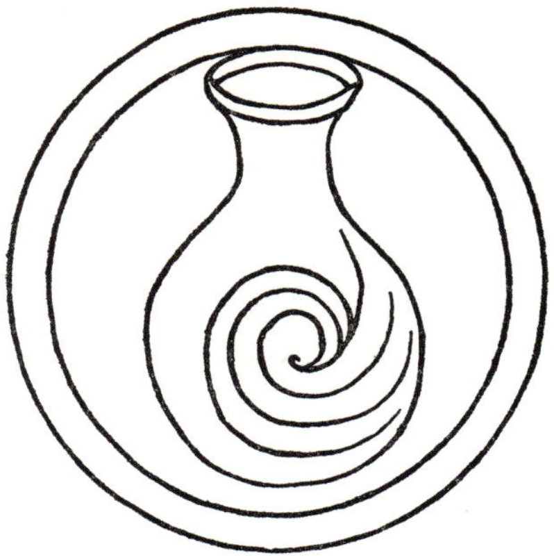

Fig. 15

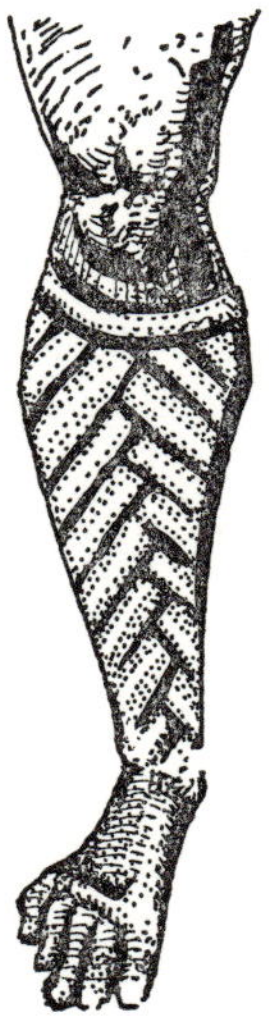

Fig. 16

as the 6th-century Moschion illustration, and the inner spiral appears to have a functional meaning. Curiously, the illustrations are stood on their heads, so to speak, so that they resemble a urine glass rather than a uterus (fig. 15).

Soranus is also the author of a *Treatise on Bandaging*, copiously provided with illustrations which have been preserved for us in the Codex Laurentianus LXXIV, 7. This codex can be traced back to Nicetas and also contains illustrations to the *Peri arthron*. These illustrations are totally naturalistic – a bandage scarcely permits any other mode of demonstration. It is still remarkable, however, that besides the schematic (organ symbols) and semi-schematic (full-figures), there are also naturalistic illustrations of purely medical themes which concentrate upon individual parts of the body, for example, the head or leg (fig. 16), when these suffice for demonstration.

Some specialists, notably historians of medicine, will certainly be familiar with what we have discussed so far. Among art experts it is widely held that the origins of book illustration are to be found during the transition from the papyrus scroll to the parchment codex, which occurred no earlier than the 1st century A.D. Now scientific illustration – and more specifically medical illustration – constitutes only a part of that which we describe as book illustration. It is quite remarkable that only recently has an attempt been made – mainly in the posthumous work of the philologist Erich Bethe – to consider the question of book and picture in antiquity, for this is after all a problem which can contribute valuable knowledge relating to the history of ancient civilization. In his survey of both extant and reconstructed illustrations, Bethe attempted their systematic arrangement into didactic and decorative pictures on the one hand, book-picture and picture-book on the other. This project is quite significant, for it leads to the inference that the didactic illustration appeared first or, in more extreme terms, the picture preceded the written word. Indeed, the traces of geometrical and astronomical illustration belonging to the category of schematic or mnemonic pictures lead back to the 6th century B.C. Accordingly, the decorative picture will be of post-Hellenic origin. Whereas the decorative book-picture, as an essentially naturalistic form of illustration, was still unknown in classical Greek literature, the picture-book is older. We are already familiar with one, namely the *Treatise on Bandaging* by Soranus. This 2nd-century work is, of course, a late example, even though it might derive from an older prototype. But there is further evidence of even earlier works, including the most beautiful of all picture-books preserved from antiquity: the Juliana Anicia Codex. We have deliberately placed this at the end of our brief summary of classical book-illustration, because this one example unites the entire complex of problems and, at the same time, has been most successfully investigated.
According to Bethe, the Juliana Anicia Codex in the Vienna National Library is the only illustrated manuscript dating from the end of antiquity which is at all

worthy of classical art. That is high praise. The codex, otherwise known as the Viennese Dioscorides, was illustrated in Byzantium, about 512 A.D., on commission of the inhabitants of Honoratae in the east Roman metropolis. The first owner was JULIANA ANICIA, a noblewoman who, in the early years of JUSTINIAN'S reign, took a great interest in medicinal plants, especially the mandrake root. The Anicia Codex survived the downfall of the eastern Roman empire in Byzantium, after which it was used by Ottoman scholars, who added notes in Arabic script. Finally, in 1569, it was purchased from a Jewish physician in Constantinople by the Austrian ambassador and brought to MAXIMILIAN II in Vienna. Nor is its history any less dramatic than that of the Florentine Nicetas Codex. Moreover, just as the latter served the iconography of surgical illustrations, the Anicia Codex enriched the pharmaco-botanical literature of the late Renaissance. Despite the name, this text is not identical with the *Materia medica* of DIOSCORIDES PEDANIUS, who lived in the 1st century A.D. (under NERO and VESPASIAN), although it contains an alphabetical extract from this standard work on ancient pharmaceutics. The illustrations derive in part from CRATEUS, physician to MITHRIDATES IV of Pontus (120-63 B.C.). As was the case with the *Peri arthron*, we have stepped back into an older era. The genealogy and cross-connections of this late classical picture-book have been the object of much coordinated historical research. We are indebted to CHARLES SINGER for a diagram which demonstrates the varied literary fate of such ancient manuscripts (fig. 17).

Since 1906,[27] the Viennese Dioscorides (Cod. med. gr. I) has been accessible as a phototype facsimile to all who have not been able to study the priceless codex in the original at the Austrian National Library. After the difficult restoration work directed by F. UNTERKIRCHNER, a new facsimile was recently produced,[28] the accuracy of which extends to the form of each individual parchment sheet and sets a new standard in quality for mechanical copying.

The fact that this codex, in common with numerous other classics of medical illustration, is not an homogenous composition, is due to its historical origin. It is only one branch of a tree, of which one root is the herbal of CRATEUS dated five hundred years earlier. SINGER believed that eleven of the illustrations could be traced directly to CRATEUS. These are the most attractive. Another clearly distinguishable group consists of strictly schematic plant illustrations, and yet another group is drawn somewhat closer to nature. Common to all is the basic conception of this alphabetically arranged medical plant atlas – which would now be termed an illustrated encyclopaedia – namely, to use pictures instead of wordy descriptions. The compiler of this atlas was one of the first medical authors to realize that a well-conceived illustration can frequently teach more than can possibly conveyed in a written text.

[27] Codices graeci et latini, cur. SCATONE DE VRIES, vol. X, Leiden 1906.
[28] Codices selecti phototypice impressi 12. Graz (Akad. Druck-u. Verlagsanstalt) 1966 ff.

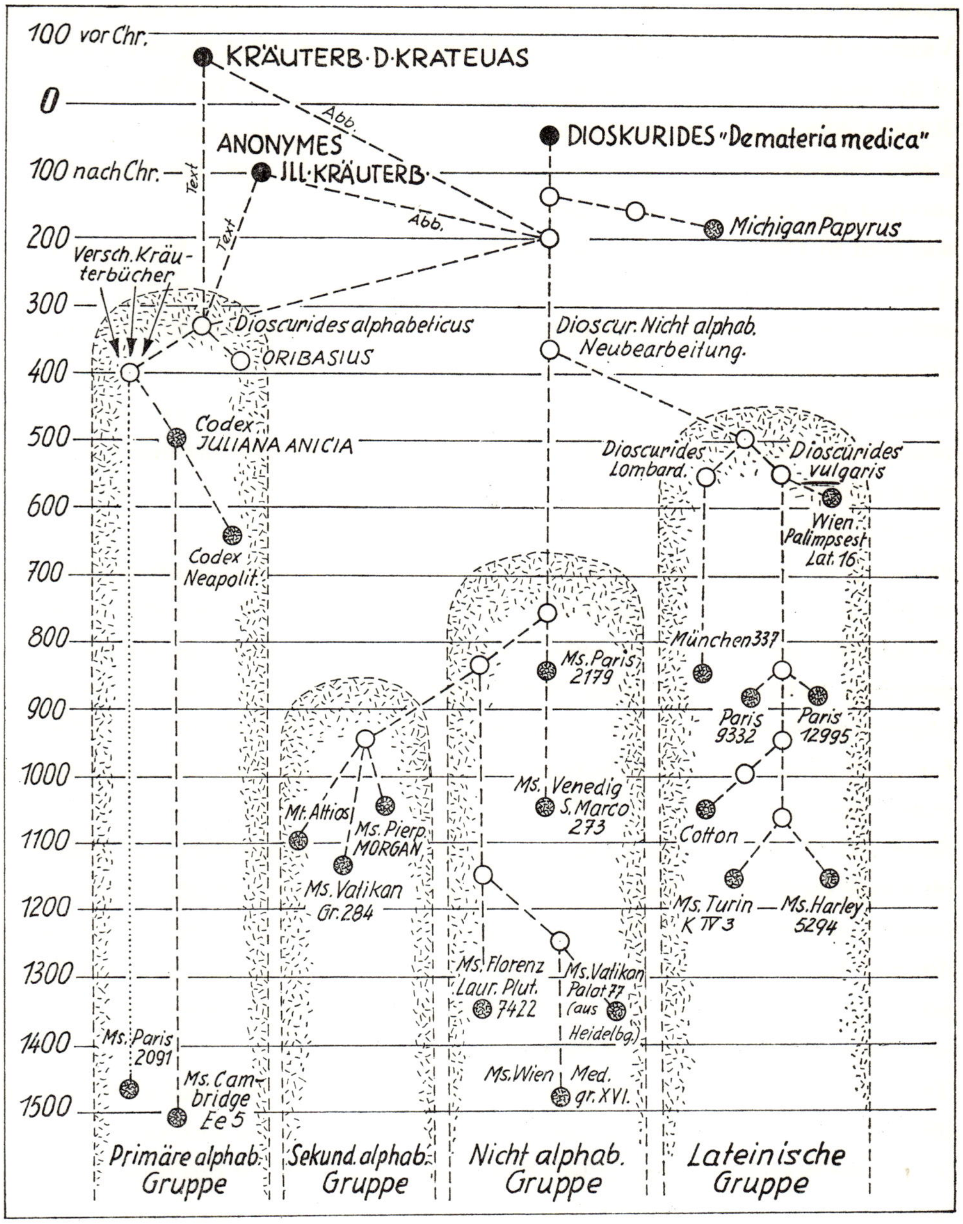

Fig. 17 The most important Dioscorides manuscripts and their probable origin. Transcribed from Charles Singer, The Herbal in Antiquity and Its Transmissions to Later Ages. *J. Hellenic Stud. 47 (1927): 20.*

Numerous animals were also originally discussed in the materia medica of DIOSCORIDES as a source of medical drugs, and the codex accordingly includes miniatures illustrating such animals. Like the pharmaco-botanical illustrations of late Byzantine books, the animal illustrations also are to be found in other manuscripts of Greco-Roman materia medica. An excellent example is the 13th-century Codex graecus 284 in the Vatican.[29]

Among the illustrations belonging to the prefatory part of the Viennese Dioscorides, which include the portraits of JULIANA ANICIA and several important physicians, notably DIOSCORIDES and GALEN, one is of special interest. Under the supervision

[29] THÉODORIDÈS, JEAN: Jahrb. Österr. Byzant. Ges. *10* (1961) pp. 21-29 – Cf. our plate XIX.

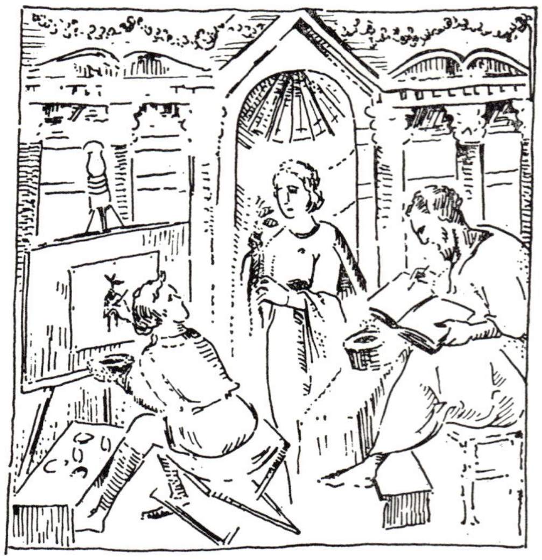

Fig. 18 An outline sketch from the badly damaged coloured original on fol. 5 of the Codex Vindob. med. graec. I ('Viennese Dioscorides'). This shows Epinoia as personified imagination, to the right of whom is Dioscorides as the author. At the easel is Crateus, the illustrator, who is drawing the mandrake held by Epinoia.

of the author, DIOSCORIDES, the artist is engaged in drawing the mandrake plant from nature (fig. 18). Even if the Byzantine miniaturist, knowing less about the historical origins of the book he was copying than we do today, represented a scene which never actually occurred, he nonetheless affirms the importance of the role played by the illustrator in producing a book. In his *Historia stirpium*, the *New Kreüterbuch* ("new herbal") of 1542, LEONHART FUCHS had his two artists, ALBRECHT MEYER and HEINRICH FÜLLMAURER, portrayed as they were preparing the illustrations (fig 19). A period of one thousand years lies between, but the motivating spirit is the same.

Our inquiry set out to define lost scientific illustrations from antiquity through the analysis of predominantly medieval illuminated manuscripts, and has led to a conclusion which can be summarized as follows: *Medical illustration was already known in antiquity and included all of the categories of modern illustration: the schematic, semi-schematic, and naturalistic.*

This concept merges harmoniously into the picture of the Greek genius revealed to us by the art of historical writing. It also fits into the mosaic of direct literary evidence and, finally, conforms to the analogical conclusions that were expected from the field of art history. Here too, the history of art has helped us to bridge the gaps in literary records and to comprehend the spirit of an epoch as an indivisible whole comprising all branches of culture, of which medicine is by no means the least important.

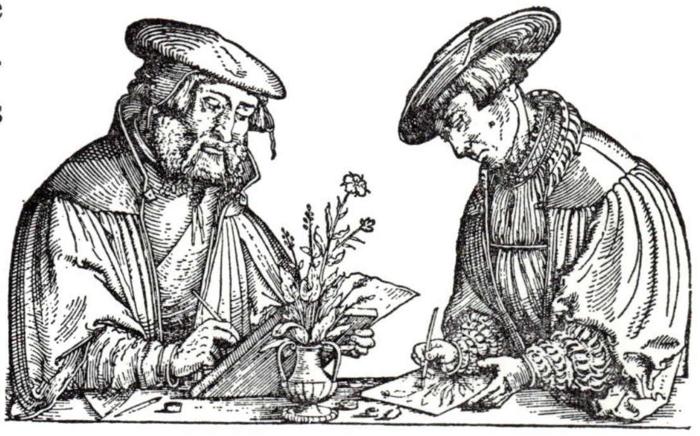

Fig. 19

The Middle Ages

Pharmaco-botanical illustration was considered at the end of the section on classical art, not only because it is at the periphery rather that at the center of actual medical illustration, but also because the whole complex of problems associated with classical illustration is embodied in this one category. Because relatively few examples of ancient graphic art have been preserved over the centuries, we shall have to concentrate more and more on selected examples which represent whole groups. This selection will necessarily become increasingly subjective, but nothing essential to our study will be omitted.

It can safely be said that a study of medieval graphic art can contribute a great deal to our understanding of the history of thought in the Middle Ages. The medieval mind accepted both *schematic* and *naturalistic* illustration. Schematization, that is the depiction of the parts of a body of information in a systematic arrangement, is more typical of this epoch than naturalism. It would be false, however, and contrary to our revised conception of a merely "dark" Middle Ages, to suppose that an illustration drawn from nature was entirely impossible. In a Theodoric manuscript from Leyden are illustrations – admittedly dating from the end of this epoch – which are amazingly vivid and show close scrutiny of nature. However, generally, didactic graphic art tends to be abstract – a tendency which finds its typical expression in scholasticism.

When authority is dominant there is little or no scope for innovation, and schematic illustration becomes equivalent to doctrine. This evaluation would be false if method were to be excessively emphasized. When the growth of medical knowledge produces new illustrations, these are conditioned by the prevailing spirit of the period. There are several types of illustration which, although the first known examples date from the Middle Ages, could possibly have already existed in Hellenism. Fundamental innovations are not to be expected; indeed, they are scarcely possible.

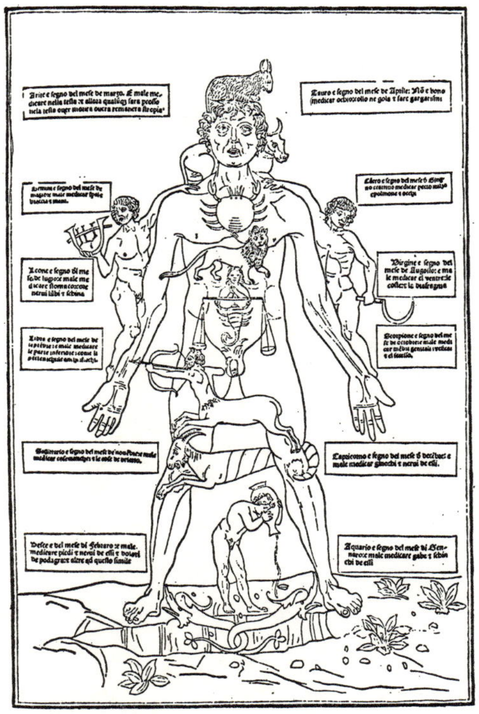

Fig. 20 Zodiac-man from the Fasciculus medicinae, *Venice, 1493.*

Reduction and stiffness are features which characterize almost all illustrations of the Middle Ages. On the other hand, medieval illustration demonstrates that both reduction and stiffness can produce impressive-looking figures, and this is as true for didactic graphic art as for other major art forms. During the last half-century, efforts have been made by art historians to establish the essential nature of the medieval formal idiom. This development can be traced from the work of such dissimilar scholars as Alois Riegl and Ernst Cassirer, through Dagobert Frey and Ernst Panofsky, down to the present generation. The search is for a broad but unified interpretation of medieval thought that can also integrate scientific illustration into art history. It has been clearly recognized that, for the Middle Ages, space and time were inseparably fused and that the passage of time was equated to a spatial journey. The qualitative attributes of such a world are essential, and it is this which binds it to antiquity and distinguishes it from the modern age. Quantitative thinking first emerges during the Renaissance: in physics and biology, theory of art and philosophy.[1] We shall also devote special attention to this transition in the history of modern medical illustration.

We have already encoutered an important part of medieval medical graphic art during our reconstruction of classical illustration: the anatomical five- and nine-figure series, the schematic organ figures, copies of ancient surgical texts, and illustrations for obstetrics books and herbals. Of all types of illustrations which are especially characteristic of the late Middle Ages the most representative are those relating to venesection.[2] One is also disposed to look for their origins in antiquity, but unfortunately the traces have become effaced. Byzantium is also a possible source. The types which are eventually printed as incunabula cannot even be traced back into the high Middle Ages. By that time, bloodletting as a therapeutic remedy had already had a turbulent history, which eventually culminated in the so-called "bloodletting dispute" of the 16th century.

Among the 15th-century venesection illustrations, the incunabula bloodletting tables, three types are to be found which still resist classification within a clear chronological line of development. Firstly, there are the naked manikins with lines indicating those points from which blood is to be let (fig. 21). These are somewhat reminiscent of the cauterization figures in medieval manuscripts, except that the individual figures of the latter are less detailed. Then there is the naked bloodletting man with the twelve signs of the zodiac, each of which covers a specific part of the body (figures 20, 22). In the third type of illustration, the signs of the zodiac have been removed from the body and placed in the margins as independent figures, the connection to their respective organs being maintained by means of a simple indication line (figures 23, 24).

The literary source of the relationship between astrology and bloodletting goes back as far as Egyptian and Babylonian medicine, but analogous illustrations from antiquity have yet to be discovered. During the later Middle Ages, graphic representation of the zodiac was sometimes combined with the names of particular organs, although not with an anatomical figure (plate IXb).[3] SUDHOFF'S oldest examples of zodiac figures date from the late 13th century.[4] Nevertheless there does appear to be one way of telling the approximate age of the zodiac and bloodletting manikins: the ram is always associated with the head, indicating that these figures

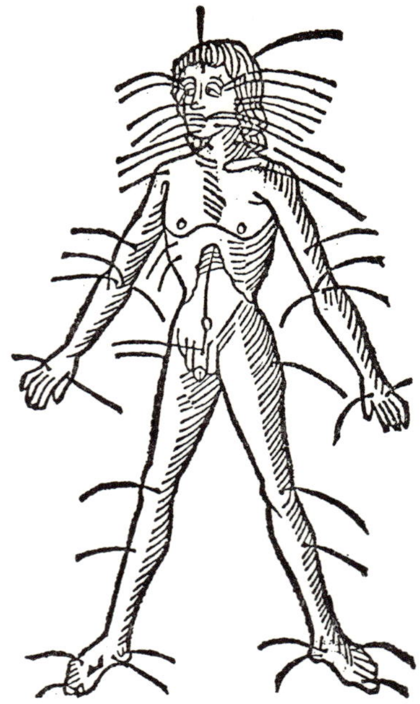

Fig. 21 Bloodletting man from a popular medical incunabulum, Heinrich Louffenberg, Versehung des Leibs, *Augsburg, 1491.*

Fig. 22 Zodiac-man from the Deutscher Kalender, *printed by Johann Blaubirer, Augsburg, 1481.*

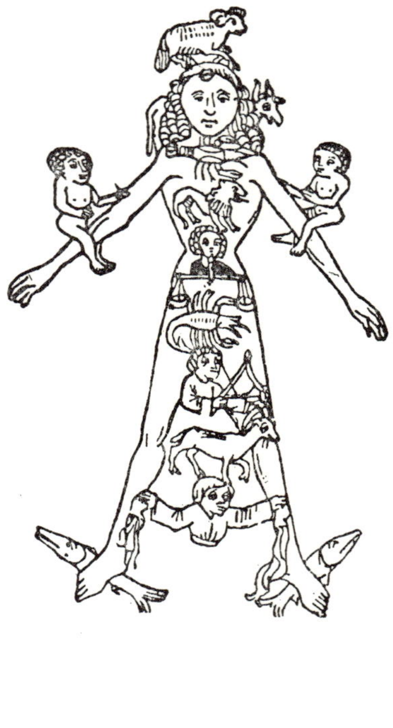

[1] This only applies in a general way. In GALEN there are the beginnings of quantitative thinking, but these remained dormant during antiquity.

[2] SUDHOFF, KARL: Männliche Eingeweidesitusbilder und Aderlassmännchen im 15. Jahrhundert. In: Tradition und Naturbeobachtung in den Illustrationen medizinischer Handschriften und Frühdrucke vornehmlich des 15. Jahrhunderts (Studien z. Gesch. d. Med. I) Leipzig, 1907, pp. 29-48. By same author: Lehr- und Merkschemata für die Beurteilung der Schwere von Verletzungen, Kauterienanwendung, Schröpfen und Aderlass. In: Beiträge z. Gesch. d. Chirurgie im Mittelalter I (Studien z. Gesch. d. Med. 10), Leipzig, 1914. The introduction to this work is contained in: Studien z. Gesch. d. Med. *11* und *12* (1918), XI-XXI. KNAPP, J. M.: Tierkreismann und Aderlassmann. Ciba-Zschr. (Basel) *22* (1935), pp. 758-61.

[3] WICKERSHEIMER, ERNEST: Figures médico-astrologiques des IXe, X^e, et XIe siècles. Janus (Leiden) *19* (1914) pp. 157-77.

[4] SUDHOFF, KARL: De westeuropäische Tierkreiszeichenmann, in: Lehr- und Merkschemata, *loc. cit.* (footnote 2), p. 205.

Fig. 23 One of the latest and most artistically perfect examples of the zodiac-man. Woodcut by Jollat signed with the Cross of Lorraine (see p. 88) and dated 1533. Printed in Paris. This figure demonstrates the close relationship between the zodiac-man and the early situs illustrations, an iconological relationship which was inevitable.

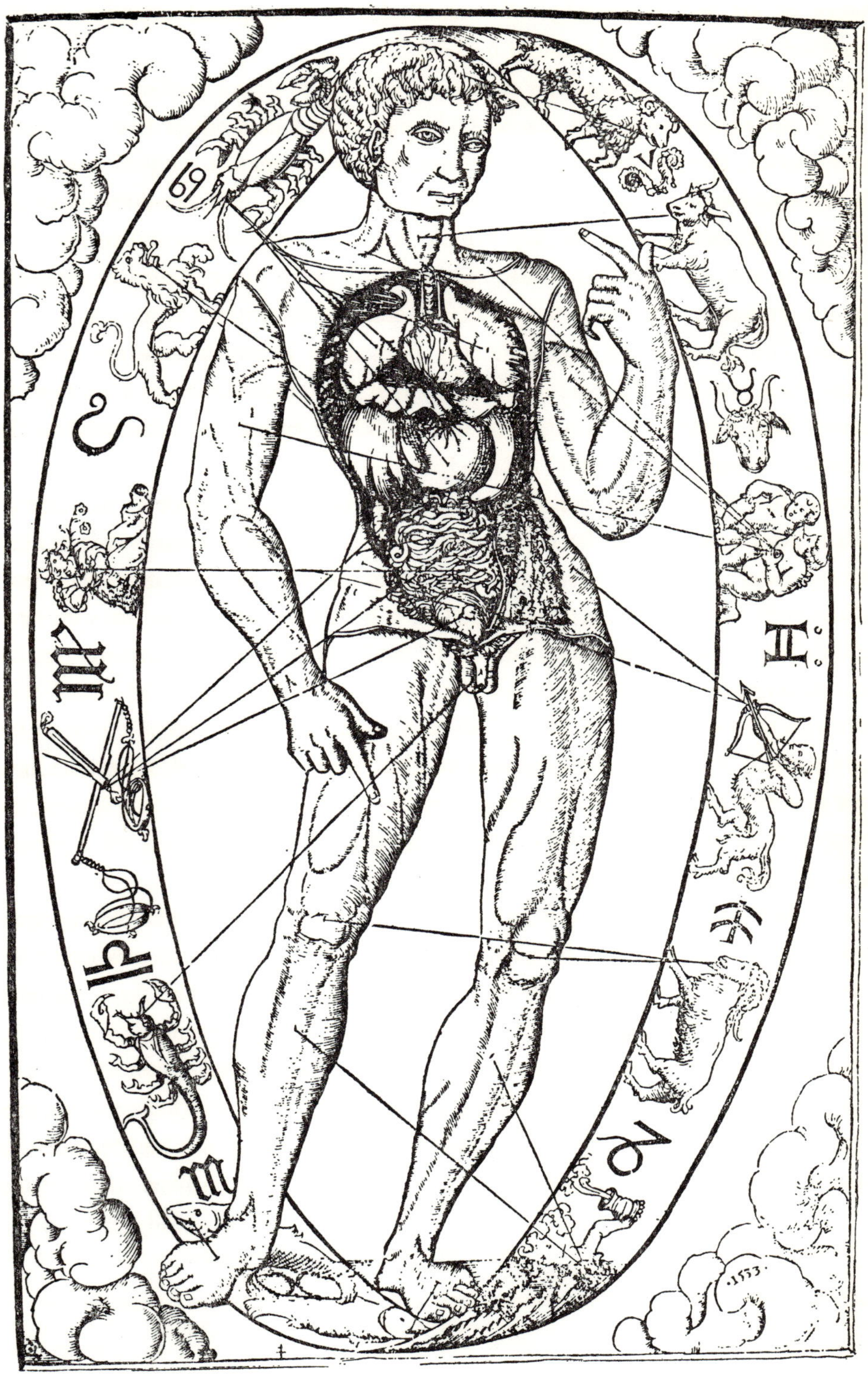

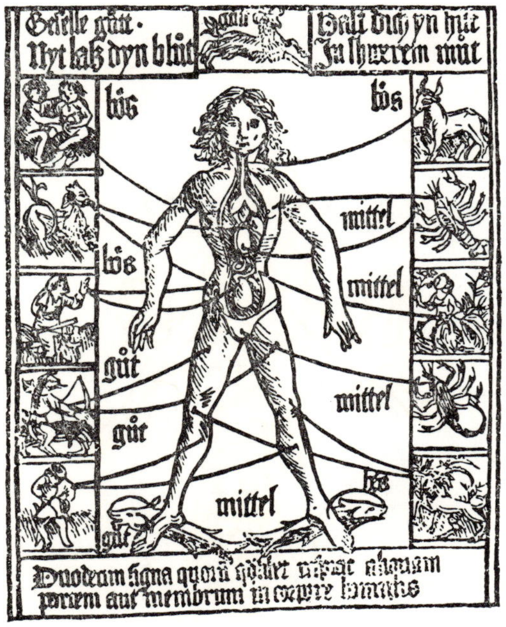

Fig. 24 Zodiac-man on a venesection plate, circa 1480, Munich, Kupferstichkabinett, Schr. 1925.

must derive from the time when Aries stood for the cosmic beginning, spring; that is, when the spring sun traversed the equinoctial line into the constellation of Aries. Such was the case between 2260 and 100 B.C. (KNAPP). It is no surprise to find ourselves once more drawn back into Greek antiquity, or even further. This source becomes even more evident when, as in our Wolfenbüttel specimen (plate X), the bloodletting man is squatting on a stool; for this clearly establishes his origin within the Alexandrian tradition.

Bloodletting tables, painted and printed, mainly belong to the practical care of health which flourished between the 14th and 16th centuries. The tables were principally employed in baths, where bloodletting was performed either regularly or on special instruction of a physician. In some fortunate cases, tables have been preserved in the public baths themselves, which allows their original place of use to be determined with some degree of accuracy.

The urine glass was the attribute of the medieval physician. It facilitated diagnosis from the urine – a process which still plays an important role in preliminary medical examination. Moreover, the glass flasks used in our hospitals for collecting urine have retained their original form.

The urine was optically examined for color, consistency (thin or viscous), and undissolved components. The color and localization of the latter, the so-called *contenta*, can be recorded in illustrations. This was done, and led to a special category of medieval illustration which flourished when bookprinting was invented. Thus, as with venesection illustrations, urinalysis illustrations subsequently passed into incunabula prints.

In urinalysis tables, simple black-and-white semi-schematic diagrams of course sufficed for specifying the location where the undissolved components could be observed (fig. 26).

Colored illustrations were employed to show discoloration of the urine; approximately twenty nuances were differentiated, from clear through yellow, orange, red, and brown, to black. The entire scale of colors is to be found in numerous preserved manuscripts, where it is represented in diverse graphic forms: incorporated in a continuous text (without the possibility of comparison); in two parallel columns on one page; and finally in the more elegant circular form of a urine-glass disk. This type also appears in many variations.[5] The oldest type shows the twenty urine glasses (*matulae*) on the branches of a tree (plate XIa) which also link groups of matulae to seven circles inscribed with terms of pathological classification. The organizational idea is graphically formed into an ornament, in a manner which is analogous to the iconography of the tree of Jesse, and was widespread during the Middle Ages. The same system is to be found in other variations, where the tree is replaced by a larger central circle[6] or else by a radial arrangement of the matulae around a disk.[7] The earliest example of this form of didactic illustration to be found

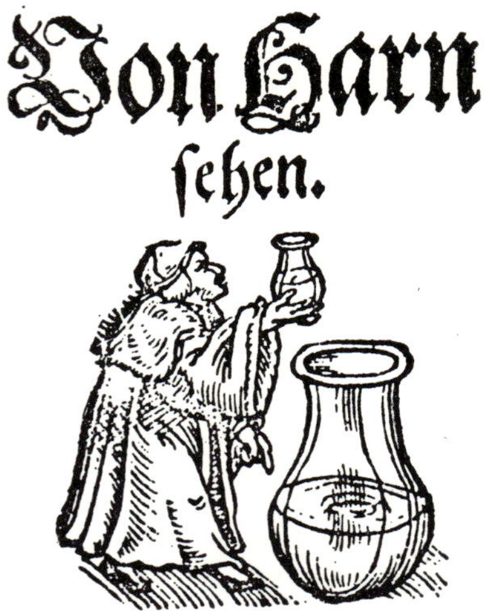

Fig. 25 Chapter heading from Walther Ryff, Practicierbüchlin bewerter Leibartznei, *Frankfort (Egenolff), 1555.*

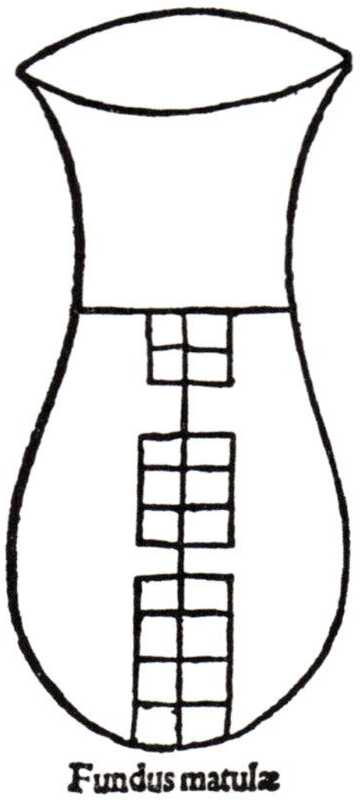

Fig. 26 Urine glass (matula), from Actuarius, De urinis, *Basel (Cratander), 1539.*

[5] Sudhoff, Karl: Die Harnglasscheibe im 15. Jahrhundert. In: Tradition und Naturbeobachtung in den Illustrationen medizinischer Handschriften und Frühdrucke vornehmlich des 15. Jahrhunderts (Studien z. Gesch. d. Med. I), Leipzig, 1907, pp. 13-18. Christoffel, Hans: Grundzüge der Uroskopie. Gesnerus *10* (1953); pp. 89-122.

[6] MacKinney, Loren: Medical Illustrations in Medieval Manuscripts. London, 1965. Fig. 6 reproduced from Codex Ashmole 391, fol. 10, Bodleiana Oxford.

[7] In Ms. 1192, University Library, Leipzig. In Sudhoff, *loc. cit.* (footnote 5), reproduced as plate IV.

reproduced in the incunabula is the urine examination table in the *Fasciculus medicinae* of JOHANNES DE KETHAM, Venice, 1491, which shows twenty-one matulae, arranged radially but opening inwards. Two of these were already colored black during printing, the rest being left for coloration by hand. Plates XIa through XId testify to the importance of this rosette-shaped diagrammatic form in medieval graphic art. Involuntarily one associates this form with the tracery in the window rosettes of Gothic cathedrals.

SUDHOFF[8] attributed the twenty-first KETHAM matula to the carelessness of the artist. More recently, however, an illustration for the Greek text of the Byzantine uroscopist THEOPHILUS[9] has been found in Bologna which, although of a different type, also contains twenty-one matulae. In this specimen, the matulae are arranged in rows below a typical late-classical scene in which THEOPHILUS is being offered a urine sample for examination. As in the Juliana Anicia Codex, the author is actually portrayed in his own work. The Bologna illustration – a late copy made in the 15th century – seems closer to the late-classical original of the uroscopic table than do the disks. It also reveals that the Byzantine urine-glass was not exclusively bulbous, but could also be of simple cylindrical shape (JOHANNES ACTUARIS, *Peri uron* II, I).

Both types, the column arrangement and the disk, appear together in an attractively conceived print dating from 1506. The mode of coloration employed is, of course, also watercolor. A carefully made copy (plate XII) is in the possession of the Madrid Universitary Library.

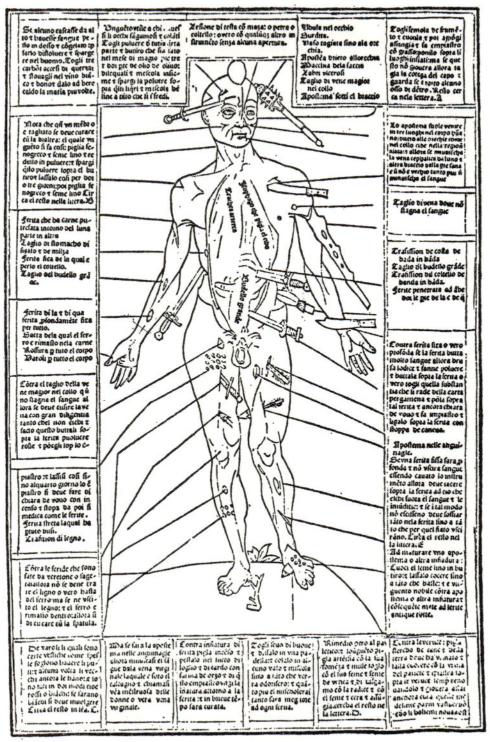

Fig. 27 Wound-man, from the Fasciculus medicinae *(Ketham), Venice, 1493.*

The figures of bloodletting men and of zodiac-men belong to a category of didactic graphic art which could be described as *reference tables*, insofar as they contain answers to specific questions connected with therapeutic treatment. In the field of diagnosis, the matula disks belong to the same category. A superficial connection also exists between these figures and a group of illustrations showing wounds, where a male figure similarly serves as the foil for a catalogue of medical opinions related to the human body and its parts.

Medieval traumatology created a popular graphic figure in the "wound-man," a diagrammatic figure containing a kind of graphic catalogue of frequent injuries. The purpose of such a figure, however, is not as obvious as that of the bloodletting man or zodiac-man. The wound-man appears at the beginning of surgical textbooks as a title-page figure – for example, in the best-known German surgical incunabula, the *Buch der Cirurgia, Hantwirckung der wundartzny* by HIERONYMUS BRUNSCHWIG (Strasbourg, 1497)[10] (fig. 57), or in the first representative textbook on cranial surgery, the *Tractatus de fractura cranei of* JACOPO BERENGARIO DA CAPRI, in the

8 SUDHOFF, *loc. cit.* (footnote 5) p. 14.

9 In Ms. 3632, fol. 51, University Library, Bologna. See plate XII.

10 Modern facsimile editions: Das Buch der Chirurgie des Hiernoymus Brunschwig. Accompanying text by GUSTAV KLEIN, Munich, 1911, contains further literature. The Book of Cirurgia by Hieronymus Brunschwig. With a Study on H.B. and his work by HENRY E. SIGERIST, Milano, 1923.

beautiful Venetian edition in quarto of 1535. In keeping with the subject matter of the book, the title page of the *Tractatus* does not depict the whole human body, but only a "wounded head" (fig. 28).

Sudhoff described the wound-man of the incunabula as a "surgical caricature of St. Sebastian," "a naked male figure thoroughly pierced in the head, torso and limbs by arrow and lance heads, daggers, knives, maces, rocks and cudgels." The fact that in most wood-engravings he is also shown with opened thoracic and abdominal cavities, which accordingly links him with the oldest anatomical illustration, has made him especially interesting for medical historians.

Comparison with the figure of Sebastian, the martyr who was pierced by arrows – who at that time was quite a fashionable subject in all the fine arts – is both pertinent and misleading. Realism, even when it impresses the observer as such, still has a hybrid quality. The true nature of this category of graphic art is revealed in some of the few extant manuscript illustrations which have preserved the character of appreciably older prototypes, such as a codex in Munich dating from about 1485,[11] or a group of extra-large-sized parchment sheets in the Kongelike Bibliothek in Copenhagen.[12] They contain medieval texts in which the wound-men were also originally featured as prominent illustrations. Moreover, their simple composition reveals that they were intended for the little-educated, nonacademic public who frequented the barbers' shops and public baths, and for whom the texts were meant to serve as educational documents, on about the same level as the level of present-day children's picture-books. Occasionally, a didactically talented surgeon might have supplemented the traditional catalogue of pictures on his own initiative, as is possibly the case with a recently published illustrated manuscript of German origin in the collection of the Wellcome Historical Medical Library in London.[13]

A similar function was served by the male and female "sickness-figures" in which the names of different maladies, frequently interspersed with anatomical terms, were related to the structure of a naked human figure. Lastly, there is the primitive picture-text figure devoted to the female genital organs and to pregnancy, in a manner quite like that of the Alexandrian five- and nine-figure series. It is still present in the printed incunabula at the end of the 15th century, and in Venice it even has a role in the transition from medieval to modern illustration: the *Fasciculus medicinae* of Johannes de Ketham (1491/93) contains – in addition to one such engraving which will be discussed later – a "sickness-man" (fig. 29) wholly in the medieval tradition.

Sudhoff is quite correct in assigning the bloodletting illustrations and their

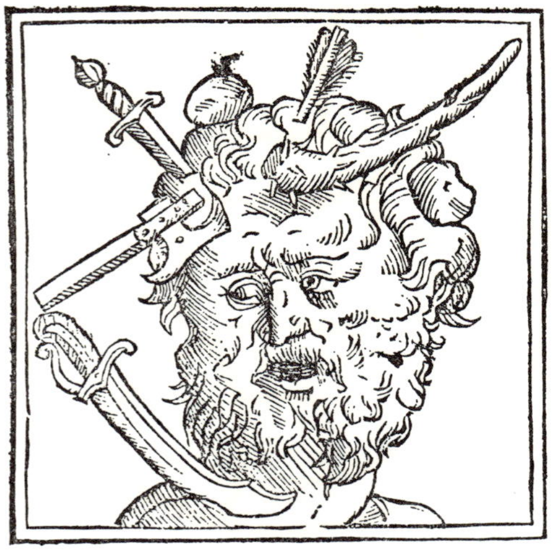

Fig. 28 Title-page woodcut, 'Wounded head', for Jacopo Berengario da Carpi's Tractatus perutilis et completus de fractura cranei, *Venice, 1535.*

Fig. 29 Sickness-figure, from the Fasciculus medicinae *(Ketham), Venice, 1493.*

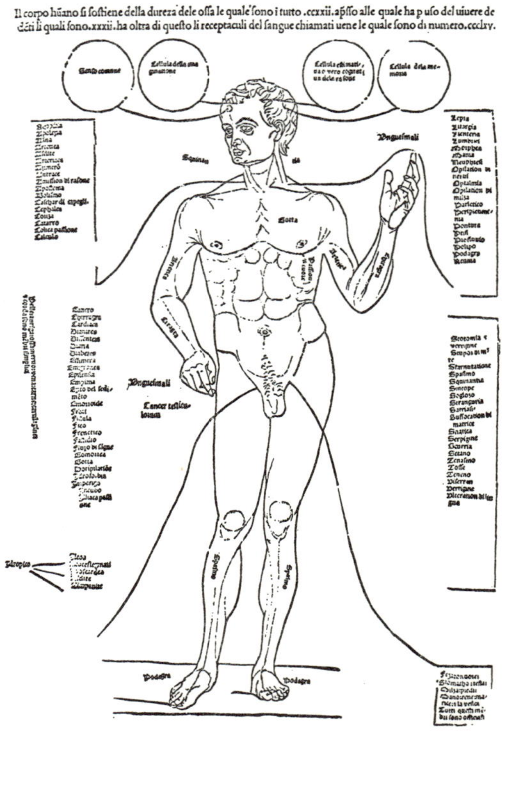

[11] Reproduced as plate VI, in Sudhoff, Karl: Der 'Wundenmann' in Frühdruck und Handschrift und sein erklärender Text. (Sudh.) Arch. Gesch. Med. *1* (1908) pp. 351-361.

[12] Sudhoff, Karl: Neue Beiträge zur Vorgeschichte des Ketham. (Sudh.) Arch. Gesch. Med. *5* (1912), p. 288 ff.

[13] Hill, Boyd, H.: J. Hist. Med. All. Sc. *20* (1965) pp. 334-357.

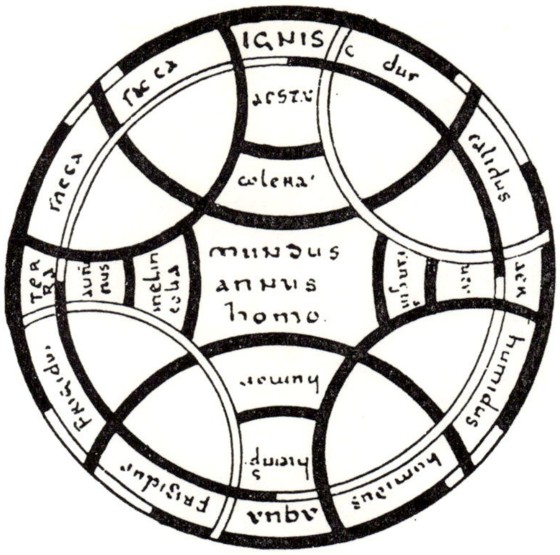

Fig. 30 Fourfold schema from the Ms. lat. Monac. 14300, Bayer. Staatsbibliothek, Munich, 8th century A.D.

unoriginal derivations, a small series of cupping illustrations[14] to the same class of explanatory or instructive diagrams as the zodiac- and wound-men. Finally, an affiliated group remains to be mentioned; namely, the tables indicating the parts of the body where wounds heal or do not heal. These diagrams are a type of wound-man whose figure is covered with wounds (or arrow-heads) and with corresponding labels, "curabilis" or "incurabilis."

These diagrams, which were a category of graphic illustration already existing in antiquity, also appear in the Middle Ages, occasionally in forms derived exclusively from abstract geometry. It is not surprising that certain late-classical doctrines in the field of biology and anthropology, such as the pathological doctrine of the four humors, should have been transformed into didactic and reference graphic art. As early as 1914, WICKERSHEIMER drew attention to the existence of medico-astrological diagrams; more recently, diagrams dating from the 8th century were discovered (fig. 30) which were developed from the circle and arc to demonstrate the interrelationship between *mundus* (four elements, four primary qualities), *annus* (the four seasons), and *homo* (four humors).[15] This confirms the suspicion that, despite the ornamental features first introduced at that time, the source of this type of medical illustration is not Arabic, but Alexandrian. It is quite plausible to assume that late-classical diagrams would naturally have been translated into Islamic designs during their passage through Arabic literature. The problem is evidently complex and requires further investigation.

A further, more widely dispersed, group of full figures related graphically to the zodiac-men and wound-men reopens the unresolved problem of the origins of such reference diagrams: I refer to the cauterization pictures. Attempts to establish their derivation from late-classical illustrations have not been completely successful, but their accompanying text has been traced back to CAELIUS AURELIANUS, so that SUDHOFF'S hypothesis of an "Alexandrian origin, with a later modification of the drawing and supplementation of the text in southern Italy under the influence of north African method,"[16] is sufficiently plausible to justify our inclusion of one example in the section on "Antiquity" (see pp. 16, 19, and plate IV); namely, the miniatures of the Oxford Codex Rawlinson 328, for which an early origin is suggested by the Byzantine-Romanesque arches and oval beds. It is necessary to return to the cauterization pictures now in order to establish their connections with medieval medicine.

During the Middle Ages, the conditions necessitating this form of therapy were generally identified by the medical doctors rather than the surgeons. We have

Fig. 31 Cauterization miniature from the Cod. lat. 13002, Bayer. Staatsbibliothek, Munich (Prüfening Codex of 1158). 'Dyocles medicus' is indicating that cauterization in this case should be performed three times on each side of the thorax and once below the navel.

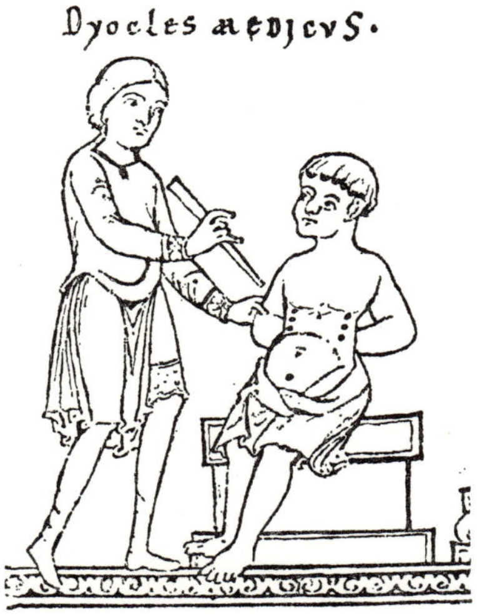

14 SUDHOFF, KARL: 'Lehrfiguren für das Schröpfen' als Abschnitt in Beiträge z. Gesch. d. Chir. im M. A., Stud. Gesch. Med. *10* (1914), pp. 125-143.

15 SCHÖNER, ERICH: Das Viererschema in der antiken Humoralpathologie. With foreword and plate by ROBERT HERRLINGER. Supplement to Sudhoff's Archiv *4* (1964). – Isidore de Séville, Traité de la nature. Ed. JACQUES FONTAINE, Bibliothèque de l'Ecole des Hautes Etudes Hispaniques XVIII, Bordeaux, 1960.

16 SUDHOFF, *loc. cit.* (footnote 1), Stud. *10* (1914): pp. 70, 80, 97, and Stud. *11* (1918), pp. XV, XVI.

already observed that these conditions were chiefly of the kind that would now fall under internal medicine and neurology. The underlying theoretical pathophysiological conceptions are in no way alien to the medical field: the predominating doctrine of the four humors with its axioms of eucrasy and dycrasy of the body fluids, and its hypothesis that a dycrasy could be restored to a eucrasy by mechanically drawing off the "sick fluids." The practice of cauterization had been a disputed, if never wholly abandoned, method of therapy during the late-classical period; it eventually regained its authority in the Arabic medical tracts of the high Middle Ages; and late-medieval European writers, who made increasing use of illustration, soon developed regular anatomical-topographical atlases for cautery. Examples of these are still to be found in the following well-preserved manuscripts which we have already encountered, or shall encouter later: Codex 13002 in the Staatsbibliothek at Munich (see pp. 11-12); Ms. Harley 1585 and Ms. Sloane 1975 in the British Museum; Codex Casanatensis 1882, and Ms. Rawlinson 328 in the Oxford Bodleian Library. SUDHOFF'S relevant catalogue[17] has already been referred to.

Plates XIII and XIV show two pages of cauterization pictures from the Ms. Sloane 1975, in which the colors are particularly well-preserved. They precede a third page of similar illustrations at the end of a codex that also contains the *Libri IV medicinae Ypocratis Platonis Apoliensis Urbis, de diversis herbis* – a copiously illustrated textbook on herbal remedies (see p. 45) – and that concludes with this three-page section. In the first picture, a master gives instructions from a prescription to an apprentice who is using a mortar. The second picture shows two physicians performing a bloody operation, evidently involving simultaneous incision and cautery, on a fettered *Epilepticus;* the skilled miniaturist has indulged his fantasy in providing realistic detail. The remaining pictures represent a compendium from a more abundant catalogue which, in other contemporary manuscripts, is frequently overworked. The maladies requiring cauterization are inscribed on small plaques distributed over the figures: *ad dolorem capitis incenditur sic, ad reuma gingivarum sic, ad epar sic,* etc. In the two pictures at the top of plate XIII, frontal and dorsal views have been combined one with another; and their correct relationship is revealed by the respective inscriptions. The already garbled prototype to this version was, however, not without a certain didactic relevance. It cannot be held against this miniaturist that one of the pair is shown clutching the hair of his partner and, in the second scene, twisting his own neck.[18]

Fig. 32 Miniature from the Ms. Harley 1585, British Museum, fol. 72ᵛ, original size. Monochrome ink drawing.

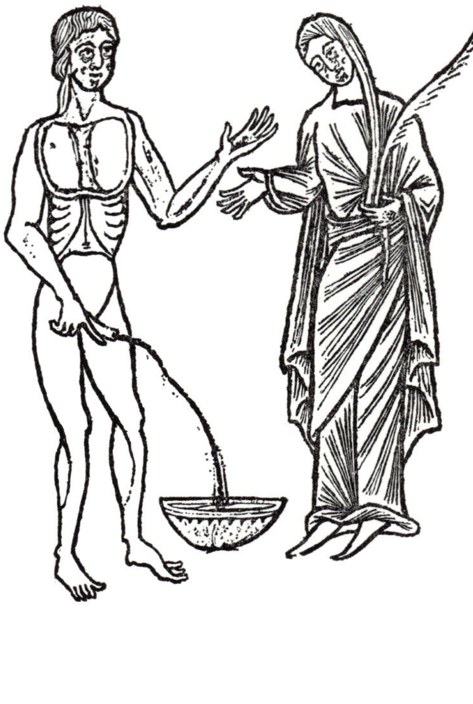

These cauterization pictures occupy an intermediate position between the venesection figures, zodiac-men, and wound-men on the one hand, and an extensive

[17] See p. 16 footnote 19.

[18] Also in Ms. Harley 1585, British Museum. This manuscript is thought to have been written in the Maas Valley, near Liège, in the third quarter of the 12th century; according to this reckoning, SUDHOFF has dated too early. See TURNER, D. H.: Romanesque Illuminated Manuscripts in the British Museum, London, 1966, for recent commentary.

group of illustrated scenes from medical practice on the other hand. Whereas the former were restricted to elementary outline forms of a virtually abstract nature, reminiscent of the Alexandrian five-figure series, the latter were represented quite naturalistically from daily life; and it was only through the work of generations of copyists that some were finally reduced to formulae. Here, too, there is nothing to contradict SUDHOFF'S hypothesis that their sources might be sought in Alexandrian medical manuscripts. This line of investigation is indicated by the Nicetas Codex. A considerable number of similar medical codices have been preserved which are opulently illustrated, and depict in small scenes the employment of drugs and physical therapeutic treatment, or illustrate surgical aid and operations. Frequently, abridgement by successive copyists has created such a distortion that only the accompanying text can render it comprehensible; occasionally, however, the illustration remains the key to a completely ruined text. The production of facsimile editions has yet to be attempted. For those who wish to gain an impression of the richness of medical graphic art in medieval manuscripts, SUDHOFF (1914-1917)[19] has published several series of illustrations reproduced as photogravures in extenso. The Vienna Codex 93,[20] of 13th-century Italian origin, and the so-called Leyden THEODORIC Manuscript (Ms. Voss. 3, Univ. Lib. Leyden), dating from circa 1375,[21] are deservedly famous. With respect to the quality of the illuminations, however, both are surpassed by a French codex containing a *Chirurgia* by ROGER OF SALERNO which, as in the case of Ms. Sloane 1977, is one of the rarities in possession of the British Museum.[22] Finally, there is a 13th-century northern Italian codex, now in the state Biblioteca Casanatense at Rome, that also belongs among the classics of medieval medical-surgical illustrations; namely, a *Chirurgia* by ROLANDI OF PARMA.[23]

Fig. 33

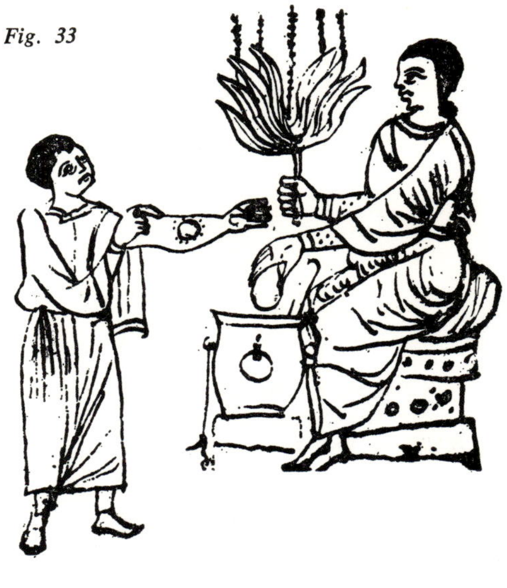

The Vienna Codex 93[24] and the London Ms. Sloane 1977 both have distinctive features: in the former, we find additional pen-and-ink drawings, while in the French miniatures in the Sloane manuscript the surgical scenes are enhanced by ecclesiastical motifs. The marginalia on the Vienna Codex, in which a "Pseudo-Apuleius" is dominant, are in part scarcely lower in quality than the miniatures in

[19] SUDHOFF, *loc. cit.* (footnote 1), Stud. *10* (1914); SUDHOFF in (Sudh.) Arch. Gesch. Med. *8* (19), pp. 378 ff. and *10* (1917), p. 71 ff.

[20] Twelve illustrations are reproduced in color in H. SCHIPPERGES 'Antike Medizin im Spiegel des Mittelalters', Therap. Berichte (Bayer) *33* (1961), pp. 201-209. – 41 illustrations in photogravure, in K. SUDHOFF: 'Szenen aus der Sprechstunde und bei Krankenbesuchen des Arztes in mittelalterlichen Handschriften III', (Sudh.) Arch. Gesch. Med. *10* (1917) p. 73 ff. and plates II-V.

[21] SUDHOFF, *loc. cit.* (footnote 1), Stud. *10* (1914), pp. 47-51 and plates VII and VIIIa with thirty illustrations in photogravure. – Two colored illustrations, in LOREN MCKINNEY: Medical Illustration in Medieval Manuscripts, London, 1965, figs. 66 and 67.

[22] SUDHOFF, *loc. cit.* (footnote 1), Stud *10* (1914), pp. 19-32 and plates II-IV, all illustrations in photogravure.

[23] SUDHOFF, *loc. cit.* (footnote 1), Stud. *10* (1914), pp. 43-46 without illustrations. – The illustrations in GIACOSA, PIERO: Magistri Salernitani nondum editi, Torino, 1902, plates 24-27. Three not very succesful colored illustrations in MCKINNEY, *loc. cit.* (footnote 21), figs. 63, 81B, 82A.

[24] SWARZENSKI, G.: Mittelalterliche Kopien einer antiken medizinischen Bilderhandschrift. Jahrb. Kaiser. deutsch. Archäol. Inst. *17* (1902), pp. 45-53. – See also the Catalogue of Vienna manuscripts compiled by H. J. HERMANN (1923).

the text proper: see figure 33, reproduced from the Vienna Codex, folio 41. The upper two-thirds of the sheet contains an ink painting of a plant called "*polinaris,*" with an explanation of its origin; Apollo created the plant and gave it to Asclepius. In the lower – originally blank – space, a late 13th-century artist has added a realistic scene in which a patient is showing an ulcer on his left forearm to a physician who is engaged in preparing the medicinal plant held before him. In addition, older illustrations based on late-classical prototypes not only display plants but also depict numerous scenes from medical practice, including not a few obstetrical scenes.

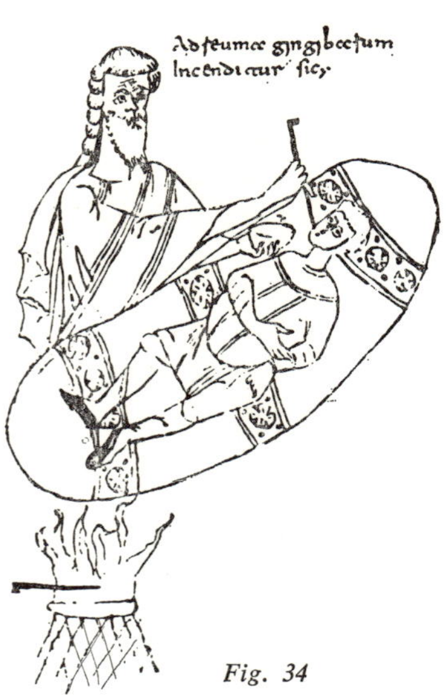

Fig. 34

There are also codices furnished throughout with pen-and-ink drawings illustrating every topic discussed. The most famous of these are the Prüfening squatting figures (see p. 11) in a Codex latinus dating from 1158. This also includes a series of cauterization pictures (fig. 31).[25] At least one century older than the Prüfening Codex is a Florentine manuscript (Cod. Laurentianus LXXIII, 41) which was originally owned by the anatomist GABRIELE ZERBI, and which contains sixteen cauterization pictures drawn in pen and ink (fig. 34).[26]

The illustrations of the Codex Roncioni 99 in the University Library at Pisa strike the observer as being even older, although they were only drawn at the end of the 12th century (fig. 35).[27] The impression gained is one of unusual closeness to Greek prototypes. A group of operation scenes, which are mainly executed in opaque ink, can be found in a copy of ROGER OF SALERNO'S *Chirurgia* in the Trinity College Library, Cambridge (Ms. 0. 1. 20). SUDHOFF has published a detailed description of this series.[27] It consists of diverse scenes demonstrating the treatments of wounds – examinations, operations, preparation and application of medicaments – in some instances with great power of expression.

Fig. 35 Pen-and-ink drawing from the fragment of a codex dating circa 1200: the Codex Roncioni 99, Biblioteca Universitaria, Pisa.

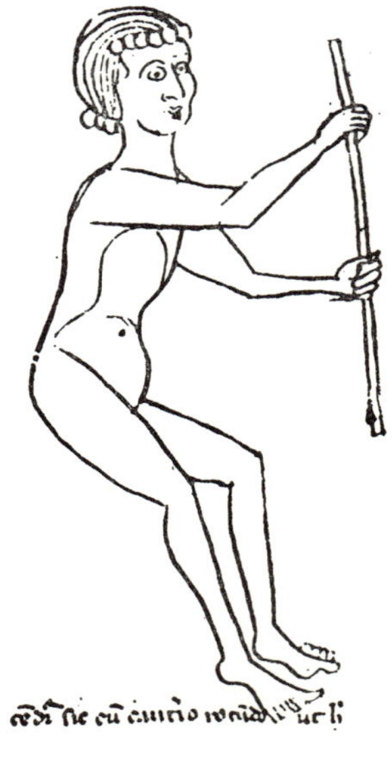

The influence of French miniature painting on the development of western manuscript illustration can hardly be overestimated. This kind of painting became pre-eminent in Europe about the middle of the 13th century. Medical illustration also profited from it, although contemporary book illustration was pervaded by ecclesiastical art. The most beautiful example of French miniature painting from the field of medical illustration is, accordingly, a hybrid derivation containing ecclesiastical and profane elements, part Christian iconography and part surgical. We are referring to the Codex Sloane 1977 in the British Museum (plate XVI). In the 13th century, surgery was to some extent still included under monastic medicine. Even where this was not the case, the Church dominated medical illustration, for the not unimportant reason that copying – the making of books – was completely in the hands of the Church. Consequently, in the French edition of the *Chirurgia* of ROGER OF SALERNO, the upper pictures on the seventeen illustrated

[25] SUDHOFF, *loc. cit.* (footnote 1), Stud. *10* (1914), pp. 95-97 and plate XXI.
[26] SUDHOFF, *loc. cit.* X (footnote 1), Stud. *10* (1914), pp. 90-91 and plates XV and XVI.
[27] For Cod. Roncioni see SUDHOFF, *loc. cit.* (footnote 1), Stud. *10* (1914), pp. 98-99 and plate XXIII. For Ms. Trinity College 0. 1. 20, see SUDHOFF, *loc. cit.* (footnote 1), Stud. *10* (1914), pp. 33-42 and plates V-VII.

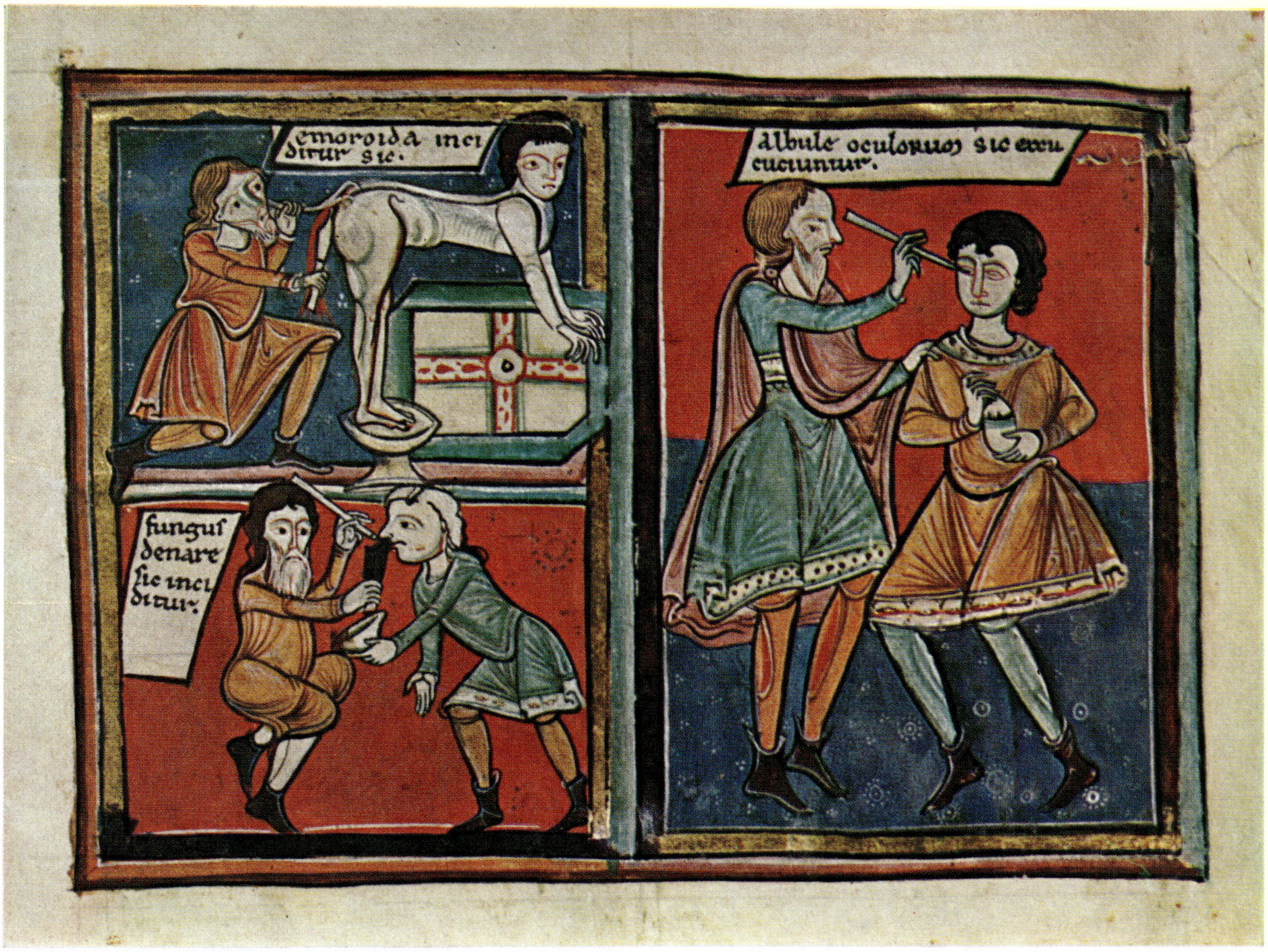

Plate III Operative treatment of hemorrhoids, nasal polyps and cataract, in the MS. Sloane 1975, British Museum, London, 12th century. Slightly enlarged from the original.

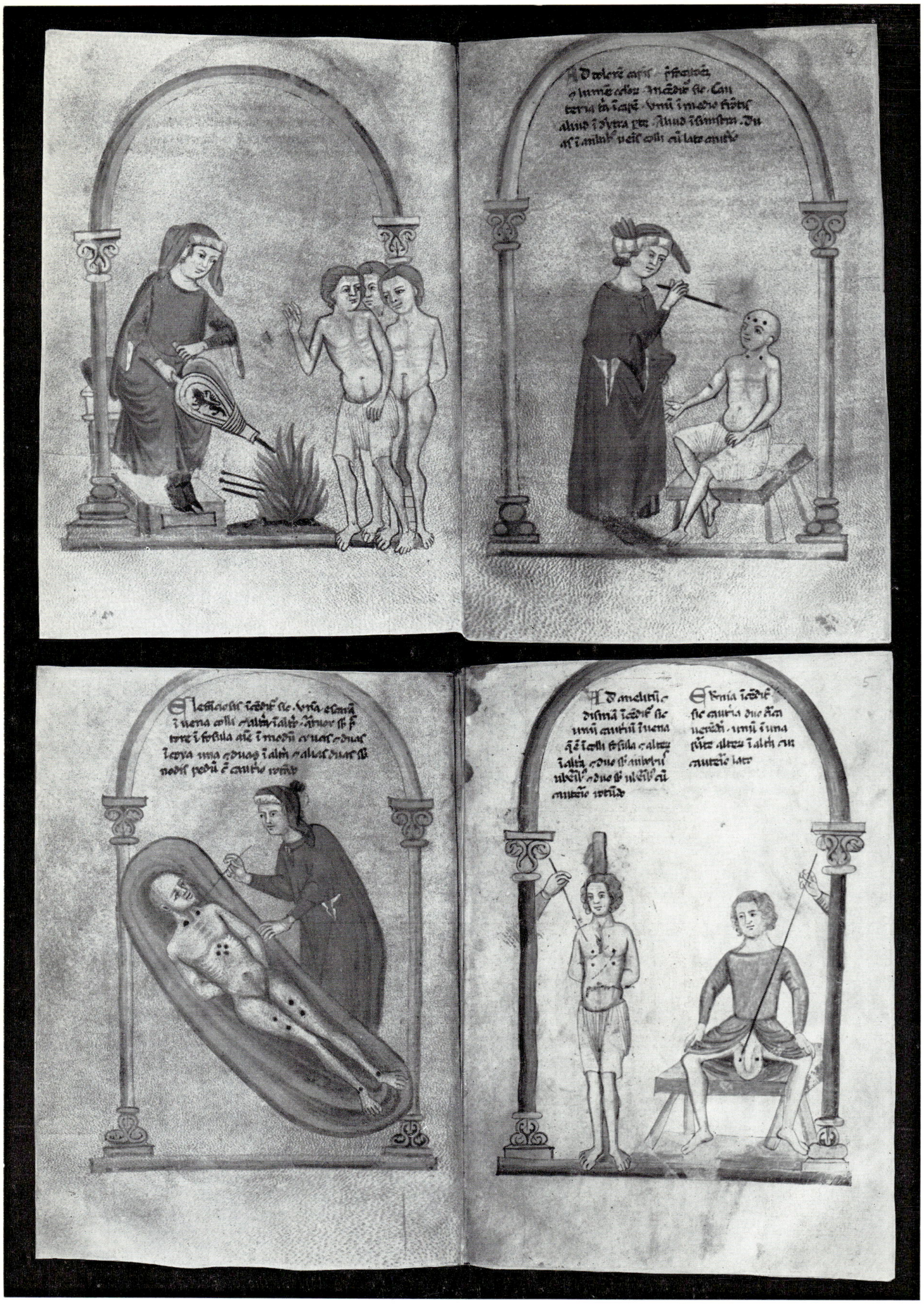

Plate IV Four illustrations from the MS. Rawlinson C 328, Bodleian Library, Oxford. They demonstrate cauterization, and at the top left, preparation of the cautery.

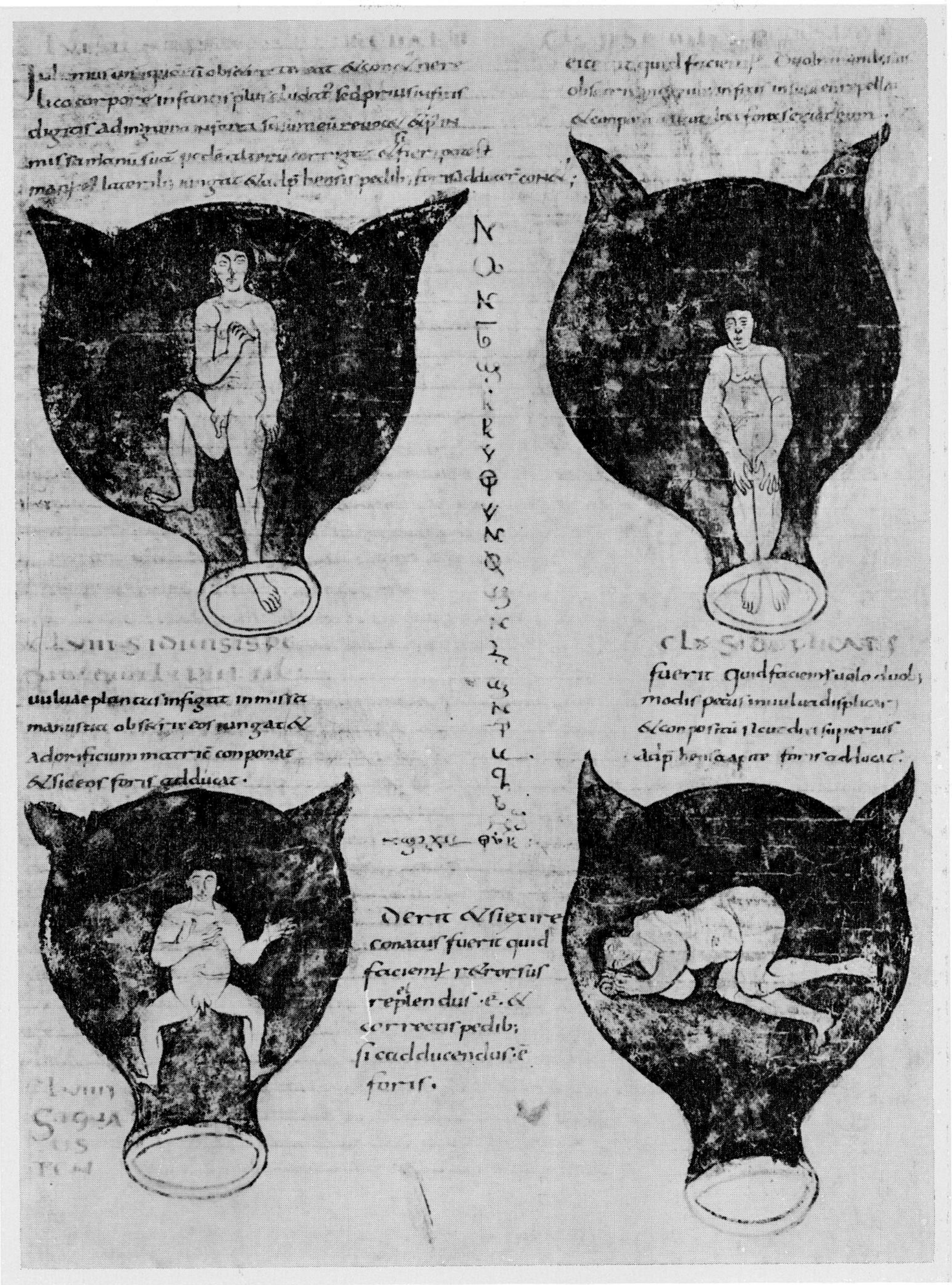

Plate V An adaption from Soranos, 2nd century A.D., of the fetus in the uterus, by Moschion, 6th century. MS. 3714, fol. 28ʳ, Bibl. Royale, Brussels, 9th century.

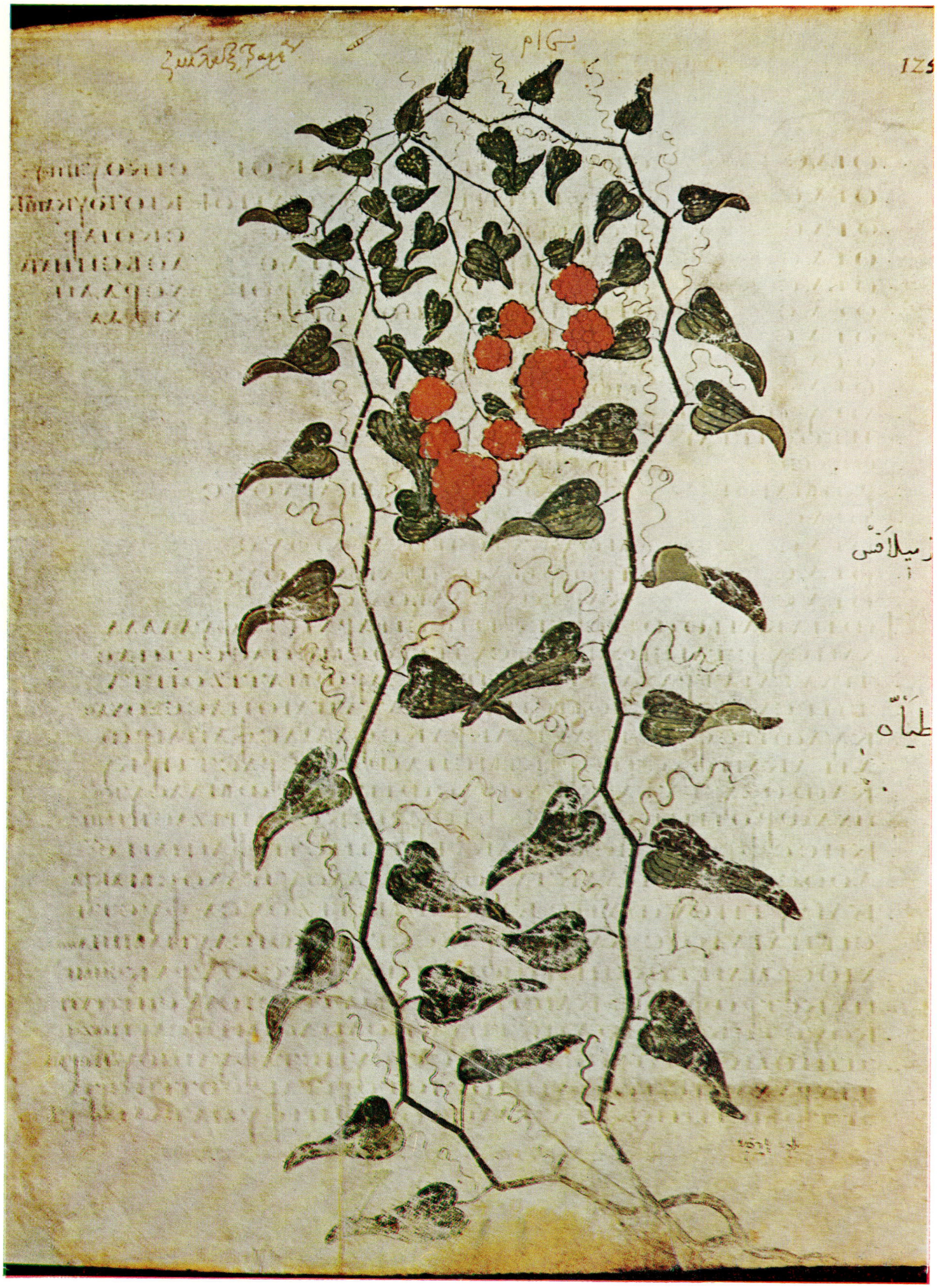

Plate VI Smilax aspera (trachea). It was valued by the ancients as an antitoxic medicament and also served as decoration for Bacchanalian feasts. From the Viennese Dioscorides, Cod. med. graec. I in the Österr. Nationalbibliothek, 6th century A.D.

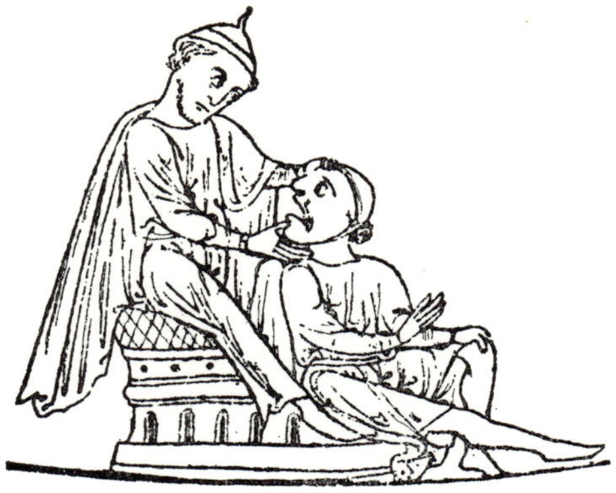

Fig. 36 Pen-and-ink drawing from a French manuscript, Codex O.I. 20, Trinity College Library, Cambridge, 13th century.

sheets present the life of Jesus, from the Annunciation to the Assumption of the Blessed Virgin, and the lower pictures present a surgical atlas of ninety-four scenes. This is a masterpiece in every respect. The colors, with blue and red dominating, are of a brilliant freshness rendered solemn by the goldleaf in the background and the framework of the biblical scenes. In the heading of the title page, Christ is enthroned between two adoring figures; under this scene, the miniaturist has portrayed himself; and then, before the name of the author – *"Mestre rogier de salerne"* – the monk has inscribed: *"Au commencement de cest livre prions dieu . . ."* Cosmas and Damian are finally portrayed as part of a scene showing a sickbed that possibly belongs to a leper. The Paris College of Surgeons was founded under the patronage of these two saints in the century that this codex was written.

The series of surgical illustrations begins with the upper extremity of the body, treating cranial surgery in the first three sheets, and then the neck. The historically trained observer will immediately recognize the familiar illustrations from the Florentine Nicetas Codex of *Peri arthron* (see p. 15), except that here the physician, patient, and apprentice are not naked, but clothed according to the fashion of the 13th century. Next comes the surgery of the thorax; the tenth sheet of illustrations concludes with the suture of a large thoracic wound, and the eleventh begins with a rib fracture which is being treated in the bath (plate XVI). The next illustrations show the major abdominal injuries and breast cancer (also plate XVI), afflictions of the male genitals, and herniotomy. Further illustrations demonstrate vesical calculus, rectal prolapse, and hemorrhoids, before the miniaturist – proceeding according to his surgical text, *"a capite ad calcem"* – arrives at the lower extremity of the body. The series ends with an illustration of leprosy. The attentive observer will discover an abundance of details, including some which are not mentioned in the text, and there can be no doubt that the artist must have had a first-hand acquaintance with surgical treatment of wounds.

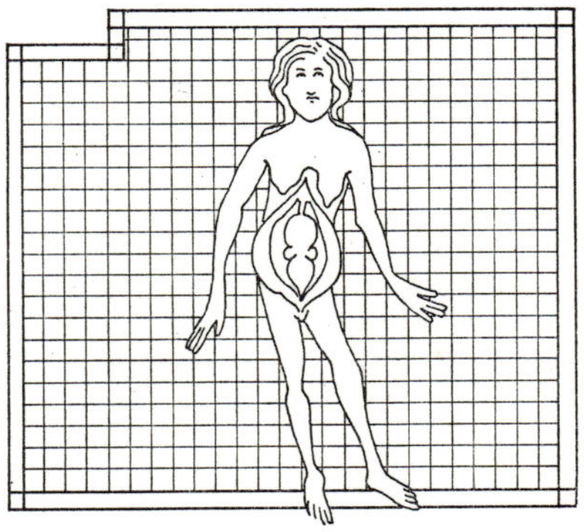

Fig. 37a

Figs. 37a, b Two miniatures from Henri de Mondeville's Anatomia Mundini, *about 1314. Ms. français 2030, Bibliothèque Nationale, Paris.*

Fig. 37b

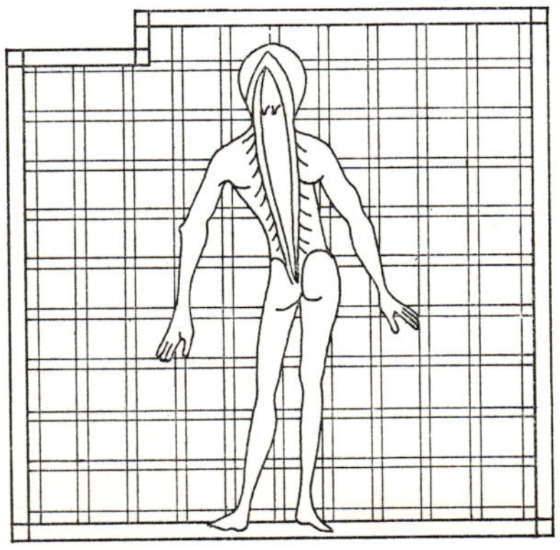

Actual anatomical illustration,[28] which, when we reach the 15th century, will force every other theme of medical science into the background, was unimportant in the Middle Ages. Most of what remains is evidently closely related to Alexandrian didactic graphic art. The explanation for this is that practical anatomy had been dead for over a thousand years. The first anatomical demonstrations to be performed in medieval Europe probably were done in Italy about the time of the publication,

[28] Historical studies of anatomical illustration began in the 19th century with LUDWIG CHOULANT: Geschichte und Bibliographie der anatomischen Abbildung nach ihrer Beziehung auf anatomische Wissenschaft und bildende Kunst, Leipzig, 1582. More oriented to art history is LORIS PREMUDA'S Storia dell' Iconografia anatomica, Mailand, 1956. CHOULANT'S work was, however, continued by KARL SUDHOFF, who published a great many articles during the course of his research, by CHARLES SINGER (The Evolution of Anatomy, London, 1925), and by MORTIMER FRANK, the English translator of CHOULANT. FRANK added to this work, which was conceived as a catalogue rather than a historical treatment of relevant problems, until the year 1917 (see the foreword to L. CHOULANT and M. FRANK'S History and Bibliography of Anatomic Illustration in its Relations to Anatomic Science and the Graphic Arts, Chicago, 1920; second edition, New York, 1945).

in 1316, of the *Anatomia Mundini*, the first anatomical textbook to incorporate new knowledge which, however tentatively, had progressed beyond that of antiquity. There are new illustrations drawn by two surgeons: HENRI DE MONDEVILLE of Montpellier, who was educated in Bologna; and GUIDO DA VIGEVANO, born in Lombardy, and later personal physician to Queen Jeanne de Bourgogne, the wife of Philip VII of Valois. Their illustrations date from circa 1314 and 1345, respectively.

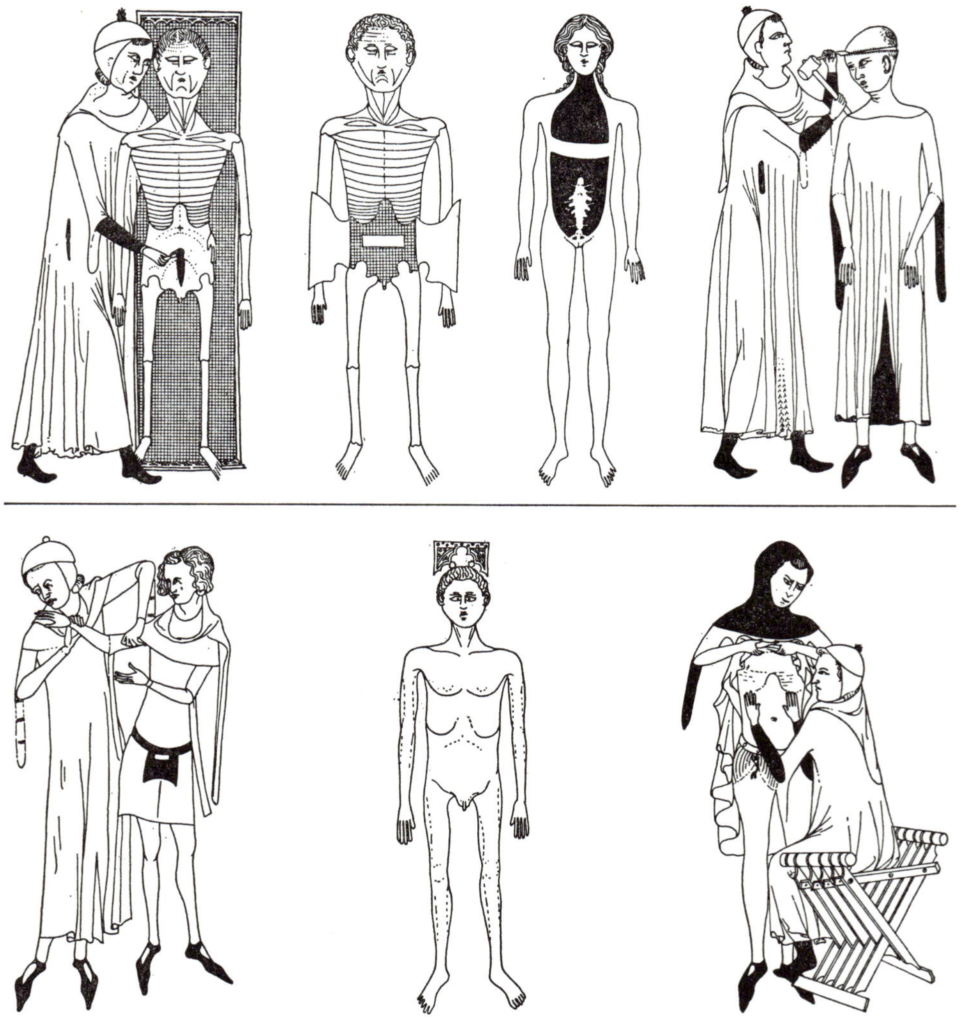

Fig. 38 Seven of the eighteen illustrations from the Anathomia *by Guido da Vigevano, 1345; Ms. 334 (ex 569), Musée Condé, Château Chantilly. Redrawn by Wolfgang Vater (Kiel).*

Of MONDEVILLE'S illustrations, only one exceptional series of miniatures remains; it is preserved in the Ms. fr. 2030 in the Bibliothèque Nationale, Paris.[29] These small pictures, more decorative than detailed, testify to the artist's break with the

[29] SUDHOFF, KARL: Abbildungen zur Anatomie des Maitre Henri de Mondeville (ca. 1260 – ca. 1320), in: Ein Beitrag zur Geschichte der Anatomie im Mittelalter, speziell der anatomischen Graphik nach Handschriften des 9. bis 15. Jahrhunderts (Stud. zur Gesch. d. Med. *4*), Leipzig, 1908, pp. 82-89 and plate XXIV. – Supplements in: (Sudh.) Archiv Gesch. Med. *8* (1915); pp. 130-133. Better illustrations than SUDHOFF'S are to be found in F. WEINDLER: Geschichte der gynäkologisch-anatomischen Abbildung, Dresden, 1908, figs. 40 - 51. We have reproduced two simple outline drawings in the margin of page 39 (figs. 37a, b).

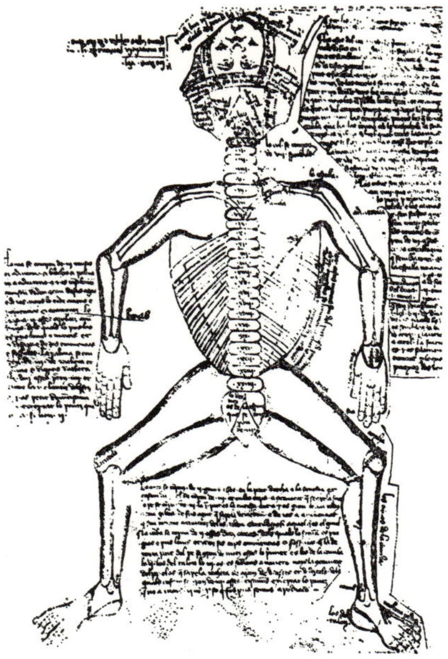

Fig. 39 Skeleton from Ms. D. II, 11, Universitätsbibliothek, Basel, folio 169ᵛ, 13th century Provençal inscription.

Fig. 40 Skeleton from the Cod. lat. 13042, Bayer. Staatsbibliothek, Munich, 14th century.

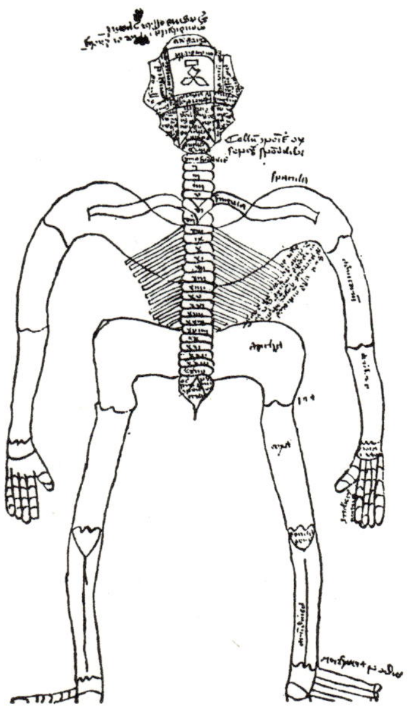

Alexandrian tradition; many of the subjects covered are clearly non-traditional. The artist employed the original plates in his lectures at Montpellier to demonstrate anatomy to his students, since it was nearly impossible at that time to demonstrate directly from the cadaver.

VIGEVANO'S illustrations,[30] eighteen full-page colored figures found in an *Anathomia* compiled for King Philip, represent genuine medieval graphic art. There is no question of naturalism – for instance, the anatomist is shown chiselling open the cranium of a live patient. A. M. CETTO'S interpretation is perfectly correct: she says, "Instead of a 'realistic' presentation which would show the cranium being opened on a naked, outstretched corpse, the artist has chosen a mode of presentation which more or less says: 'Imagine a human body. The anatomist is chiselling open the cranium of the dead man at the point that I am indicating, and this is being performed with the instruments I have reproduced here.' "

As far as the topographical pictures are concerned, it is immediately clear that the artist has worked from earlier designs. Most interesting in this respect is the seven-lobed uterus. The first illustration in figure 38 shows the casual manner in which the artist has drawn the frontal and top views on one plane. Only two of the pictures break the clearly delineated bounds of traditional form: in one artistically drawn scene, the physician is palpating his patient's abdomen; in the other, he is feeling his patient's pulse, which from the aspect of medical history is quite remarkable, for the physician has a practiced double-hold on the radius and brachium. The realistic presentation is intentional and also well-executed. In 1345, the year of origin of this truly regal codex, which is now at the Musée Condée in the Château de Chantilly, GIOTTO had been dead for less than ten years.

As previously mentioned, prior to the appearance of the two innovators MONDEVILLE and VIGEVANO, anatomical illustration depended largely on the thousand-year-old Alexandrian tradition. Since MONDEVILLE and VIGEVANO were not copied, the situation had not changed even by the early 15th century. There are only three variants which seem worthy of note: first, the skeleton-figure from the Provençal manuscript in the Municipal and University Library of Basel, which has already been discussed in connection with the ancient squatting figure series (Ms. D. II, see plate II); second, two viscera figures in the Royal Library at Stockholm, which were first reproduced by SUDHOFF in 1915 and which date from the late 15th and early 16th century, respectively; and third, a handful of examples of what SUDHOFF has termed the "skeleton with the black abdomen and gaping symphyse."[31]

The Provençal skeleton from the end of the 13th century seems on the one hand to belong to the series of "squatting figures," by virtue of the characteristic open

[30] WICERSHEIMER, ERNEST: (Sudh.) Arch. Gesch. Med. *7* (1914), pp. 1-26. – PREMUDA, *loc. cit.* (footnote 27), pp. 36 ff. and tables XIX-XX. – CETTO, A. M.: Ciba Symposium (Basel) 5 (1957), Heft 4, pp. 124-126 – ḤUARD and GRMEK, *loc. cit.* (footnote 21, p. 16), colored plate IV/V.

[31] SUDHOFF, KARL: Ein Skelettbild in einer Handschrift der Bibliothèque Mazarine aus dem Anfang des 14. Jahrhunderts, in: Studien *4*.

position of the legs; on the other hand, the face – simulating a dorsal view – is shown upside down. It is the only figure in the manuscript that has a surrounding text, a feature which also distinguishes it from the traditional series (see figure 39). A rough pen-and-ink drawing in the Munich codex Ms. 13042 of the Bavarian State Library, reproduced in figure 40, represents the same type. SUDHOFF has misunderstood the essential nature of this figure when he states that it represents "the dorsal aspect of a cadaver with the head drawn back to the maximum into the neck."[32] Rather, this is a typical example of medieval symbolic graphic art, and the principles of its formal development will shortly be discussed. The simultaneous representation of two discrepant objects, in this case the face and the back of the neck, belongs to the tradition of medieval artistic representation.

Similarly, the viscera figures in Stockholm[32] (plate XVII) also fall into the category of traditional medieval art. It is inadmissible even to describe these fascinating illustrations with the eyes of a modern anatomist, let alone criticize them according to our sense of "false" or "correct." The fundamental perception which caused the artist to represent a sagittal section through the head and torso remains obscure. But, apart from an association with butchers' shops, it is possible that the author was attempting to realize a specific didactic purpose: nowhere else is the symmetry of the head and the asymmetry of the visceral components so clearly demonstrated in one illustration. This device would be quite worthy of LEONARDO.

Finally, in KARL SUDHOFF'S "skeleton with the black abdomen" we have a masterpiece of anatomical iconology. However, while these skeletons may seem to represent a step forward – if only a small one – in anatomical illustration, it is quite possible that the improvement in the rendering of details may have resulted chiefly from the fascination that the skeleton, as a symbol of death, held for the medieval mind. SUDHOFF suggested[33] that to settle this question would require systematic research into the symbolic use of skeletons in medieval art and, indeed, even into symbolic representations of death in ancient art.

Today, a survey of the relevant literature published since SUDHOFF made his suggestion reveals that some of the elements integral to his comprehensive catalogue have been compiled, but the "most exhaustive inquiry" initially advocated by SUDHOFF has still to be undertaken. No other sector of medical illustration has been so obviously subject to a formative influence from outside medical science as the representation of the human skeleton, which is simultaneously a symbolization of death. Yet, it remains one of the most astonishing phenomena in the history of medicine that not until 1538 was an anatomical object as accessible as the bones of the human body drawn "correctly" – that is, from nature – in medical literature, although medical illustration had long been

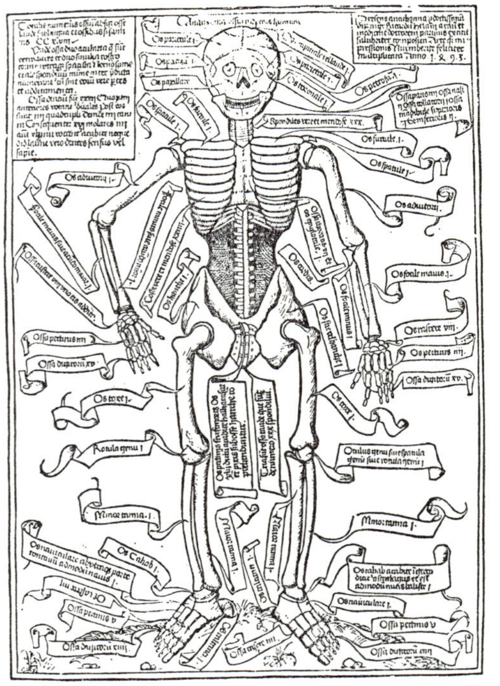

Fig. 41 The Nuremberg skeleton of 1493, probably (according to Sudhoff) from a French design.

Fig. 42 Detail from folio 116v of Cod. 3599, Bibliothèque Mazarine, Paris, first half of the 15th century.

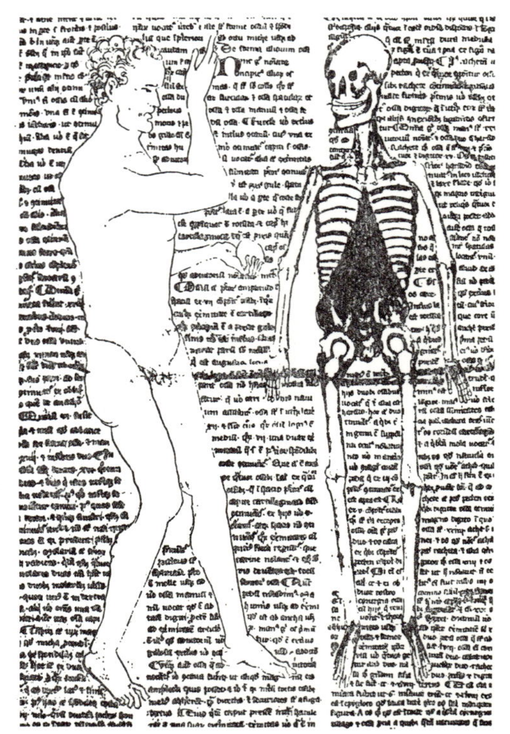

[32] SUDHOFF, KARL: Die graphische Weiterbildung der anatomischen Fünfbilderserie aus Alexandrinerzeit und eine anatomische Serie aus Stockholm. (Sudh.) Arch. Gesch. Med. *8* (1915), p. 132.
[33] Footnote 2 on p. 60 in (Sudh.) Arch. Gesch. Med. *1* (1908).

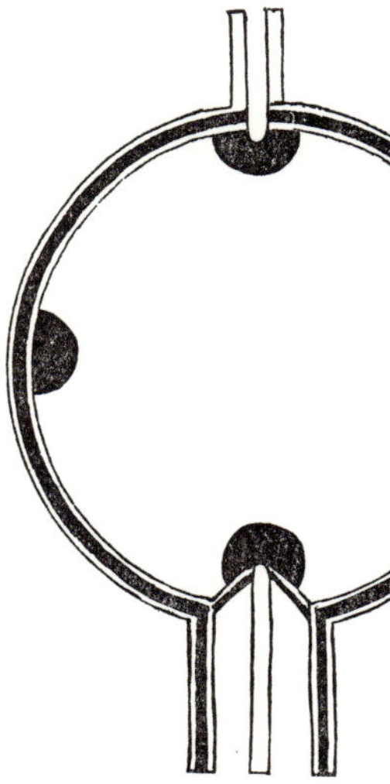

Fig. 43

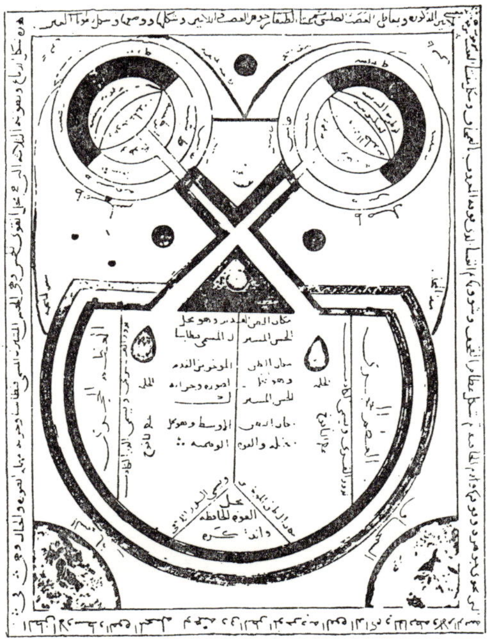

Fig. 44

Fig. 45

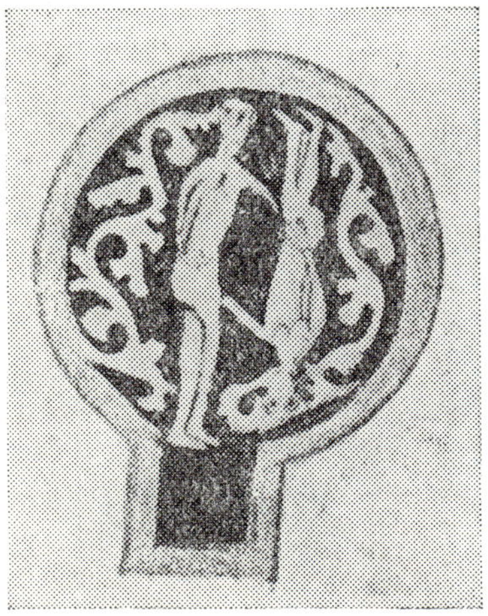

Fig. 43 Diagram of the stomach conceived in stark geometric form, Ms. Ashmol. 399, Bodleian Library, Oxford. The circular form suggests an Arabic modification of a late classical design from which our figure 6, from the Cod. Roncioni 99, Pisa, could be a purely Latin derivative.[34]
Fig. 44 Brain-eye scheme from Ms. 924, Yeni Cami-Library, Istanbul, drawn by 'Jaḥjā of Mosul,' circa 1560.[35]
Fig. 45 Uterus with twins, from the Cod. lat. 161, Bayer. Staatsbibliothek, Munich. (The complete series is reproduced in WEINDLER, FRITZ: *Geschichte der gynäkologisch-anatomischen Abbildung, Dresden, 1908, figs. 17-19.)*

technically capable of doing this. What is more, there is no better proof for the theory that naturalistic medical illustration – medical illustration in the sense of a scientific documentation – was not *needed* before 1500, than the total nonexistence of naturalistic skeleton figures even at the end of the 15th century. The causes lie in medical history and not in the history of graphic art. Like its sister sciences of geography and botany, medicine long relied on a traditional body of illustrations, which were perpetuated as a kind of secret doctrine for several centuries after the artistic style of secular illustrations had turned in new directions.

The Nuremberg "skeleton with the black abdomen" reproduced in figure 41 dates from 1493. SUDHOFF has convincingly established its origins within a French tradition, by first tracing it to a similiar type dating from 1454, in the Ms. français 19994 of the Bibliothèque Nationale, then to a copy of rather poor quality in the Ms. latin 7138 belonging to the same library; at the end of this series, we find a skeleton which is drawn into the middle of the last sheet of an early 14th-century anatomical manuscript which is now in the Bibliothèque Mazarine of the Institut de France (fig. 42). This skeleton, however, which faces a naked man, simultaneously represents death, so that one is tempted to ask if death *alone* is not implied. If so, the "skeleton with the black abdomen" would be nothing more than an offspring of those innumerable representations of death found within the context of medieval Christian iconography, and it could not be regarded as a purely anatomical illustration.

It is well known that "Arabian" medicine – employed in the same descriptive sense as "Latin" – was the main path along which the medical knowledge of late antiquity, especially GALEN'S work, was conveyed into the late Middle Ages. Moorish medicine – that is, the sum total of medical knowledge of Spanish Islam in the 12th and 13th centuries – was important in this process because it was the most important of the vehicles by which this transmission took place. Had the transmission of texts from antiquity to the late Middle Ages taken a course different from that of the corresponding illustrations, we would be faced with a unique phenomenon in the history of civilization.

It is all the more surprising, therefore, that SUDHOFF and all who followed in his

[34] A comparison can be also made in this sense between the brain-eyes-nose schemata of both codices, which is even more pertinent. See our fig. 10 and SUDHOFF'S illustration in: Arch. Gesch. Med. 7 (1914), p. 183.
[35] Cf. SUDHOFF, KARL: (Sudh.) Arch. Gesch. Med. *8* (1915) pp. 1-21. Distinctly Islamic is fig. 5 on color plate 1 in SUDHOFF.

steps have either conceded little importance to the role of Islam in medieval medical illustration, or overlooked it completely. Only in the study of illustrations to ophthalmic medicine (HIRSCHBERG,[36] SUDHOFF[37]) did the connections become obvious to medical iconologists. SUDHOFF would have liked to classify these wholly within the Alexandrian tradition, but he finally became uncertain. The study of medieval medical illustration gives rise to the suspicion – which, in the case of some manuscripts not yet considered in this context, gradually crystallizes into certainty – that the medical illustration of late antiquity underwent morphological changes during its passage through Islamic culture. These changes seem to be quite obvious and distinctive (see figure 43). The occurrence in the uterus of motifs characteristic of Moorish art, for instance, can otherwise scarcely be explained (fig. 45). Unfortunately, our general knowledge of Islamic graphic art during this period is not adequate for us to be certain that we are standing on firm ground from the point of view of art history.[38] Moreover, we must not be tempted to overrate such general characteristics of Islamic formal expression as geometric abstraction and a predilection for stylizing organic elements.

With regard to illustrations of medical instruments, there is apparently no tradition reaching back to late antiquity. The earliest known illustrations are in Islamic sources; however, these early pictures date from a period when Moorish art was greatly given to geometric ornamentation. The well-known illustrations of surgical instruments[39] in the manuscripts of ABŪL'L-QĀSIM (ABULCASIS), an Arabian surgeon at the court of Cordoba in the 10th century, are so distorted that they can only be identified in conjunction with illustrations found in later manuscripts of this type. What we have been pursuaded to term "distorted" can, of course, be at least partly understood as stylization for aesthethic purposes. SUDHOFF spoke depreciatingly of "colorful delusion."

Scenes from surgery and obstetrics are by no means infrequent in Arab manuscripts. These scenes confirm what has long been known in the history of art: that the antipathy of the Koran to illustration is not absolute. Medical illustration exemplifies this fact extremely well.

Finally, turning to botanical illustration, we note that its history follows the same course as that of medical illustration proper. In the early Middle Ages there is a decline in Hellenistic naturalism; then, under the intellectual influence of scholasticism, there is a blind reliance on traditional authority; then, finally, there is the late entrance of a new realism, leading up to what is commonly called the

[36] HIRSCHBERG, JULIUS: Geschichte der Augenheilkunde, II/I, Leipzig, 1905.
[37] SUDHOFF, KARL: Studien *1* (1907), pp. 21-26: (Sudh.) Arch. Gesch. Med. *8* (1915), pp. 1-21.
[38] See DIRINGER, DAVID: The Illuminated Book, London, Faber and Faber, 1958.
[39] SUDHOFF, KARL: Beiträge z. Gesch. der Chirurgie im Mittelalter II. Stud. Gesch. Med. 11/12, 1918, pp. 16 ff. – SCHIPPERGES, HEINRICH: Schmerzbekämpfung in der arabischen Chirurgie durch schmerzhafte Applikation, in: Therapeutische Berichte (Bayer Leverkusen) *35*, 1963, pp. 92-93. – HAMARNEH, SAMI: Drawings and Pharmacy in Al-Zāhrāwi's Tenth-Century Surgical Treatise, in: U.S. National Museum (History and Technology), Bulletin, *288*, 1961, pp. 81-94.

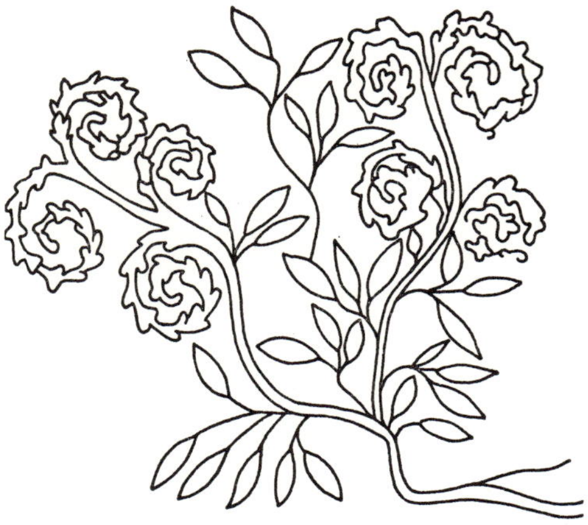

Fig. 46 'Heliotropium.' Ms. Pluteus 73.41 (Pseudo-Apuleius), *Florence, Bibl. Laurenziana, 9th century. Redrawn from Singer.*

Fig. 47 'Eleotropion.' Ms. Sloane 1975 (Pseudo-Apuleius), *folio 28*[r], *British Museum, London, end of 12th century (see plates XIII-XIV). The colors are purely decorative and quite unnatural. Plant and leaves are light green, the background dark blue and gold, the frame red.*

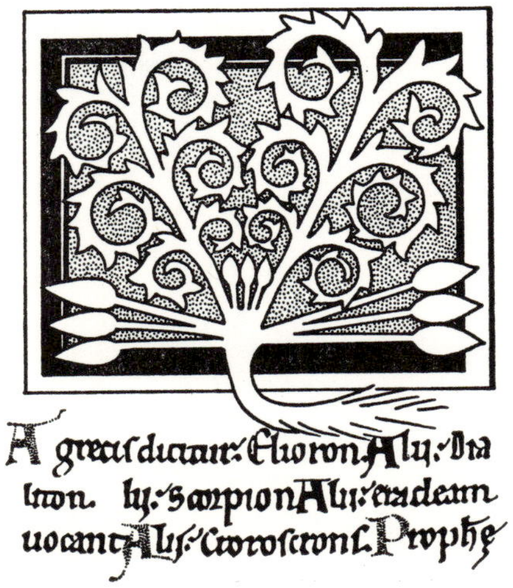

"Renaissance." In the study of botanical illustration, the trends that can be seen in medical illustration appear even more clearly, since, in contrast to anatomy and surgery, no restrictions are imposed by the subject matter.

The artistically excellent illustration in the 6th-century Juliana Anicia Codex is followed by poorer work in manuscripts such as the Codex Neapolitanus (which is now housed in the National Library at Naples). This example dates from the 7th century, when the prototype was still in Constantinople; it was followed by others, up to the more or less indirect imitations of the 14th and 15th centuries. In the high Middle Ages there was extensive illustration of botanical materia medica, probably based on prototypes from antiquity and, in part, on Roman prototypes which are no longer identifiable. After first losing their naturalistic character through repeated copying, the original designs were altered time and time again in the Middle Ages, and the botanist is only partly able to identify such a simplified plant. This is especially true for the plants belonging to the flora of the eastern Mediterranean and Near East, which served no practical purpose in the herbals of northern Europe, and which were handed down from one generation to another only because they were part of the traditional doctrine, naturally without any improvement being made in their delineation.

Again, botanical illustrations, like medical illustrations proper, also underwent special treatment at the hands first of Arab artists and then of European pre-Renaissance artists.

Experts[40] have traced Arabic botanical illustrations to late-antique sources. Accordingly these illustrations reveal little that is specifically Islamic, although one should reflect on what has just been said of Islamic illustration with reference to illustrations of medical instruments.

More interesting is the change in pharmaco-botanical illustration that took place in the pre-Renaissance – or whatever one wishes to term this period that reached its height in the 14th century.[41] Just as many other kinds of art experienced a tendency towards naturalism at that time, several botanical illustrations also show plants that are more easily identified than in earlier or later illustrations. LOTTLISA BEHLING made a thorough study of botanical motifs in the ecclesiastical art of this period, in the chapter "Die blühende Kathedrale" ("the blossoming cathedral") of her book *Die Pflanzenwelt der mittelalterlichen Kathedralen.*[42] Here she refers in passing to the influence of ALBERTUS MAGNUS, which can be detected in the

40 NISSEN, CLAUS: Die botanische Buchillustration; gives a list of the literature published up to 1950; supplemented by NISSEN himself in his introduction to "Kräuterbücher aus fünf Jahrhunderten," Zurich, Munich and Olten, 1956.

41 WHITE, LYNN jr.: Natural Science and Naturalistic Art in the Middle Ages, in: Am. Historical Rev., *52*, 1947, pp. 421-435. This work scintillates with regard to comprehensive references, especially to works written in German. We shall make frequent reference to them.

42 Cologne and Graz, 1964.

naturalism that is found in the work of the builders of the Cistercian abbey at Altenberg near Cologne, to mention only one example. This naturalism was soon to be permeated with a symbolism that in our terminology is customarily called "medieval."[43]

The illustrations for a 12th-century pharmaceutical herbal with a text beginning "Circa instans" – which exists in numerous copies, variants, and hybrids – show considerable variation in quality and in developmental tendencies. NISSEN detects in Codex Hamilton 407 at the Berlin State Library, a Burgundian manuscript of the "Circa instans" dating from the early 14th century, a much more naturalistic style of illustration than that found in later transcripts of the same text. Irrespective of the technical qualities of the various related manuscripts, the illustrations for the "Circa instans" texts in general are "in a sense, the first scientific illustrations of plants to be actually drawn from nature since DIOSCORIDES or even CRATEUS" (SUDHOFF).[44]

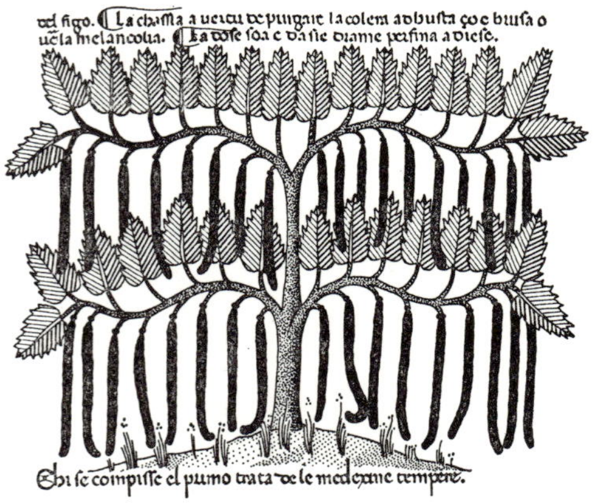

Fig. 48 Scholastic pharmaco-botanical illustration in Ms. Egerton 2020, folio 10ᵛ, British Museum, London, end of 14th century.

From the naturalism of the pre-Renaissance, which resulted from a new reliance on the evidence of the five senses – a pertinent formulation applied by MAX HERBERGER in connection with ALBERTUS MAGNUS – there leads a direct, if sometimes narrow, path to late Gothic panel painting, which shows a preference for botanical subjects. In this period avant-garde trends are found in practical ecclesiastical painting rather than in the academic scientific drawing which would include illustrations of medical texts. Because they are drawn so accurately, the plants of the charming little "garden of Eden" from the Upper Rhine (circa 1410), or of the Ghent Altar (1432),[45] or even those of GHIBERTI'S door frames for the baptistry of the cathedral in Florence stand in notable contrast to most pharmaco-botanical illustrations of the 15th century. Exceptions confirm the rule.[46] When the first botanical incunabula left the printing presses in Rome and Mainz, their illustrations gave no indication of the naturalism found in contemporary panel painting. Initially they were wholly in the tradition of that specialized iconography practised by 15th-century copyists who were more interested in the symbolic content of a picture than in its faithfulness to nature.

Fig. 49 Early naturalism in Ms. Egerton 2020, folio 11ʳ, British Museum, London, end of 14th century. In the actual codex this illustration faces fig. 48.

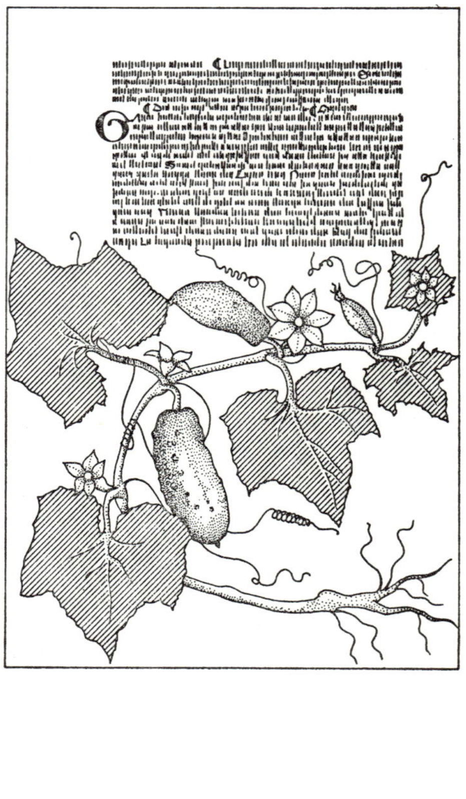

Research, which is very active in this field, has uncovered three different pharmaceutical incunabula printed before 1490:

1. The *Herbarium Apulei Platonici ad Marcum Agrippam,* Rome 1481/83. This work was published by a physician to the papal court, JOHANNES PHILIPPUS DE

[43] Perhaps the term "scholastic," implying the authoritarian and dogmatic aspect of scholastic thinking, would be better for the phenomena in question.

[44] MEYER-STEINEG, TH. and SUDHOFF, KARL in: Geschichte der Medizin im Überblick mit Abbildungen, Jena, 1928, p. 222.

[45] BEHLING, LOTTLISA: Die Pflanze in der mittelalterlichen Tafelmalerei, Weimar, 1957.

[46] Above all, the Ms. Egerton 2020 in the Brit. Museum, the so-called *Carrara Herbar* from the end of the 14th century, two centuries later in possession of ALDROVANDI. See figs. 48 and 49. – PÄCHT, OTTO: J. Warburg and Courtauld Inst., XIII (1950), pp. 30-31. See especially footnote 1, p. 30, which gives an interpretation of the phenomenon of the naturalistic decorative sculpture in Gothic cathedrals that differs from that of L. BEHLING (see above).

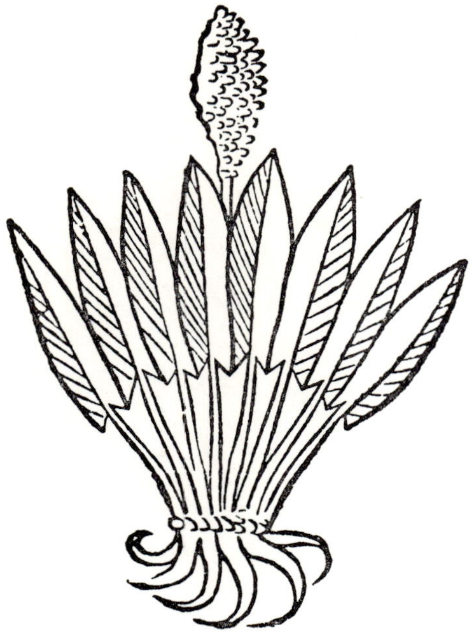

Fig. 50 Acetosa, from the Herbarius Maguntie impressus, *Mainz (Schöffer), 1484.*

Fig. 51 Acetosa, from Hortus sanitatis deutsch, *Mainz (Schöffer), 1485. This illustration is drawn from nature.*

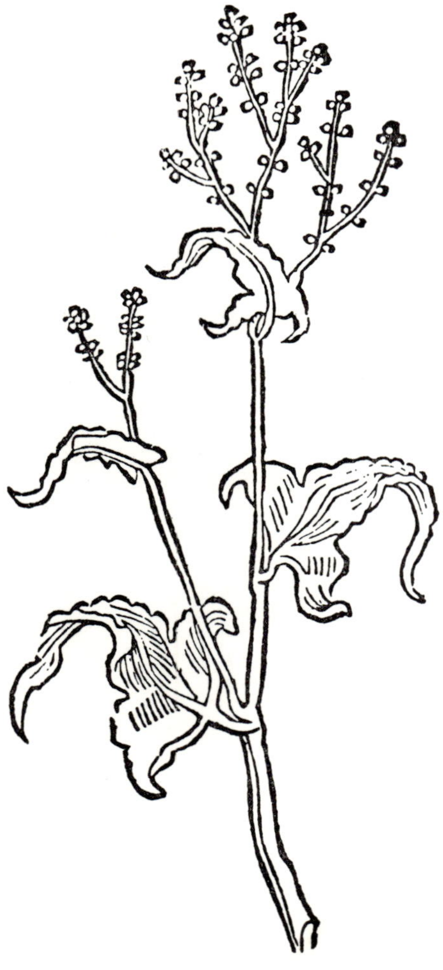

LIGNAMINE, who also produced a small dietary, "De unoquoque cibo et potu." He is said to have been both printer and publisher.[47]

2. The *Herbarius Maguntie impressus*, 1484, printed by PETER SCHÖFFER in Mainz, is one of the most precious German incunabula. This work has provoked a great deal of discussion by scholars from CHOULANT to KLEBS and NISSEN.[48] A manuscript pertaining directly to the book has not yet been found. It appears to be an original composition from the 15th century, but contains absolutely no innovations. The illustrations belong to the "Circa instans" figures. It was a solid success, and during the following eighty years innumerable reprints were produced in Germany, Holland, France, and Italy.

3. The so-called *Gart der Gesundheit* was also printed by PETER SCHÖFFER in Mainz and appeared on March 28, 1485. In contrast to the *Herbarius*, which is in quarto, this is a folio volume; it contains more than twice as many illustrations. Its origin is more complex, in that one sixth of the 368 illustrations of medical plants did not derive from previous illustrations, but were new ad hoc drawings. Significantly, they represent indigenous spring-flowering plants.[49] The wood-engraving technique frequently employs hatching (that is, marking with fine, closely spaced lines) and thereby anticipates the accomplished use of hatching that will be made later in the first "modern" anatomical illustrations. The artist is believed to be ERHARD REWICH of Utrecht, who was possibly also the so-called "Hausbuchmeister" ("master of the *Housebook*"), an early copperplate engraver who spontaneously used natural models. The rapid success of *Gart der Gesundheit* in the bookselling trade resulted in a race among publishers, which SCHÖFFER lost to competitors in Augsburg and Strasbourg. Basel, Besançon, and Ulm followed within the next two years.

These incunabula of pharmaco-botanical illustration have been discussed in some detail, because they represent for the historian a kind of prelude to an exciting event that has fascinated all book-loving physicians from CHOULANT on: the transition from "medieval" scholastic medicine to the medical texts produced by the age of Renaissance Humanism.

47 The manuscript suspected to be the direct prototype was only re-discovered in 1930; namely, Codex 97 in the Biblioteca Cassinensis, on Monte Cassino near Salerno. Critics have partly disputed the close relationship between the Cassinensis manuscript and the Roman incunabulum. Facsimile edition: The Herbal of Pseudo-Apuleius from the ninth century manuscript in the Abbey of Monte Cassino (Cod. Cass. 97) together with the first printed edition, edited by F. W. T. HUNGER, Leiden, Brill, 1935.

48 Best treatment in NISSEN, CLAUS: Kräuterbücher aus fünf Jahrhunderten, Zurich, Munich, Olten, 1956, p. 29 ff. The various German incunabula prints of the "Herbarius" and the "Hortus sanitatis" are reproduced in SCHRAMM, ALBERT: Der Bilderschmuck der Frühdrucke, Leipzig, 1922, continued by the Kommission für den Gesamtkatalog der Wiegendrucke.

49 SCHUSTER, JULIUS: Secreta Salernitana und Gart der Gesundheit, in: "Mittelalterliche Handschriften," Festgabe (60). HERMANN DEGERING, Leipzig, 1926, pp. 203-235. – BEHLING, LOTTLISA, *loc. cit.*, footnote 45, excursus: Pflanzendarstellungen in dem handschriftlich illustrierten Herbarius des Vitus Auslasser von 1497 und in der Inkunabel des Mainzer Gart der Gesundheit von 1485. Even a century earlier than this, the miniaturist of the *Carrara Herbar* (see footnote 46) went into the abbey garden and painted from nature. His own illustrations now stand in delightful contrast to the traditional figures of the *Circa instans* repertoire, which he simply copied in part.

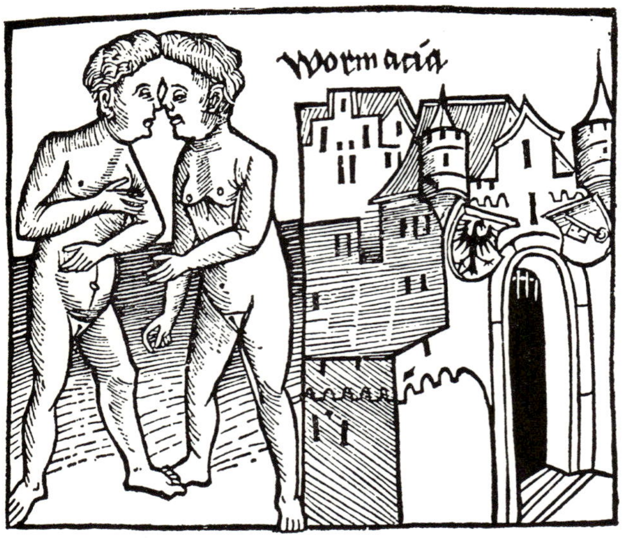

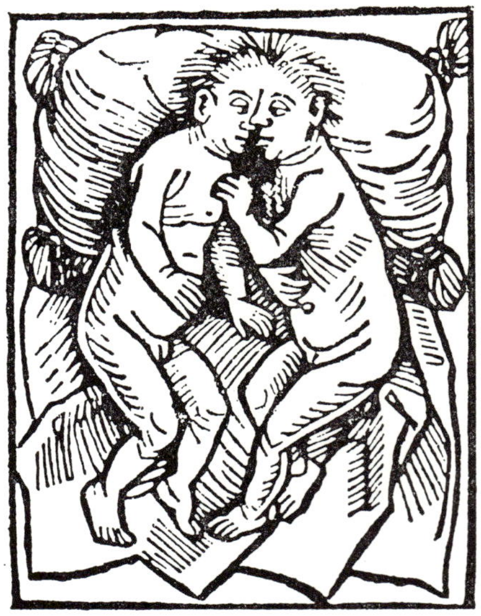

Figures 52 and 53 Woodcut illustrations from two pamphlets printed after the birth of Siamese twins in Bürstadt near Worms, in 1495. Only the drawing on the right, from a pamphlet by Sebastian Brant, seems possibly derived from firsthand observation.

By contrast, the illustrations to be found in other early printed works dealing with other aspects of medicine[50] do not ever cross the border into the "modern age," and only in individual cases do they approach it. In many respects teratological illustration – the depiction of gross birth deformities – is an interesting example of early printed work. On September 10, 1495, Siamese twins who were joined at the forehead were born at Bürstadt near Worms. E. Holländer has reproduced no fewer than five different pamphlets recording this event in his study, "Wunder, Wundergeburt und Wundergestalt," 1921. The most faithful representation is by Sebastian Brant, the author of "The Ship of Fools." According to one of the pamphlets, King Maximilian I, the main figure of the memorable Worms Imperial Diet of that year, saw the twins and gave them ten florins. Our examples illustrate the undocumentary manner in which the children are represented in most of these pamphlets, quite in the sense of medieval formal expression, and on occasion in a decidedly abstract form. They are shown standing together, larger than the houses that symbolize the city of Worms, outside which the unnatural birth occurred, or converging on each other like two fighting athletes. Only in one pamphlet, which was dedicated by Brant to the "Roman King," does the artist attempt to present a realistic picture, showing the children lying on a pillow and sheet; it would appear that an original sketch has been freely copied. Teratological illustrations drawn from nature are not encountered until the 16th century. The often exaggerated pictures of what Konrad von Megenberg called "strange human beings," which appear regularly after Bämler's incunabulum of 1475, do not actually belong to medical illustration and have a tradition reaching back to Pliny.

Fig. 54 The Worms twins in a pamphlet by Hans Sporer, Erfurt, 1495.

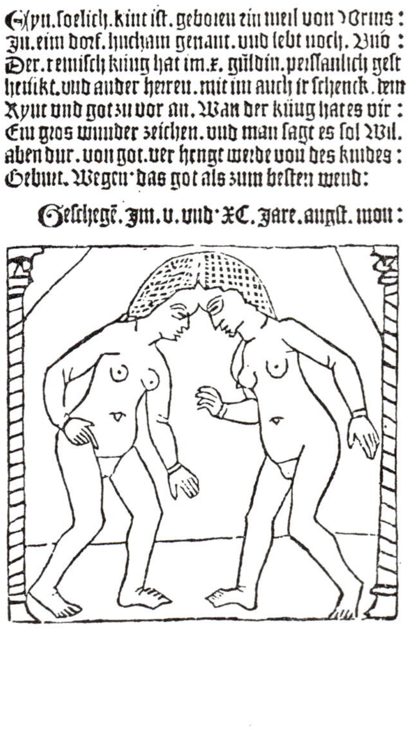
Eyn.soelich.kint ist.geboren ein meil von Wrms:
In.eim dorf.huchaim genant.und lebt noch.Und:
Der.remisch kunig hat im.x.guldin.persanlich gest
heufikt.und ander herren.mit im auch ir schenck.dem
Kynt und got zu vor an.Wan der kunig hat es vir:
Ein gros wunder zeichen.und man sagt es sol Wil.
aben dur.von got.ver hengt werde von des kindes:
Gebuirt.Wegen das got als zum besten wend:

Geschegē.Im.v.und.XC.Jare.augst.mon:

Surgical illustrations from the early days of printing appear sometimes on broad-

[50] The best survey is still in Sudhoff, Karl: Deutsche medizinische Inkunabeln, (i.e. Stud. Gesch. Med. Heft 2/3), Leipzig, 1908. Copious picture material in a compilation by Schramm, see footnote 48, above.

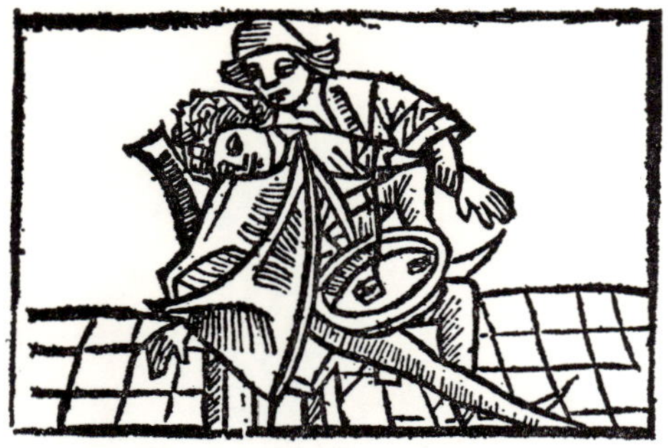

Fig. 55 From a bloodletting calendar by the Basel municipal physician Johannes Wonneker, Workshop of Ysenhut, Basel, 1493. This scene surpasses the mass of contemporary illustrations in the liveliness of the print cutter's transposition from his traditional model. The patient undergoing venesection is shown in the very act of collapsing, as though the artist wanted to give an eyewitness report.

sides – single-sheet calendars or venesection tables[51] – and sometimes as book illustrations in the incunabular literature typified by the "Bartholomaeus Anglicus."[52] There is also a realistic surgical scene, drawn in the late Gothic manner, in a plague incunabulum by HANS FOLZ, Nuremberg, 1482. Considering the magnificant and varied miniatures produced during the 13th, 14th, and early 15th centuries, there are very few surgical illustrations to be found in the incunabula.

The most extensive series of surgical illustrations is contained in the first illustrated textbook to be printed in this field: HIERONYMUS BRUNSCHWIG'S *Cirurgia* of 1497. This incunabulum, whose title-page woodcut has already been mentioned in our section on "wound-men" (see p. 29), has always interested bibliophiles. Through the reprints of G. KLEIN, Munich, 1911, and H. G. SIGERIST, Milan, 1923, this work has become widely known. The woodcuts are in the late Gothic or "early German" style, and their stage of development corresponds approximately to that of the work of an artist from the Upper Rhine who often signed his works "E.S." The illustrations are more decorative than explanatory. With a few thematically justified exceptions (fig. 57), the author reproduces scenes with the physician and his retinue on the one hand, and with the physician and his patient on the other. In all there are 49 full-page and 3 half-page illustrations from a total of 272 printed pages[53] – practically every fifth page thus carries a large woodcut. Some of the printing blocks were used twice or, in a few cases, even more often. The majority of the full-page illustrations, however, are each produced from two half printing blocks that form one scene. The variation is so skillful that twenty-nine of the forty-nine

[51] For example, Ysenhut, Basel, 1499, illustrated in SUDHOFF: Stud. 2/3, fig. 4. Counterpart in PETERS, fig. 39.

[52] Haarlem, 1485, illustrated in SUDHOFF: Stud. 2/3, fig. 14.

[53] There are many variations; our page numbering corresponds to the facsimile editions by KLEIN and SIGERIST.

Fig. 56 Woodcut from Ein fast köstlicher spruch von der pestilenz, *compiled by 'Hans Folcz barbirer,' Nuremberg, 1482. The surgeon is opening an axillary bubo.*

Fig. 57 Title page for Hieronymus Brunschwig, Cirurgia, *Strasbourg (Grüninger), 1497.*

Fig. 58 Refracturing a crookedly healed leg. From Brunschwig, tract. III, cap. 2, folio 98v.

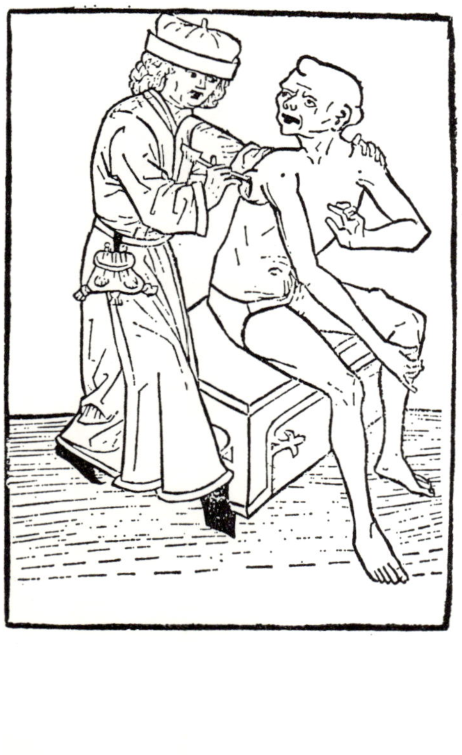

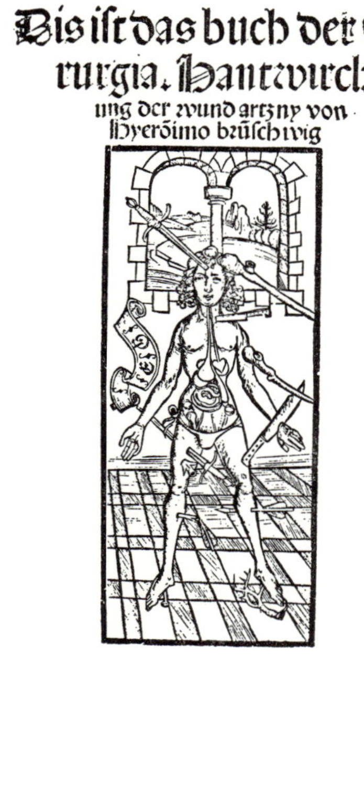

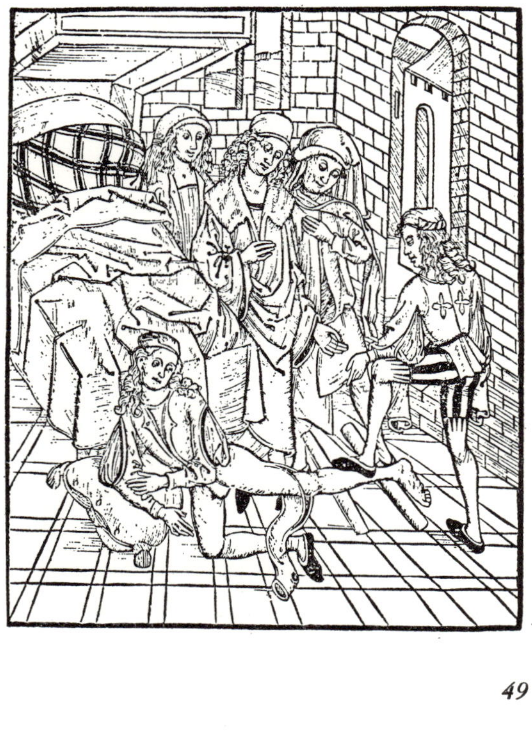

plates, more than half of this opulent series, consist of such combinations. Finally, a trick that was to find many adherents was evidently employed here for the first time: a small window was cut out of a block in such a way that a new detail could be inserted for the next impression, thereby introducing a further variation into the illustration. In the course of running off the single editions, the inserted piece of wood occasionally shifted. In fact, the compositor at the workshop of GRÜNINGER in Strasbourg was generally rather careless in the combination of his half-plates,

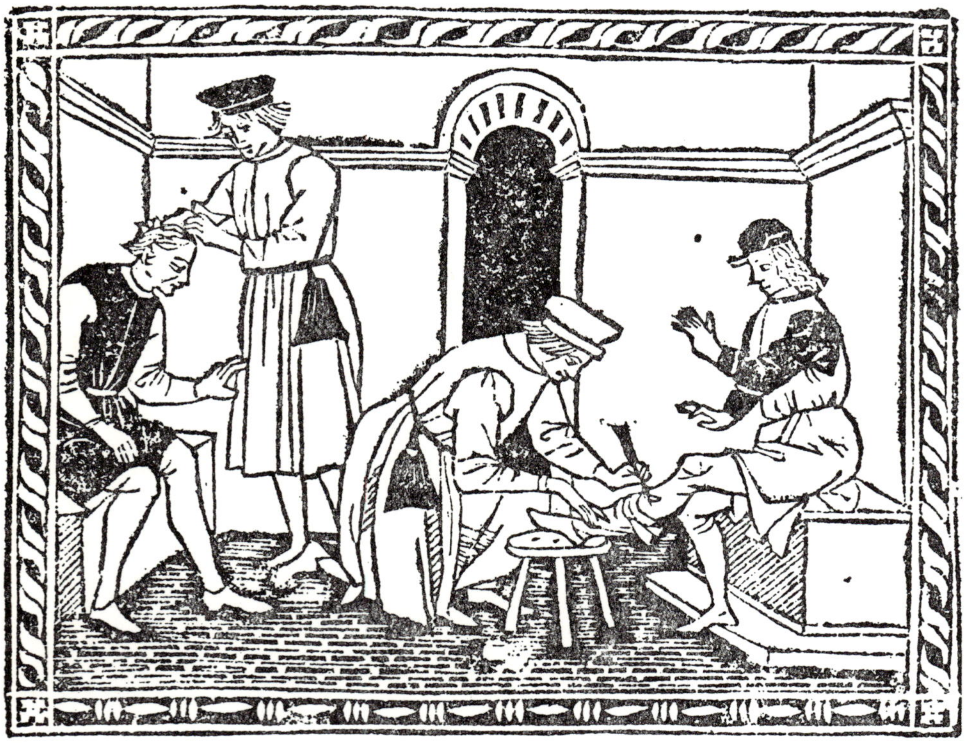

for the perspective of the floor patterns had only been partially prepared by the artist for this trick. In other books GRÜNINGER also used printing blocks which had been sawed into sections.

A Florentine incunabulum of the *Thesaurus pauperum*, by PETRUS HISPANUS, contains illustrations already representative of early Renaissance art, which, in view of the place and time (1497), is quite understandable. Compared with the Strasbourg woodcuts, they appear quite "modern" (see figure 59).

Also part of medical illustration in the wider sense of the term are the religious title-page woodcuts for plague and syphilis tracts, which flourished during this epoch. Towards the end of the 15th century, a type of illustration developed which is as commensurate with a large fresco on the wall of a church as with the new art of the woodcut with its linear formal expression. Enthroned above the clouds is an image of Christian authority, be it God or the Blessed Virgin. Positioned somewhat lower, conforming to the hierarchical order, are figures of angels or saints, or symbolic depictions of religious scenes: perhaps a Pietà, the saints Sebastian and

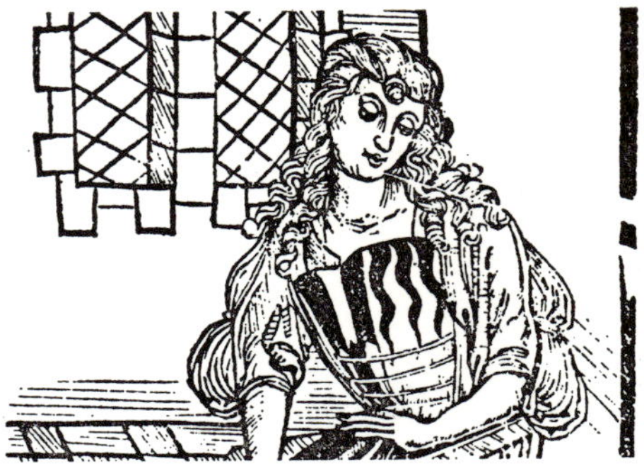

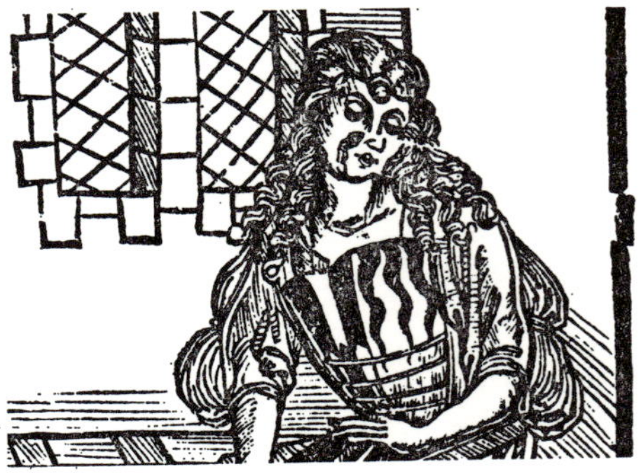

Figures 60, 61

Fig. 59 Double scene at the surgery. From Petrus Hispanus, Theasaurus pauperum, *Florence, 1497.*

Figures 62, 63

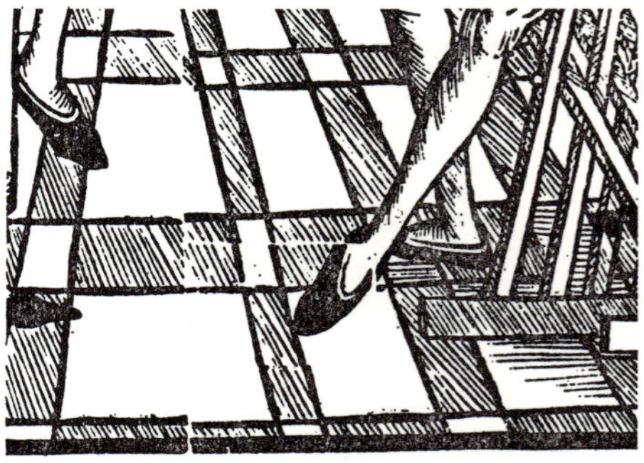

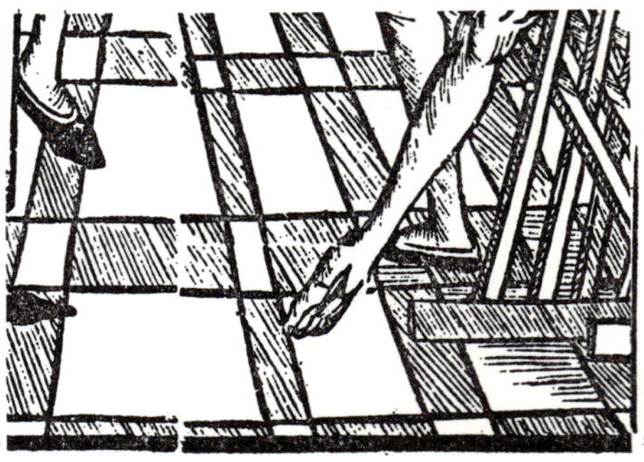

Fig. 64

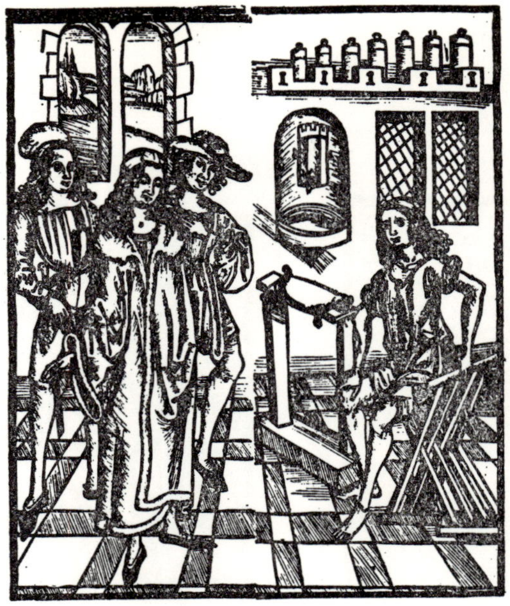

Fig. 65

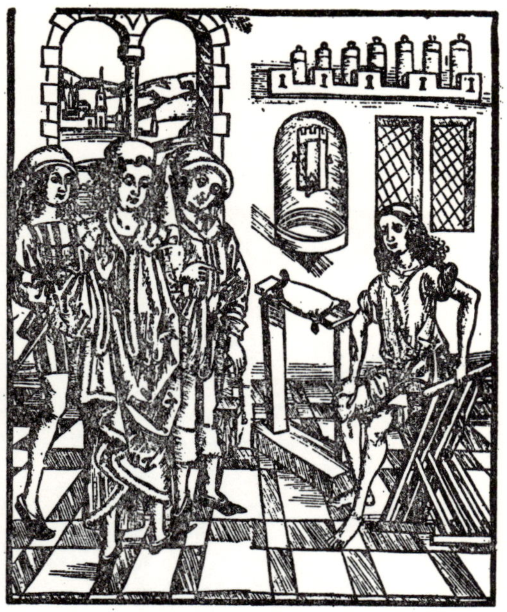

Fig. 66

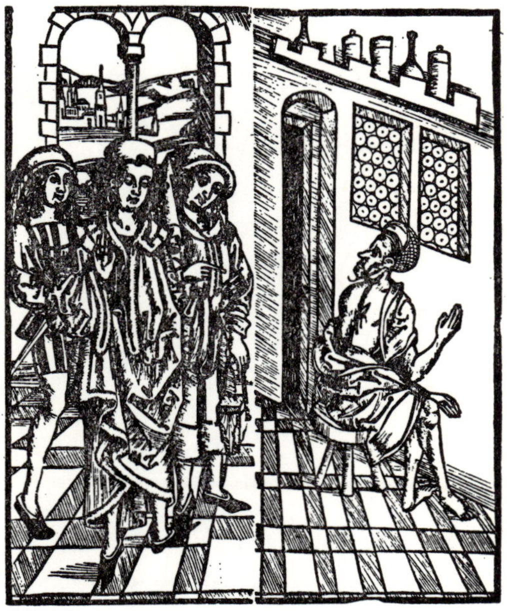

Figures 60 to 63 Details from Brunschwig's Cirurgia, *1497. Top left, from folio 101 and folio 68; bottom left, from folio 54 and folio 41ᵛ. In each case, a small piece has been cut out of the block so that a new piece can be inserted. The inserted piece in figure 61 shows a nose wound; in figure 63, a foot wound.*

Figures 64 to 68 Five pages from Brunschwig's Cirurgia, *1497, composed from two wood blocks. Figures 64 and 65 have the right half in common; figures 65, 66, and 68, the left half. Figure 67 combines two wood blocks of unequal size.*

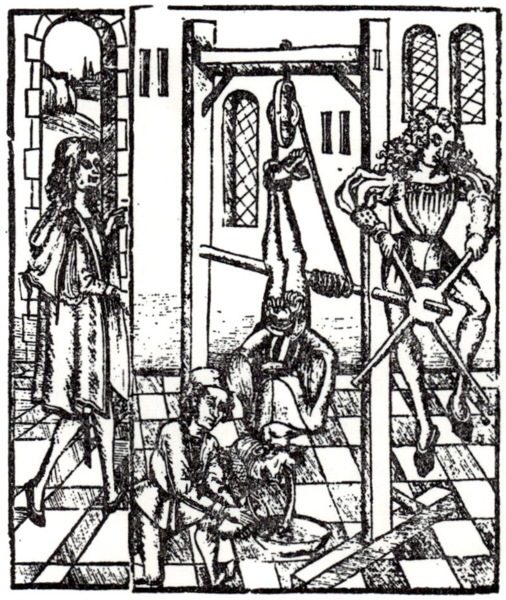

Fig. 67

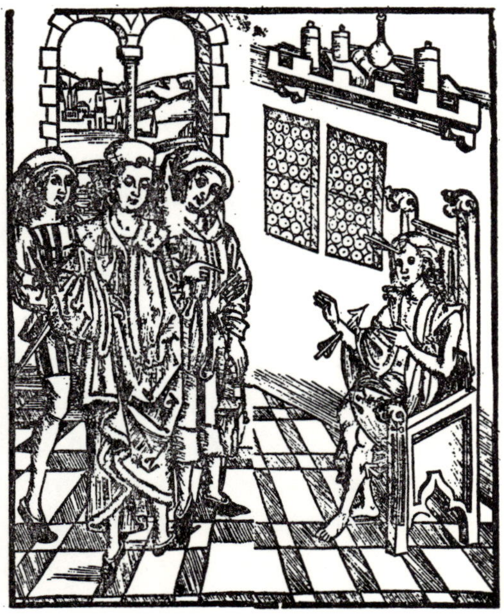

Fig. 68

Fig. 69

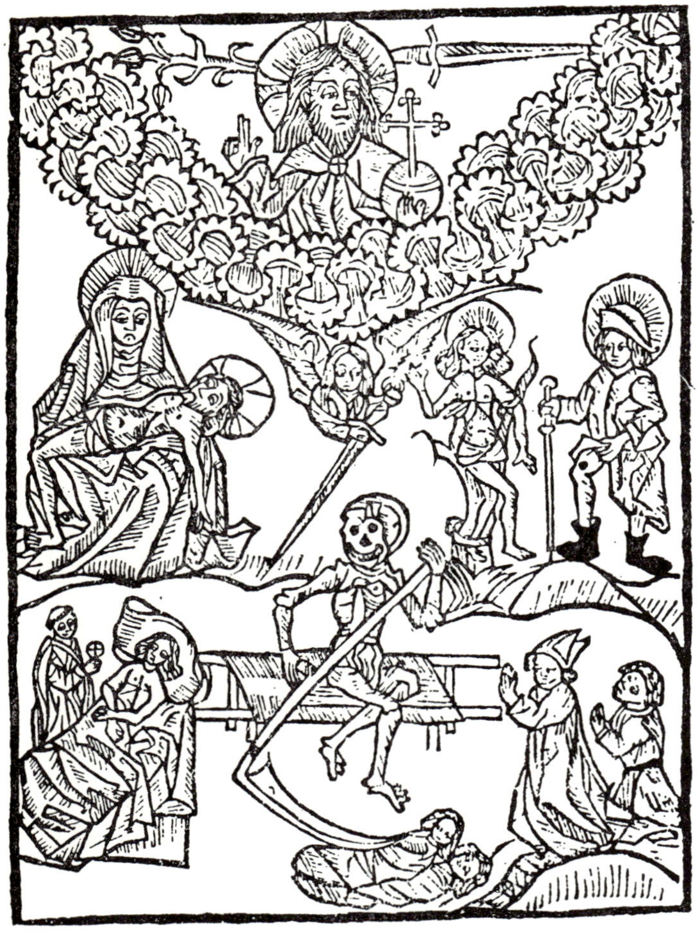

Fig. 70

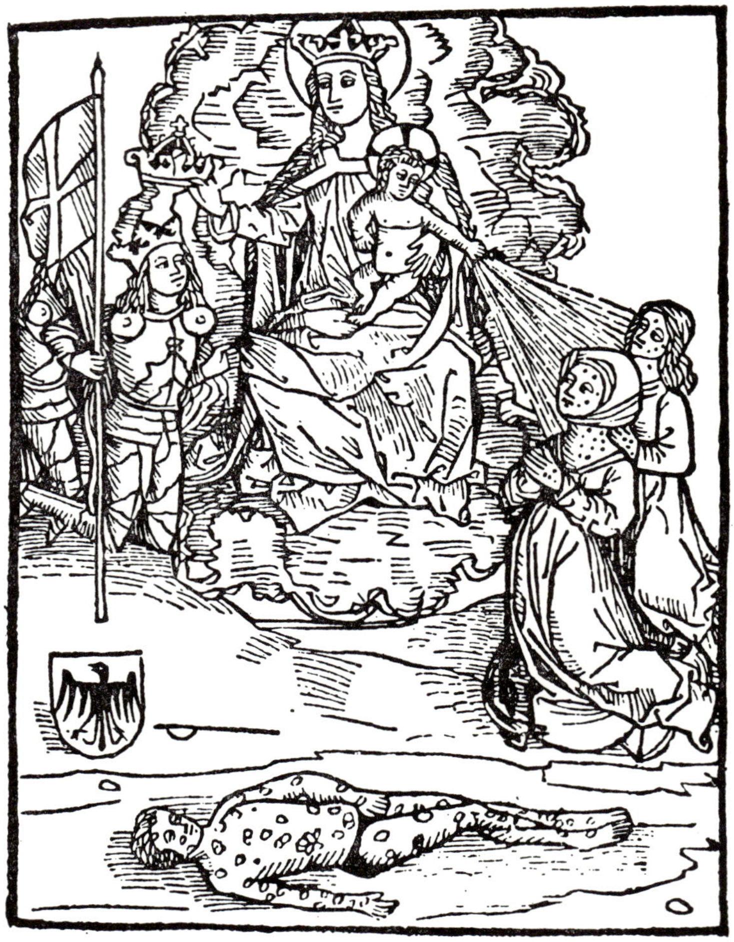

Roch, or adorational figures receiving the divine benediction. At the lowest of the three levels, the invalid is depicted in all his misery, in a manner which is entirely medieval. Both woodcuts reproduced here reveal a stirring power of expression in their detail (figs. 69, 70).

The saints Cosmas and Damian were also represented in the title pages of incunabula, which merely required simple adoption of the figures already found in miniatures and altar panels. Their secular counterparts, above all the physician engaged in uroscopy, appear on numerous occasions in incunabula. The most famous of these pictures is the first of the illustrations in KONRAD VON MEGENBERG'S *Buch der Natur*, Augsburg, 1481; it belongs to Book I, "Vom Menschen," and shows a naked man between his two "doctors" – the doctor of the body and the doctor of the soul. Another early printed work, a book of comfort for invalids with the somewhat clumsy title, "Versehung Leib, Seel, Ehr und Gut" – a regular "Doktorbuch" of the kind still to be found today in Germany and other countries – is decorated with a title-page woodcut showing a man at the end of his earthly life lying on a sick-bed, where he is similarly attended by "doctors." These artists of the pre-Dürer period in Germany express themselves in a language that

Fig. 69 Title-page woodcut for the Regimen zu deutsch *of Philipp Culmacher, Leipzig (Martin Landsberg), not dated but earlier than 1500.*

Fig. 70 Title-page woodcut for the Tractat von dem ursprung des Bösen Franzos *of Josef Grünpeck, Augsburg (Hannss Schawr), 1496.*

Fig. 71 Physician at the sickbed, from a Buchkalender for the year 1483, printed by Johann Bämler in Augsburg.

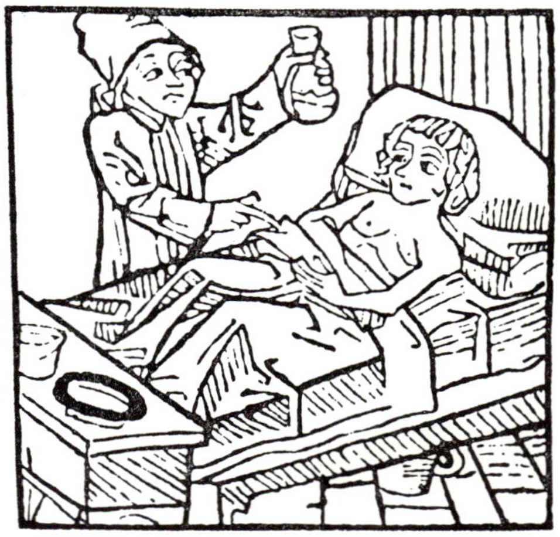

is still quite medieval.

A final type of medieval illustration includes the numerous genre scenes with medical subjects, which are to be found regularly in popular treatises such as Heinrich Louffenberg's *Versehung des Leibs*, a compilation of rules for health dating from the beginning of the 15th century and first printed in Augsburg in 1491. These scenes depict urinalysis, surgeons performing venesection, pregnancies, women in childbed, child-rearing, the plague, and the physician at the sick-bed. This type of illustration also includes the miniatures contained in the margins of venesection

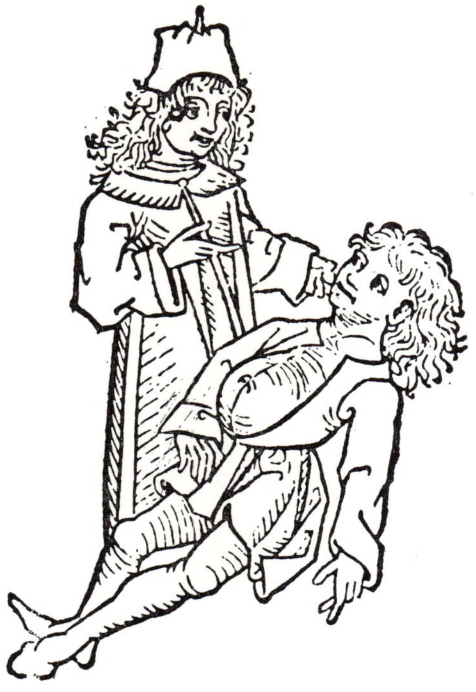

Fig. 72 Physician and patient with ascites, from the Hortus Sanitatis, *printed by Jacob Meyenbach in Mainz, 1491.*

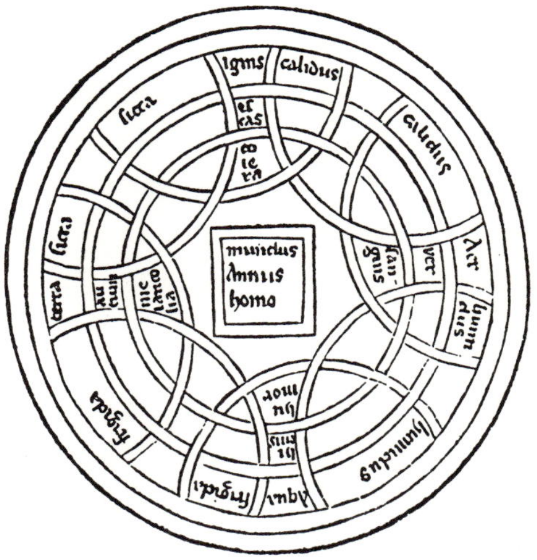

Fig. 74 A 15th-century copy of a late-classical 'mundus-annus-homo' diagram, from the workshop of the Strasbourg printer Johann Mentelin.

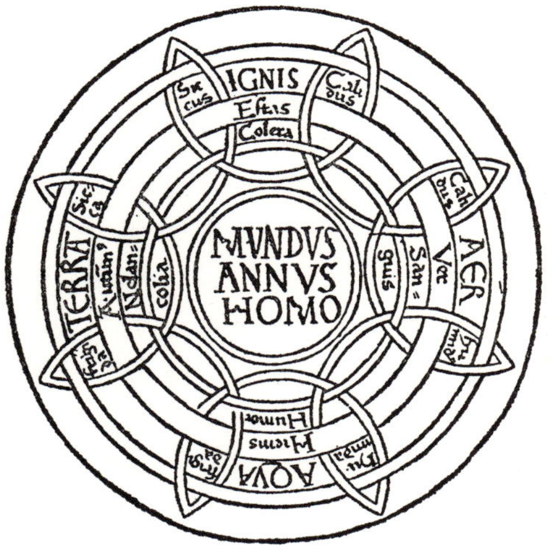

Fig. 75 The same diagram in an artistically modified form from the workshop of Zainer in Augsburg, 1472.

Fig. 73 Medieval diagram of the cerebral ventricles drawn into a realistic portrait. From Ludovicus de Prussia, Trilogium animae, *Nuremberg (Anton Koberger), 1498. Koberger was Albrecht Dürer's printer.*

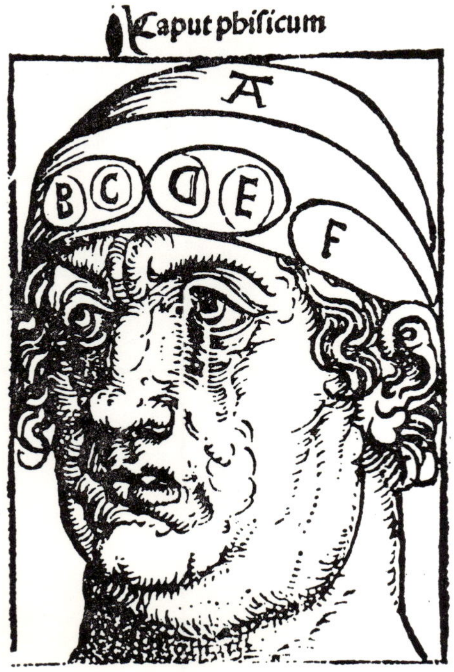

tables or calendar sheets, which we have already discussed in connection with surgical illustrations (see pp. 48-49). These small scenes are conceptually closely related to those in the Leyden Theodoric manuscript mentioned at the beginning of this chapter (see p. 25; three scenes from this manuscript are reproduced in plate XV).

The wide range of medical graphic art in incunabula is again demonstrated by the woodcuts reproduced on this page: the one extreme is shown in the small medical scene, masterfully executed and full of realism, which has been taken from the artistically eminent *Hortus sanitatis*, Mainz, 1491 (fig. 72). The two versions of the "mundus-annus-homo" diagram (figs. 74, 75) from an 8th-century Munich codex (fig. 30) exemplify the other extreme, representing a geometrical type of diagram which had been in use for perhaps a millenium. Between these examples is a "Caput phisicum" from a Nuremberg incunabulum by Dürer's printer, Anton Koberger. This is a hybrid composition – half portrait, half diagram. Walther Sudhoff undertook a classical inquiry[54] into the tradition of this type of illustration in 1913, but overlooked this aggressive Koberger incunabulum. It is clear that a great range of historical styles are to be found in the illustrations of medical incunabula.

[54] Sudhoff, Walther: Die Lehre von den Hirnventrikeln in textlicher und graphischer Tradition des Altertums und Mittelalters. (Sudh.) Arch. Gesch. Med. *7* (1913), pp. 149-205.

Origins of the Indication Line

Although the anatomical illustrations that were produced by early printers usually contained few innovations, there was one new feature that did quickly become prominent in the illustrations of anatomical incunabula. That feature was the indication line. It is employed as one of the methods of elucidation, albeit tentatively and clumsily, in the *Fasciculus medicinae* of KETHAM (1491/93); but the other possible way of explanation, by labeling the figure directly, was used simultaneously (see fig. 88). The threadlike indication lines in figure 88 resemble those that are found in venesection table of the type reproduced in figure 21; these tables, of course, have a tradition going back to medieval hand-produced versions. The Venetian wood-engraver of the KETHAM plates of 1491 missed the opportunity of replacing the illuminator's freehand stroke of the pen with a straight line; but two years later, in the 1493 edition, most of the lines are straight. This tendency toward the use of straight lines influences the whole composition: the legends are now squeezed into the margin in geometrical order (fig. 89). A "sickness-figure" in KETHAM'S *Fasciculus* is also provided with indication lines leading to descriptive legends in the margin (fig. 29).

When we reach the period of the post-incunabula (that is, early printed works produced after 1500), we find that indication lines from now on are as a matter of course drawn with a ruler. The same development took place in the work of Strasbourg printers as in the work of the DE GREGORIUS brothers in Venice: whereas the skeleton in the BRUNSCHWIG *Cirurgia* of 1497 (fig. 78), which was engraved for GRÜNINGER'S workshop, still has threadlike indication lines, the engraver of SCHOTT'S print of 1517[1] (fig. 79) drew all the indication lines for the skeleton and viscera figures with a ruler.[2] (The viscera figure will be discussed in the next chapter, pp. 61 ff.) The Strasbourg artist lacked the Venetian artist's sense of composition, however, and he arranged the legends according to the directions of the indication lines instead of lining them up horizontally.

GRÜNINGER'S skeleton of 1497 has a pedigree which was drawn up by KARL SUDHOFF (see pp. 41-42). The direct prototype of this illustration was the Nuremberg skeleton reproduced in figure 41. When the two illustrations are placed side by side (figs. 77-78), the dependence of the Strasbourg skeleton on the Nuremberg skeleton becomes evident. The source of the indication lines in the Strasbourg figure also becomes clear: it is as if banderoles – that is, scrolls – are still being implied. The banderoles that had appeared in 15th-century manuscripts were quite clearly borrowed from panel painting. Considered from the point of view of

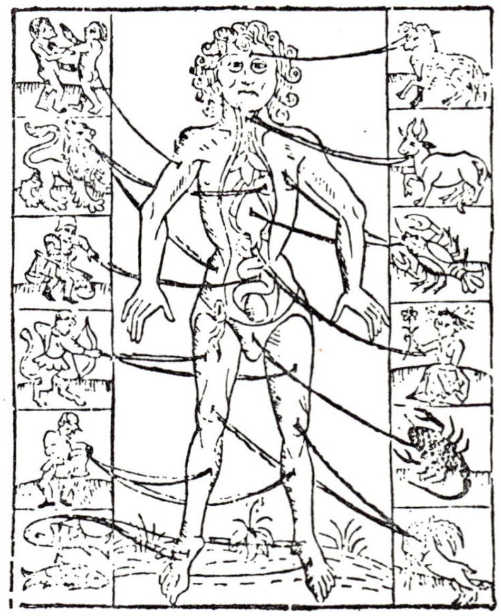

Fig. 76 'Zodiac-man' in the Deutscher Kalender for the year 1483, from the workshop of Knoblochtzer in Strasbourg.

[1] CHOULANT, LUDWIG and MORTIMER FRANK: History and Bibliography of Anatomic Illustration, New York/London, 1962, pp. 162-166.

[2] SCHOTT employed both illustrations as folding plates in GERSSDORFF'S "Feldtbuch der wundartzny," 1517. They were made for this purpose. In the following year, 1518, they were taken over by GRÜNINGER'S workshop, where they were used in a deceptively successful recutting for an edition of LORENZ PHRYES'S "Spiegel der Artzny," and they have become much better known in the PHRYES version than in their first printing. See BENTZING, JOSEF: Bibliographie der Schriften des Colmarer Arztes Lorenz Fries, in: Philobiblon (Hamburg) 6 (1962). Heft 2, p. 129 ff.

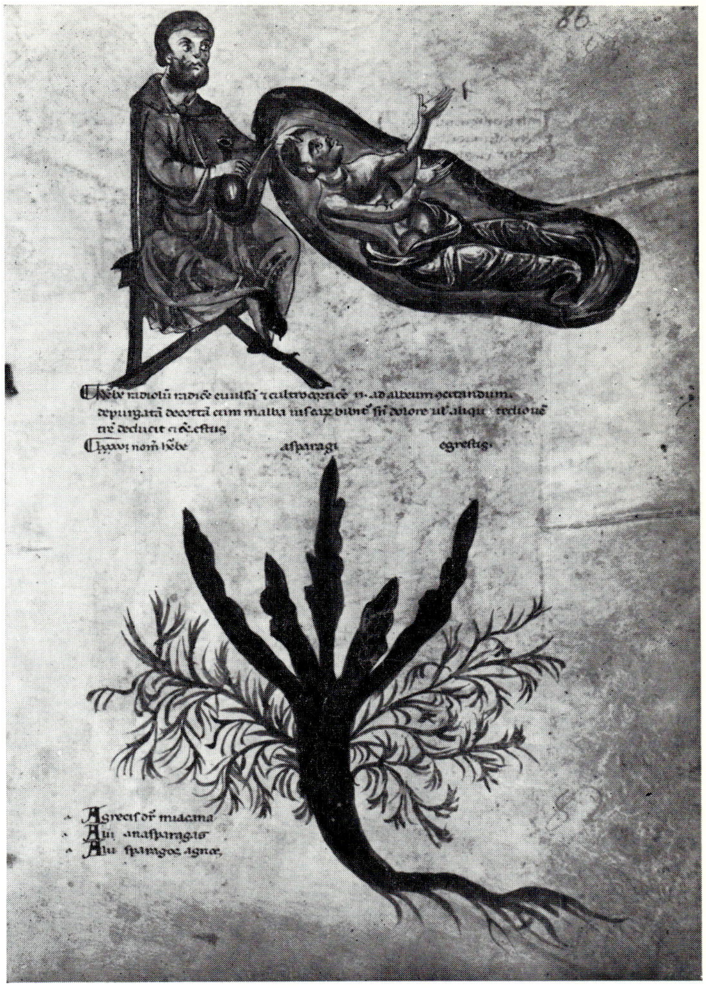

Plate VII A sheet from the Cod. lat. 93 in the Österr. Nationalbibliothek, Vienna. Among other items, the codex contains a richly illuminated manuscript of Apuleius, De medicaminibus herbarum liber. *The manuscript is held to be a copy inscribed and painted from the 6th-century original, in the first half, or about the middle of the 13th century in southern Italy. The notable feature of this late classical illustrated book is the juxtaposition of medicinal plants and medical scenes depicting their use. Our example (fol. 83) shows above a physician relieving the pain of his patient by the laying on of hands in conjunction with the administration of drugs. The plant underneath can still be clearly identified as the asparagus.*

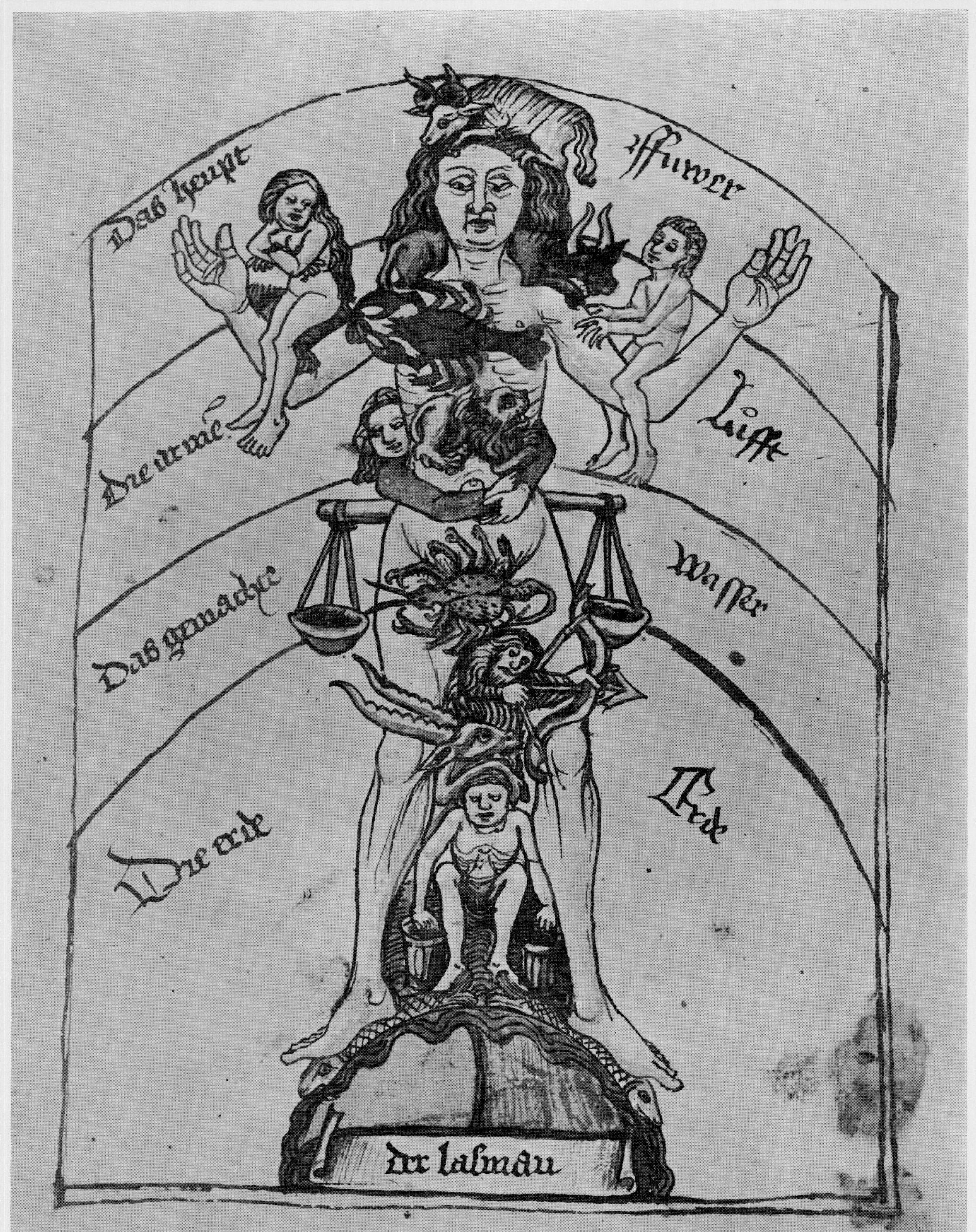

Plate VIII 'Zodiac-man' f
a MS. (M. d. 2) in the
Universitätsbibliothek,
Tübingen, 15th century.

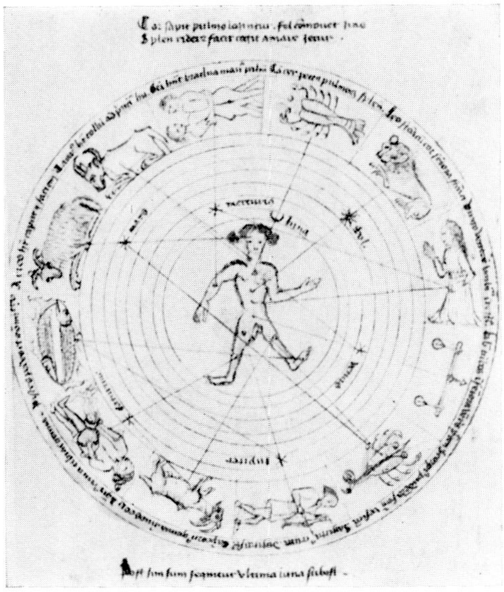

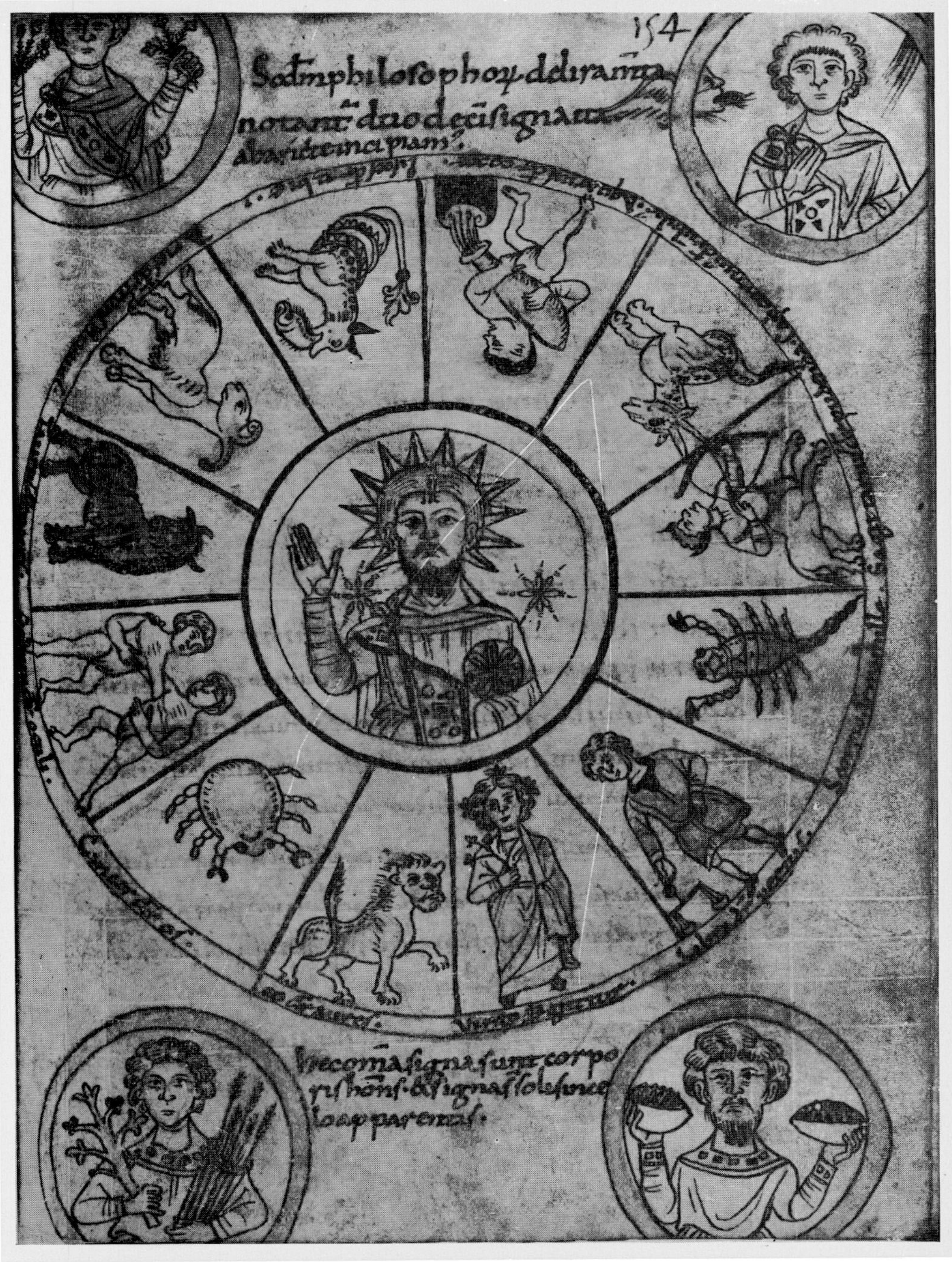

Plate IXa 'Zodiac-manikin' in the traditional medieval schema. From a Latin manuscript of the Ketham type, circa 1400. Now in the Bibliothèque Nationale, Paris, as MS. lat. 11229. The 7 planets are inserted between the manikin and the signs of the zodiac, cf. Sudh. Arch. 2 [1909], 98.

Plate IXb Christ as Salvator mundi in the zodiac. The 12 astrological symbols are represented with their names and respective organs. The four seasons are placed in the corners. MS. lat. 7028, Bibliothèque Nationale, Paris.

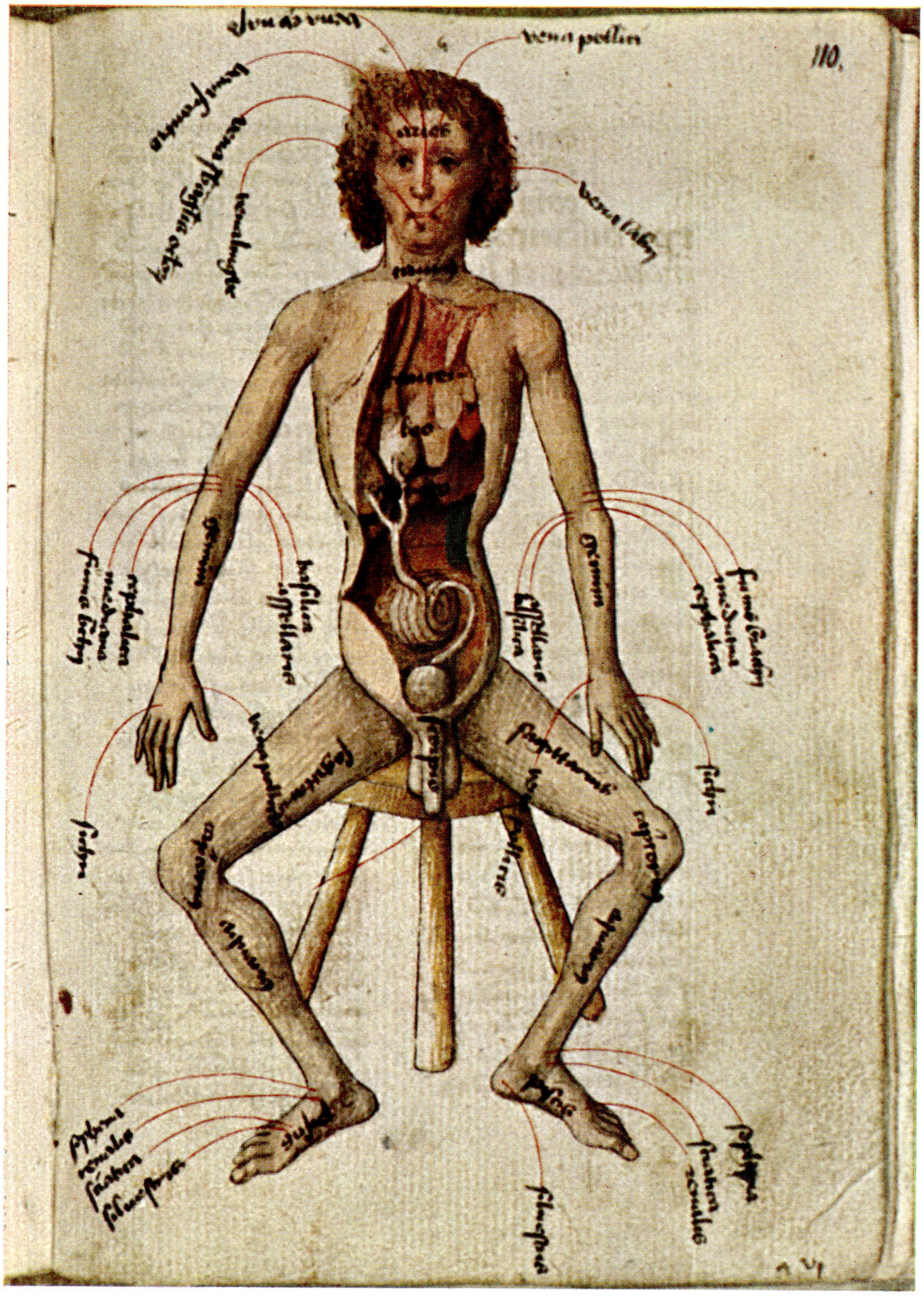

Plate X 'Bloodletting man' from the MS. 18. 2. Aug. 4° in the Herzog-August-Bibliothek, Wolfenbüttel. Numerous similar figures found in the works on venesection printed during the 16th century are in this tradition, which has been traced back to the Alexandrian 'squatting figures' *(cf. p. 10).*

Fig. 77

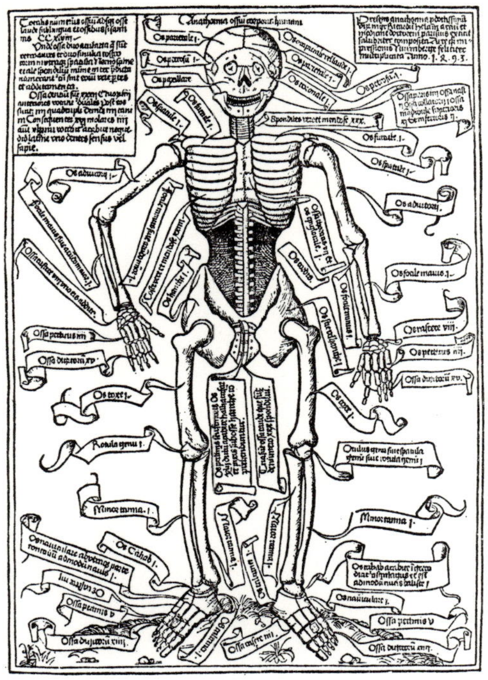

Fig. 78

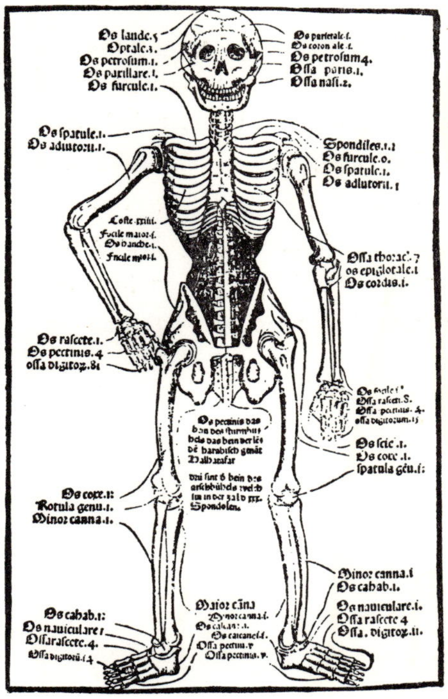

Fig. 79

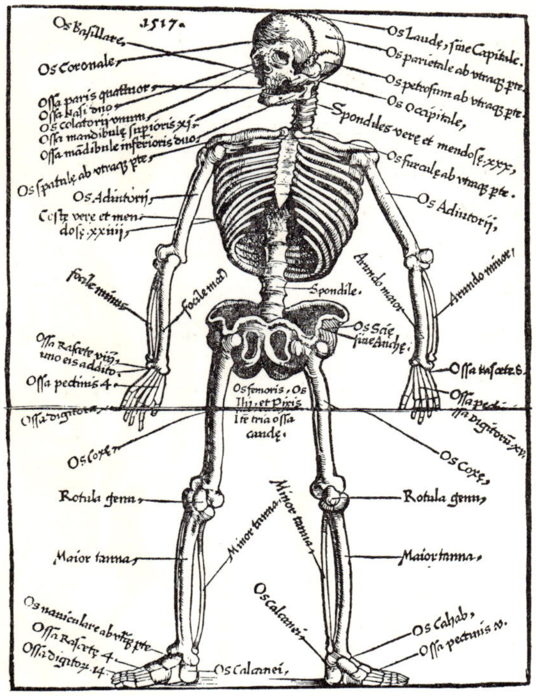

Figures 77 to 79 Development of the indication line: three skeletal diagrams from southern Germany. Ricardus Helain, Nuremberg 1493; Brunschwig, Strasbourg 1497; Hans von Gerssdorff, Strasbourg 1517.[3]

Fig. 80 Diagram of the thoracic and abdominal viscera, from Hans Peyligk's Philosophie naturalis compendium, *Leipzig, 1499.*

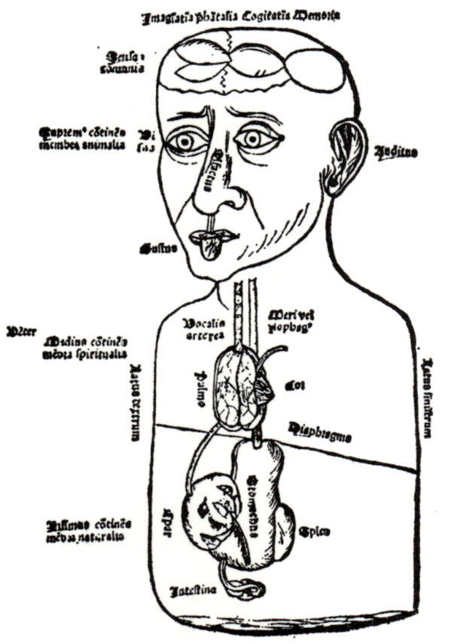

art history, they reflected the desire for movement that was often so strong in late medieval art. Here, having outlived their purpose, they stand testimony to the fact that medical illustration of the closing Middle Ages had one of its roots in ecclesiastical art.

Banderoles bearing legends or labels thus appear to be the immediate ancestors of our indication lines. A previously mentioned hypothesis – that the cautery became a pointer and may have been another direct ancestor of the indication line (see p. 19) – cannot be proved. However, like the use of a hand with a pointer in Italian manuscripts of about 1300, and like the adoption of the banderole itself, this use of the cautery as a pointer does show that illustrators were continually faced with the problem of identifying specific points on a full-figure illustration, and that the solutions they arrived at were remarkably similar in their logic.

The use of indication lines, however, was a fairly late development.[4] The simplest, and almost certainly the earliest, method of identifying parts of the body was merely to write the name on the part in question, or as close beside it as possible. This method, which is demonstrated in figure 80 on this page, worked well as long as the labels were short and the parts to be labeled were relatively few – and as long

[3] There was apparently no skeleton available in Strasbourg in 1517, for this illustration "is literally sculptured from stone by Master NICKLAUS, Sculptor of Zabern;" i.e., it is probably a design for a relief on a gravestone.

[4] SUDHOFF also commented very cautiously on the age of the venesection figures, which evidently had "indication lines" from the beginning, but he found none which he could date with certainty before 1400. SUDHOFF: Studien I, p. 29/30 and Studien 11/12, p. XVII.

as the precise location of particular items was not of great concern. This system had been used from time to time throughout the Middle Ages (see the labeling of the organ diagrams on pp. 13-14), and by the end of the 14th century it was general practice. Arabic illustrations were also sometimes labeled in this way. It is not surprising, therefore, that this kind of labeling predominated in incunabula and post-incunabula, for instance in KETHAM, in PEYLIGK'S *Philosophie naturalis compendium*, or in REISCH'S *Margarita philosophica* (Strasbourg, 1503), A refinement of this method was introduced several decades later (see p. 115) when engravers began to label parts only with letters – "A," "B," "C," etc. – rather than with words; a key to the meaning of the letters was then supplied by the author somewhere in the text.

The End of Scholastic Illustration

Between about 1500, the period of the early printed works which have been considered so far, and the explosive development in anatomical illustration which set in at the end of the 1530's, there was a turning-point in the history of medical illustration which requires explanation.

As early as 1949, my art-history teacher, OTTMAR KERBER,[1] encouraged me to contribute to the discussion of medical history some "Fundamental Ideas about Anatomical Illustration Around 1500."[2] Subsequently, the pair of illustrations which had served as my model were employed by WERNER LEIBBRAND[3] in a comparative study of the histories of art and of thought. An understanding of the relation between art history and the history of thought is essential to an understanding of the transformation from medieval to modern illustration and is, therefore, the pivotal point of this chapter. My original model has proved itself useful and can be of further service here.

Anatomical illustration before LEONARDO and VESALIUS is still regarded as primitive or – as American scholars like to say – pre-Vesalian. However, the historical break we are interested in occurs not between VESALIUS'S *Fabrica* of 1543 and its predecessors, but several generations earlier. G. RATH is certainly correct in his recent demand for an adequate treatment of those anatomists who were already advancing towards a regeneration of anatomy before VESALIUS and – what is more – towards a criticism of GALEN, their most celebrated master in antiquity. RATH, however, is concerned with the texts, while we are referring only to the illustrations.

1 KERBER, OTTMAR: Meister Francke und die deutsche Kunst um 1400, Kallmünz, 1939.

2 HERRLINGER, ROBERT: Grundsätzliche Gedanken zu anatomischen Abbildungen um 1500, in: Grenzgebiete der Medizin *2*, 1949, pp. 561-63.

3 LEIBBRAND, WERNER: Heilkunde. Eine Problemgeschichte der Medizin, in: Orbis Academicus II/4, Freiburg/Munich, 1953, figs. 6 and 7.

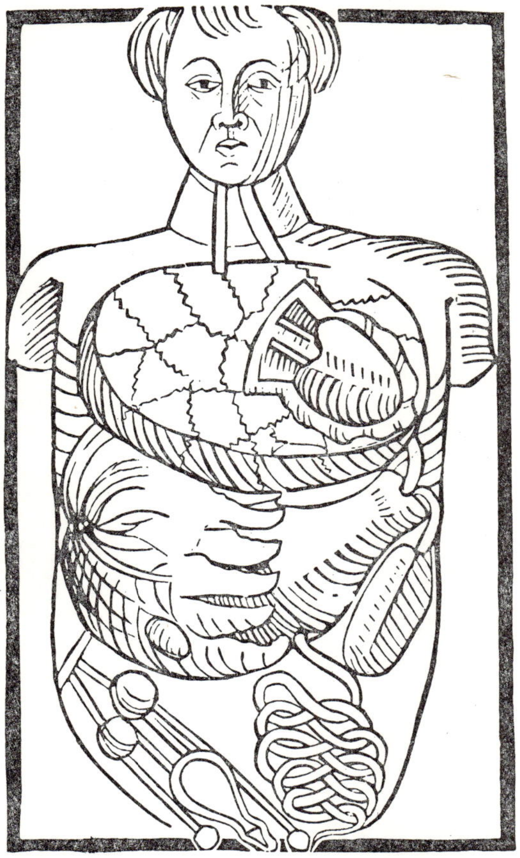

Fig. 81 Diagram of the thoracic and abdominal viscera, from Magnus Hundt, Anthropologium, *Leipzig 1501.*

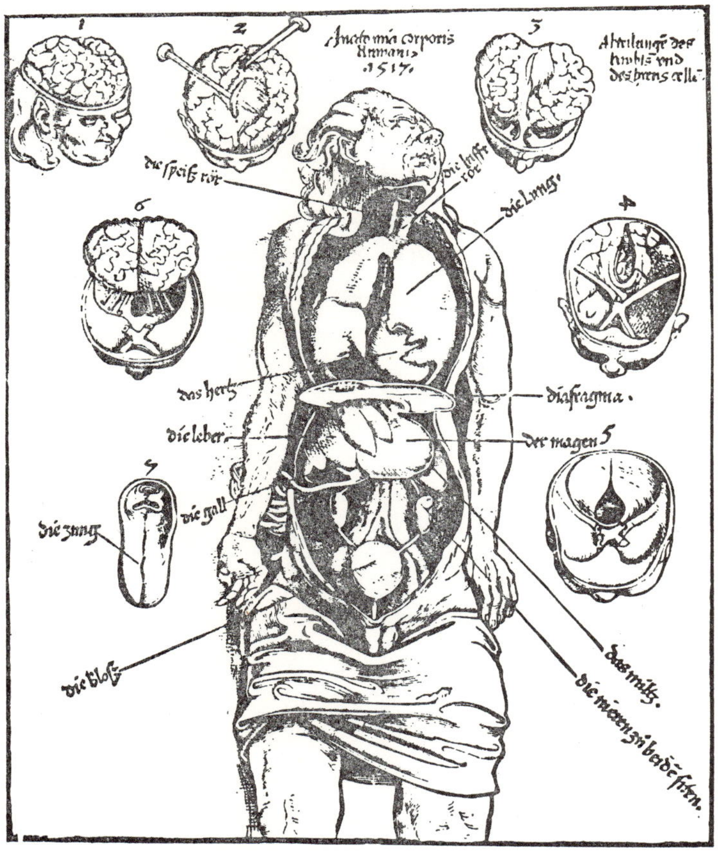

Fig. 82 Situs of the viscera from Lorenz Phryes (Fries), Spiegel der Artzny, *Strasbourg, 1518.*

We can most easily analyze the break in style by describing the developments in medical illustration that took place in the two 16th-century centers of European medical publishing: Strasbourg and Venice. Although the example provided by Strasbourg came later, it is the more impressive. The first "modern" anatomical illustration in German literature – a situs of the viscera – appears on two sheets printed by the Strasbourg publisher JOHANNES SCHOTT in 1517. The counterpart of this illustration is the skeleton already discussed on pages 54 and 59. Executed by the engraver HANS WÄCHTLIN of Basel,[4] this viscera figure has an obscure history.[5] It is reproduced above next to a figure from 1501: a visceral scheme from the *Anthropologium de ho(mi)nis dignitate, natura, et p(ro)prietatibus* by the Bachelor of Medicine and later theologian MAGNUS HUNDT of Leipzig. The sixteen-year interval between the two quite different representations of the same theme can be reduced to one year if HUNDT'S diagram is replaced by the visceral figure from a

[4] CHOULANT had thought it to be by HANS BALDUNG GRIEN.
[5] See footnotes 2 and 3 on pp. 54 and 59. The corresponding skeleton was produced under totally different circumstances, a fact that has not previously been taken into consideration. The situs was originally drawn for an anatomy compiled by the Strasbourg physician WENDELIN HOCK.

Leipzig picture encyclopedia from 1516 (fig. 83). This illustration is printed in the anonymous *Compendiosa capitis phisici declaratio,* and is derived from HUNDT'S figure. It is known that the anonymous author was actually JOHANN PEYLIGK, son of the mayor of Zeitz and later professor of law. This small compendium of natural science was for him nothing more than a youthful indiscretion committed during his basic studies in art. As was observed above, it had already appeared in 1499 under the title *Philosophie naturalis compendium,* with a visceral figure of far inferior quality (fig. 80) and a series of organ illustrations (figs. 84-85) which can be regarded as the oldest woodcuts relating to this subject. Two years later, HUNDT'S publisher copied them all, with the exception of the thorax-abdomen diagram, which is his – or HUNDT'S – own work.

SUDHOFF was apparently not yet in a position to determine the place in art history of these illustrations.[6] He saw the Leipzig woodcut as merely deriving from drawings originating "in antiquity" which "in the course of centuries, had become schematized as a result of continual redrawing." SUDHOFF supposed that PEYLIGK and HUNDT had "compounded"[7] their illustrations from those late antique organ diagrams which we have already encountered in medieval manuscripts (see p. 13). It appears to me that this compounding must have occurred, if at all, at a much earlier date. CHOULANT[8] says of HUNDT'S illustrations: "They contain the most complete pictorial representation of all the viscera so far undertaken, to a degree not found in their predecessors or even Ketham, and a clear survey of pre-Berengarian anatomy – the essence of how the positions and forms of the parts were conceived in the 15th century." PHRYES'S – i.e. WÄCHTLIN'S – situs of 1517/18 is described by CHOULANT as being "much better than all previous anatomical illustrations known to us"; "the representation is original, being particularly novel and remarkable in respect of the brain; drawing and engraving, especially of the non-anatomical components, are beautifully executed."

The American anatomist and interpreter of LEONARDO, MCMURRICH (1930), regards the WÄCHTLIN-PHRYES illustration as a modification of the figure by MAGNUS HUNDT, an improvement "clearly based on Peyligk and Hundt." He interprets HUNDT'S illustration as follows: "In the thorax, the greater part of the cavity is occupied by the lungs by virtue of their position on top of the diaphragm, and the heart is characteristically prominent; in the abdomen, the stomach lies obliquely, and the kidneys and bladder are reproduced, but curiously displaced to the right." But is there really a connection between PHRYES'S situs and HUNDT'S diagram? This can hardly be maintained even with respect to content, and it is difficult to

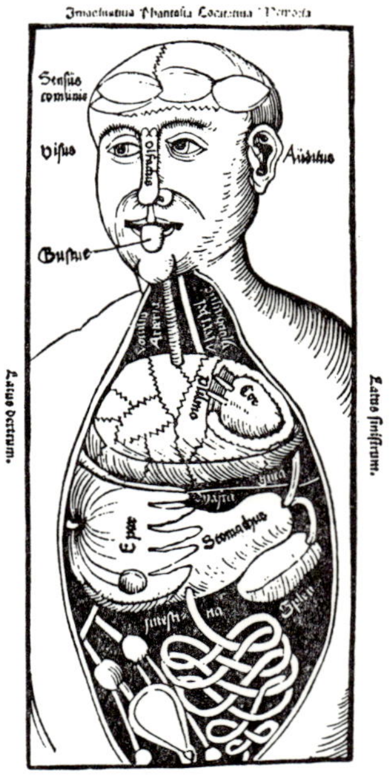

Fig. 83 Diagram of the thoracic and abdominal viscera in Peyligk's Compendiosa declaratio *of 1516 (cf. fig. 80).*

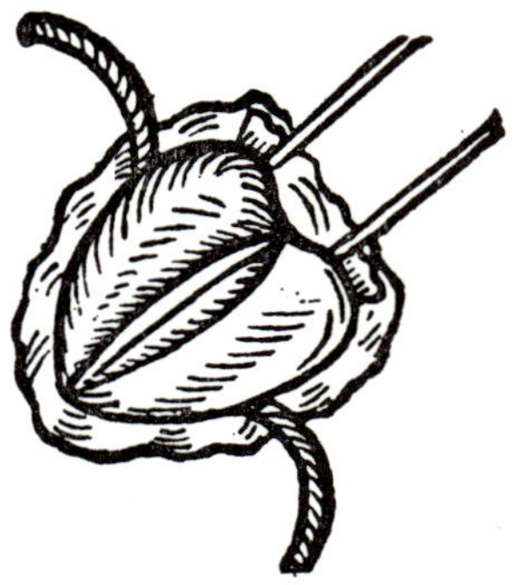

Figures 84 and 85 Two figures from Peyligk's Compendium, *1499.*

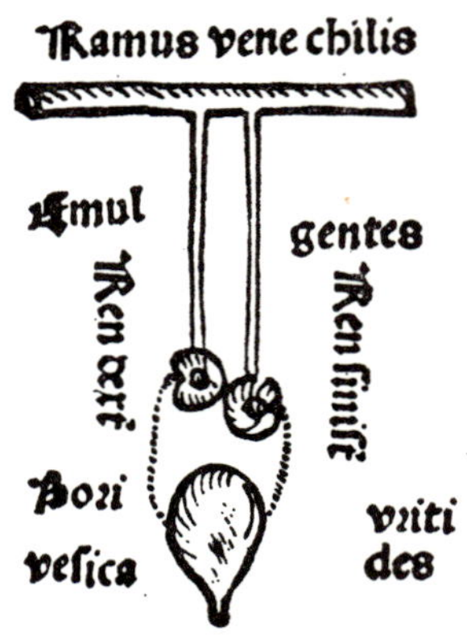

[6] Nor was L. FLECK, who, in an interesting but little-known study, recognized some of the problems involved. FLECK, LUDWIG: Zur Frage der Grundlagen der medizinischen Erkenntnisse, in: Klin. Wochenschrift *14*, 1935, pp. 1255-1259. – This is even more true of GARRISON. GARRISON, F. H.: The Principles of Anatomic Illustration Before Vesalius, New York, Hoeber, 1926.

[7] SUDHOFF, KARL: Geschichte der Anatomie an der Universität Leipzig, in: Stud. Gesch. Med. *7*, 1909, p. 121.

[8] CHOULANT, LUDWIG: Geschichte und Bibliographie der anatomischen Abbildung nach ihrer Beziehung auf anatomische Wissenschaft und bildende Kunst, Leipzig, 1852, p. 24.

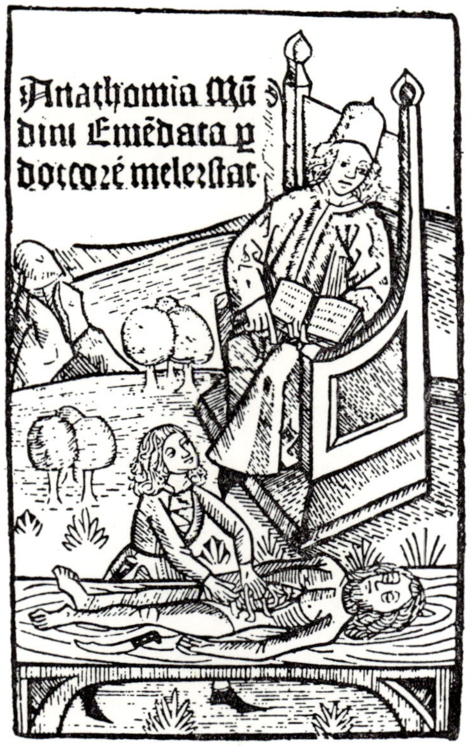

Fig. 86 Title-page woodcut for Martin Pollich, Anathomia Mundini, *Leipzig (Landsberg), circa 1495.*

Fig. 87 Title-page woodcut for Arnald von Villanova, Speculum medicine, *published by Martin Pollich, Leipzig (Landsberg), circa 1495.*

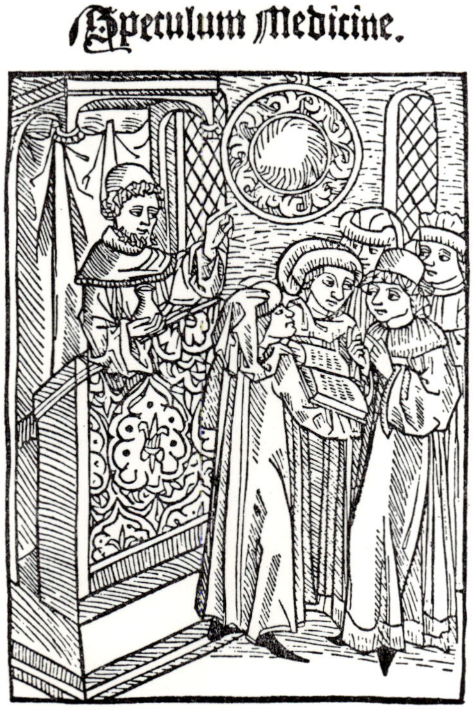

appreciate what McMurrich understands by "modification." It seems clear that, quite apart from content, we are faced with a fundamentally different type of pictorial representation. While this is immediately obvious to the art historian, it appears that medical historians have only recently become aware of the difference.[9] Hundt's figure is entirely medieval; that of Phryes, wholly modern. It is hard to believe that a period of only sixteen years lies between them, or that so short a period could embrace a whole epochal transition. In order to explain this, a brief digression into the sphere of aesthetics is required.

In the history of the visual arts north of the Alps, the transition from medieval to modern panel painting was accomplished by about 1400. In quite general terms, panel painting is to be understood as painting which represents space as though the observer and the figure occupy it at the same time. Space is sustained by the figure depicted in it. The beginning of panel painting is thus the turning point in artistic vision, where the artist abandons his standpoint outside an abstract picture constructed by him according to specific – that is, medieval – rules of form, in favor of a standpoint within the space he is representing. The discovery of central perspective is not the cause of this event, but rather its consequence. Nor is the intrusion of landscape into painting the cause – we still find gold ground-color long after this occurred, whereas landscape background already existed in medieval compositions.[10]

Figures 86 and 87 are clear examples of the difference between the medieval and the modern treatment of pictured space. Figure 86 is a representation that is completely medieval in its formal idiom, although it dates from approximately 1495. It is intended to show an anatomical demonstration. Now, no one would maintain that such demonstrations took place in a field with a landscape in the background and tufts of grass in the foreground. Here, each element of the whole picture has its own specific meaning in the manner of a formula: the chair signifies a lecturing chair, but it would be wrong to think it is meant as a real lecturing chair; the landscape is not a landscape in the objective sense, but signifies a neutral background consisting of the formulae "rock," "tree," "tuft," and so forth, fundamentally in the same manner as in metaphorical language. The woodcut is the frontispiece of a Mondino anatomy edited by the "doctor melestat," i.e. Martin Pollich from Mellerstadt in Franconia.

Figure 87, the title page for a *Speculum medicinae* by Arnaldo de Villanova, was also published by Martin Pollich about 1495, but is altogether different: this illustration shows the interior of a university lecture room which is more or less well-drawn in a naturalistic manner. The room is a fact of reality; the standing figures are in relationship to one another; and we, as observers, find ourselves in

[9] The argument presented here is based on the 1949 article by the present author (footnote 2, above).
[10] The question of how far it is permissible to think in psychobiological terms in explaining this phenomenon – perhaps taking into consideration developmental studies concerning children's perception of physical objects – is not raised here, however tempting this might be for a medical man.

the same room, just as a painter with his easel, or a photographer with his camera, occupies a position within the space of his picture.

A person who is able to appreciate this fundamental difference, apply it to the great works of art he is familiar with, comparing perhaps a Byzantine mosaic and a Baroque mural painting, and then return to the situs pictures by MAGNUS HUNDT and LORENZ PHRYES, will now see these two illustrations with quite different eyes. HUNDT'S "situs"[11] does not actually try to show what the viscera really look like; e.g., the formula symbol for "intestine" appears to the right of the symbols for "kidneys" and "bladder." It is not a matter of all this being false, for the categories of "correct" and "false" do not belong to the basic substance of such a formal idiom. At the most they can be applied to certain details – for instance, it is false to represent the liver with five lobes; or, there is no actual "passage" from the stomach to the spleen – but the basic statements of the situs figure, which are topographical, are neither "false" nor "correct" to a knowledgeable modern observer, because it was really not the intention of the designer to represent true-to-life topographic anatomical details.

It is admissible, however, to evaluate the artist's execution of the task which confronted him. This particular problem was solved by HUNDT'S illustrator in an aesthetically pleasing form, as is obvious when the illustration is compared with other known illustrations at the same stage of development and style, for instance, the "situs figure" in PEYLIGK'S *Compendium* (fig. 80).

The situs figure from PHRYES'S *Spiegel der Arzteny* represents something completely different. As we have already emphasized, a period of only sixteen years separates this from HUNDT'S illustration. It is even more surprising that the two illustrations reproduced in figures 86 and 87 should derive from works of the same publisher – indeed, from the same workshop, that of MARTIN LANDSBERG in Leipzig. The explanation for this is that early bookprinters began to reproduce on paper everything that their new technical skills permitted: century-old manuscript texts and illustrations, as well as recent works. Thus by about 1500 the transitional point between the medieval and the modern formal idiom had been passed – without, however, the medieval elements having been completely eradicated, at least as far as practical graphic art is concerned. DAGOBERT FREY has quite rightly drawn our attention to the "shifts and dislocations in time" which, even in closely related fields, become obvious here.[12]

The PHRYES illustration is just as modern in its basic conception as the contemporary illustrations of LEONARDO. Moreover, it has recently been suggested by SIGRID ESCHE that the representation of the brain in this figure could not have been conceived without a knowledge of LEONARDO'S sheets. The PHRYES situs

Figures 88 and 89 Illustrations of the 'tabula tertia de muliere' in the first and second editions of Johannes de Ketham, Fasciculus medicinae, *Venice 1491 and 1493.*

[11] The term "situs," which has been commonly used since SUDHOFF, reveals the misunderstanding.
[12] FREY, DAGOBERT: Gotik und Renaissance als Grundlagen der modernen Weltanschauung, Augsburg, 1929, p. XVIII.

Fig. 88

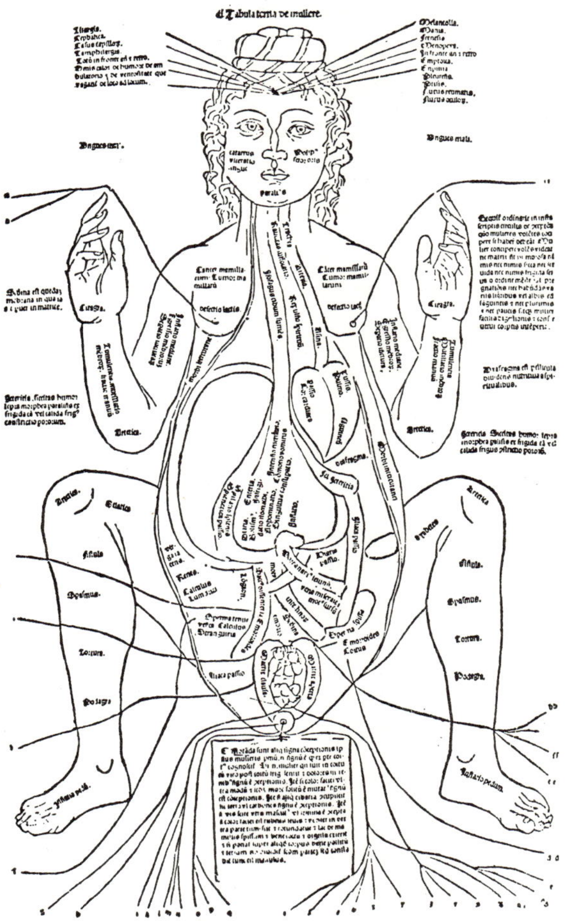

Fig. 89

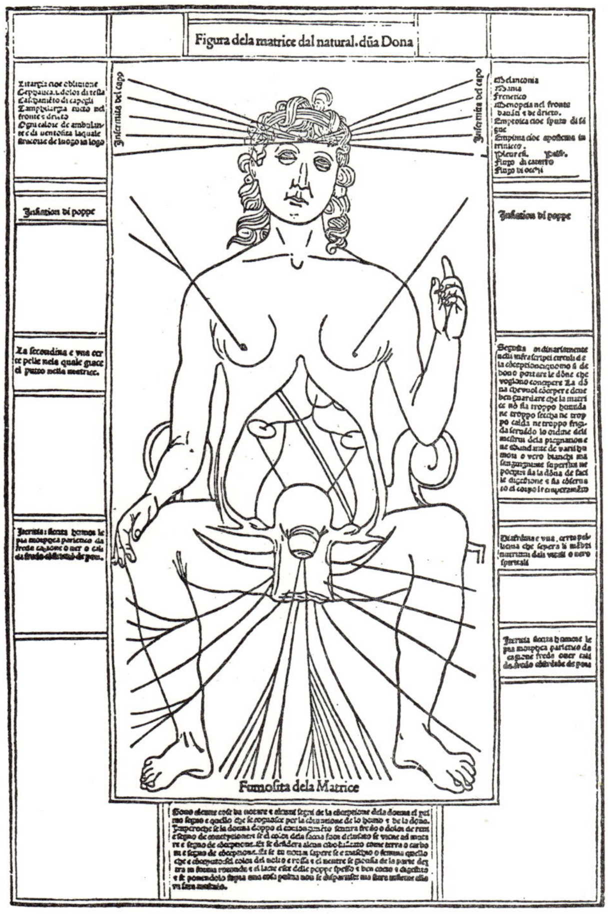

figure actually does contain errors, for it does attempt to illustrate "correctly": among the errors are the deficient intestine displaced to the right, the representation of the kidneys and their vessels, and so on. From this point forward, there is a direct line of development to modern textbook illustration; more and more errors are gradually eradicated until a scientifically accurate illustration is achieved.

PHRYES'S situs figure now gains a quite different status in the history of anatomical illustration: as far as we can determine at this time, it is really the first German anatomical illustration to be conceived in terms of the modern formal idiom. This means that it can never be traced from the tradition of medieval manuscripts, and that regardless of the errors it contains, it can already be measured against the standards which we now generally apply to modern scientific or medical illustration.

The same kind of abrupt transition from a scholastic to a realistic style of illustration that we have just described as taking place in Strasbourg also took place in Venice, the other European center of medical publishing. The first printed edition of KETHAM'S *Fasciculus medicinae*, published in Venice in 1491 by the DE GREGORIUS DA FORLI brothers, contained illustrations that were clearly in the medieval tradition, modeled on those that had appeared in the handwritten prototype. (This prototype was published in 1907 by SUDHOFF, who presented it as a representative work of its kind and provided it with a moving introduction.[13]) A main feature in this work was the "tabula tertia de muliere" (figure 88), illustrating female anatomy, which CHOULANT described as "a rough representation of the thoracic and abdominal viscera in quite arbitrary outline and without any relation to nature." Two years after the first printed Latin edition appeared, an Italian edition was published, in a smaller format that necessitated the making of new woodcuts. These new illustrations – which were used again in the second Latin edition in 1495 – included an entirely redesigned figure showing female anatomy (fig. 89). This is the sheet that represents our transition from medieval to modern illustration. The scholastic figure from 1491 must have irritated the eyes of the artistic Venetians to such a degree that they immediately abandoned it. After this the female figure actually sits in an armchair, so that the traditional position corresponds to a real situation. The position itself, of course, can be traced all the way back to the Alexandrian squatting figures (see p. 10) or to even older representations of the figure.[14]

At exactly the same time, in Milan, the forty-year-old LEONARDO, who had just completed his "Last Supper" for the refectory of Santa Maria delle Grazie, drew up his first plan for an anatomical textbook. The oldest sheet of his sketchbook of anatomical figures drawn from nature bears the date 1489 (fol. 42^r of Fogli B with two details of the skull). The date of the large folding sheet containing the female situs (Quaderni L 12^r), which LEONARDO repeatedly corrected during the course of his studies, cannot be precisely determined. The best judge of the subject material, SIGRID ESCHE-BRAUNFELS, is not prepared to date it earlier than 1503/05. The uterus has an unfortunate similarity to the organ outline of the KETHAM figure dating from 1492/93.

The phenomenon of the gap between the modern scientific terminology of the textbooks and the corresponding graphic art presented in these books remains a mystery, despite all the information we have gleaned about the subject. One reason for the gap, however, could be the still existing dependency of late medieval science on its Arabic traditions. Islamic illustration (see pp. 37-39) is characterized by the same inherent tendency toward abstraction as the so-called "medieval" formal idiom. Scholars expert in this branch of Arabic studies have not yet been able to supply a thorough account of the influence of Arabic illustration – and its antipathy to pictorial representation – on late medieval medical literature.

[13] SUDHOFF, KARL: Weibliche Situsbilder von ca. 1400 bis 1543, in Stud. Gesch. Med. *1*, 1907, p. 79 ff.
[14] Cf. WELLS, L. H.: The "Great Mother" and Some Early Medical Illustrations, in: J. Hist. Med. *15*, New Haven, 1960, pp. 59-63.

Leonardo da Vinci

Although LEONARDO did not publish any of his anatomical illustrations during his lifetime, he was one of the outstanding masters in this field, as all historians after CHOULANT have recognized.

When the large facsimile editions of LEONARDO'S sketchbooks were published, around the beginning of the present century,[1] his anatomical work attracted attention mainly because of the amazing technical knowledge it revealed.[2] A discussion immediately arose concerning how far VESALIUS had been influenced by LEONARDO; the academic exchanges between HOLL and JACKSCHATH, and between ROTH and HOLL, provoked heated controversy throughout the first decade of this century. In the years since then, scholars have been concerned largely with determining the degree to which LEONARDO'S drawings are "correct" or "false," and this has been a recurrent theme of special studies[3] – for instance, studies concerning his knowledge of hemodynamics (blood circulation),[4] or concerning the critical ordering of his work according to anatomical criteria[5] – but the importance of LEONARDO'S role in the history of scientific illustration is now becoming increasingly recognized.[6] The most recent studies undertaken in this field give priority to the question of technical originality, and emphasize the methods that LEONARDO invented or adopted for illustrating anatomical features in a clear and understandable way. Many of the problems that cause difficulty to anatomical illustrators can be discussed with reference to his anatomical sketches. LEONARDO solved many of these problems in a surprisingly modern manner, and because of their fundamental importance we will examine his solutions in detail.

LEONARDO began his anatomical studies by turning to printed texts. Consequently, among his early sketches – which may have been made while reading MONDINO or the then recently published works of ZERBI – there are sketches of three brain ventricles, of pores in the interventricular septum of the heart, of some unrealistic connecting tubes between the liver and the spleen, and of distinctly unrealistic musculature in the abdomen. Even these derivatory sketches show some of the technical devices LEONARDO used in his attempt to represent – initially in a manner plausible to himself – anatomical textbook knowledge that in part had never been illustrated.

When LEONARDO noticed that the textbooks did not always conform to his own observations, he finally decided upon the same course of action which VESALIUS was to take half a century later: namely, to write his own textbook.

1 KNOX 1852, LANGER 1867, RICHTER 1883.

2 SABACHNIKOF and PIUMATI 1898-1901; Feuillets inédits, Paris, Rouveyre, 1901; VANGENSTEN, FONAHN and HOPSTOCK 1911-16.

3 FAVARO 1919 ff., BILANCIONI 1919 ff., ARGENTIERI 1939, BUCHER 1946, ELMER BELT 1954, and others. For titles and further references, see the bibliography in BRAUNFELS-ESCHE, SIGRID: Leonardo da Vinci, Das anatomisch Werk, Stuttgart, 1961; and CIANCHI, RENZO: Bibliografia degli Scritti Vinciani di anatomia e materie affini (1550-1963), in: Leonardo da Vinci, Il trattato della Anatomia Roma, 1962.

4 MCMURRICH 1930, KEELE 1592.

5 MCMURRICH 1930, O'MALLEY and SAUNDERS 1954, HUARD 1961, PAZZINI and others 1962.

6 HOLL 1905, KLEBS 1916, BENESCH 1943, HEYDENREICH 1945, HERRLINGER 1949 ff., and especially ESCHE 1954.

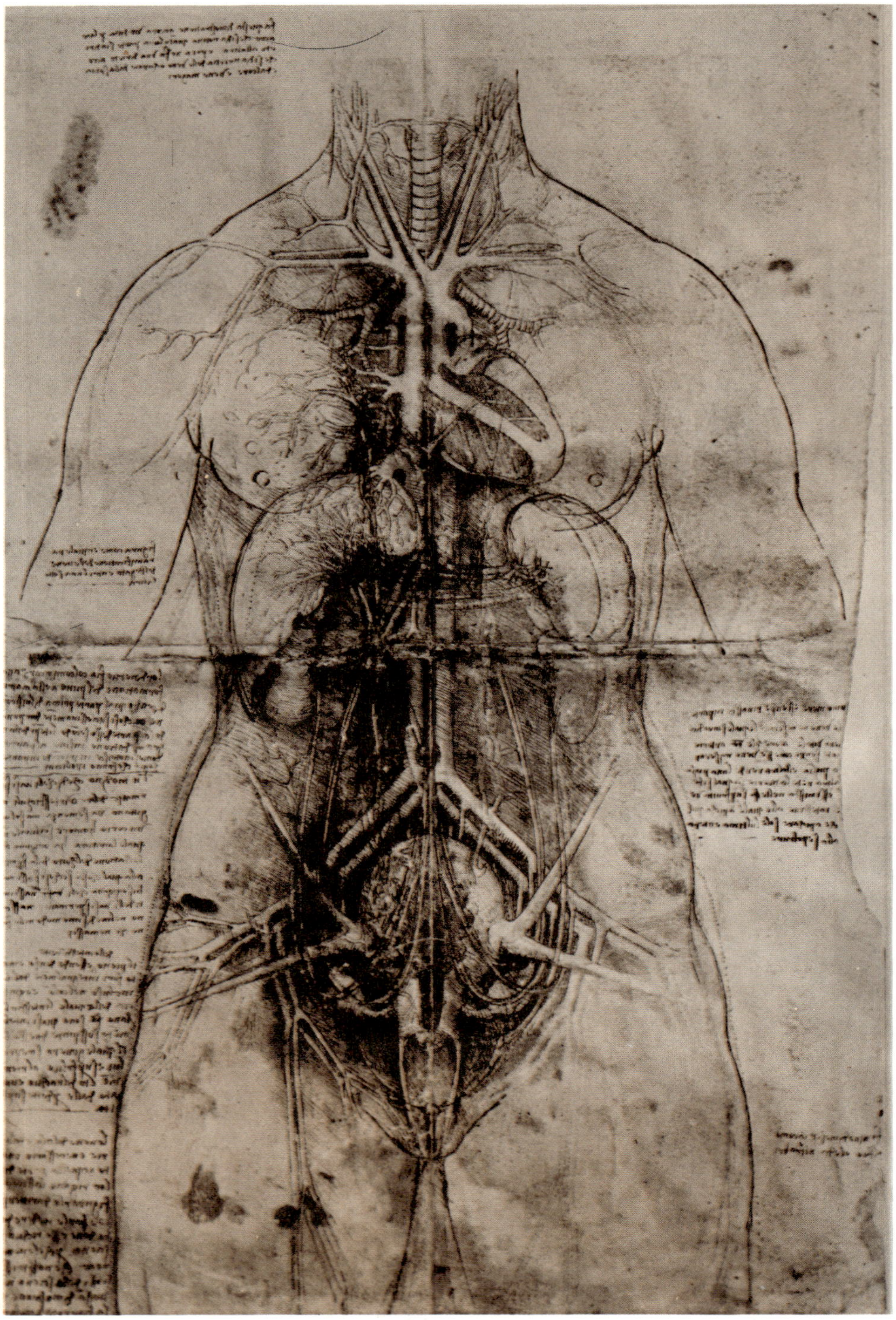

Fig. 90 Quaderni I 12^{v}. A 'transparent' torso. Leonardo's notes, here and on other sketches, are written backwards; he deliberately used mirror-writing in his personal notebooks.

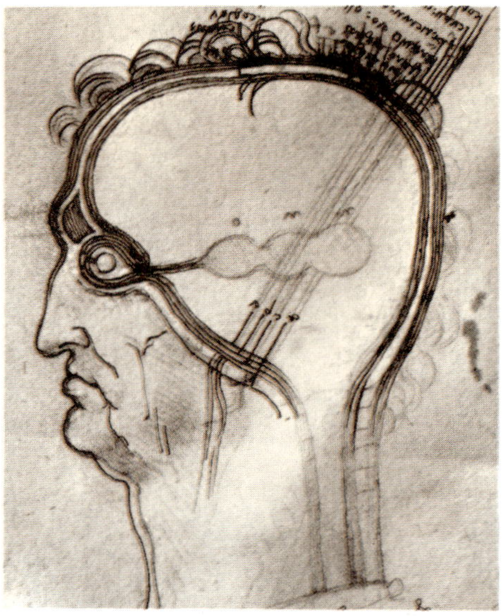

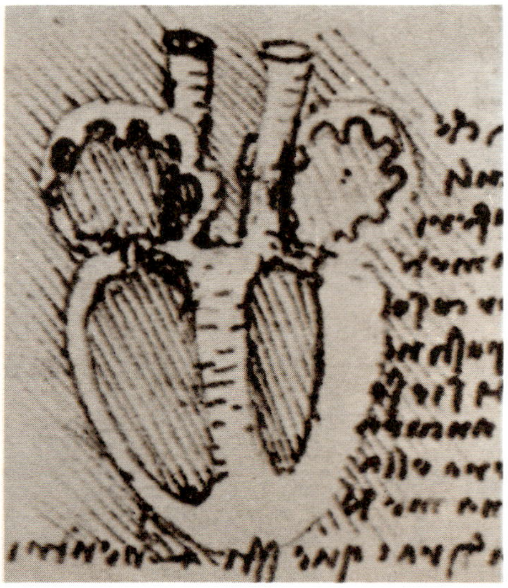

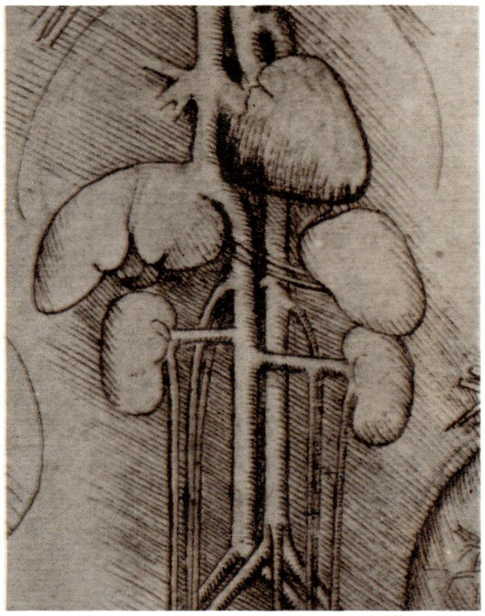

Figures 91 to 93 Three sketches based on medical texts. (Quaderni V 6^{r}; Quaderni I 3^{r}; Quaderni III 10^{v}) Produced between 1495 and 1505.

Fig. 94 Drawings for a systematic representation of the skeleton. Fogli A 13^{r}, circa 1510.

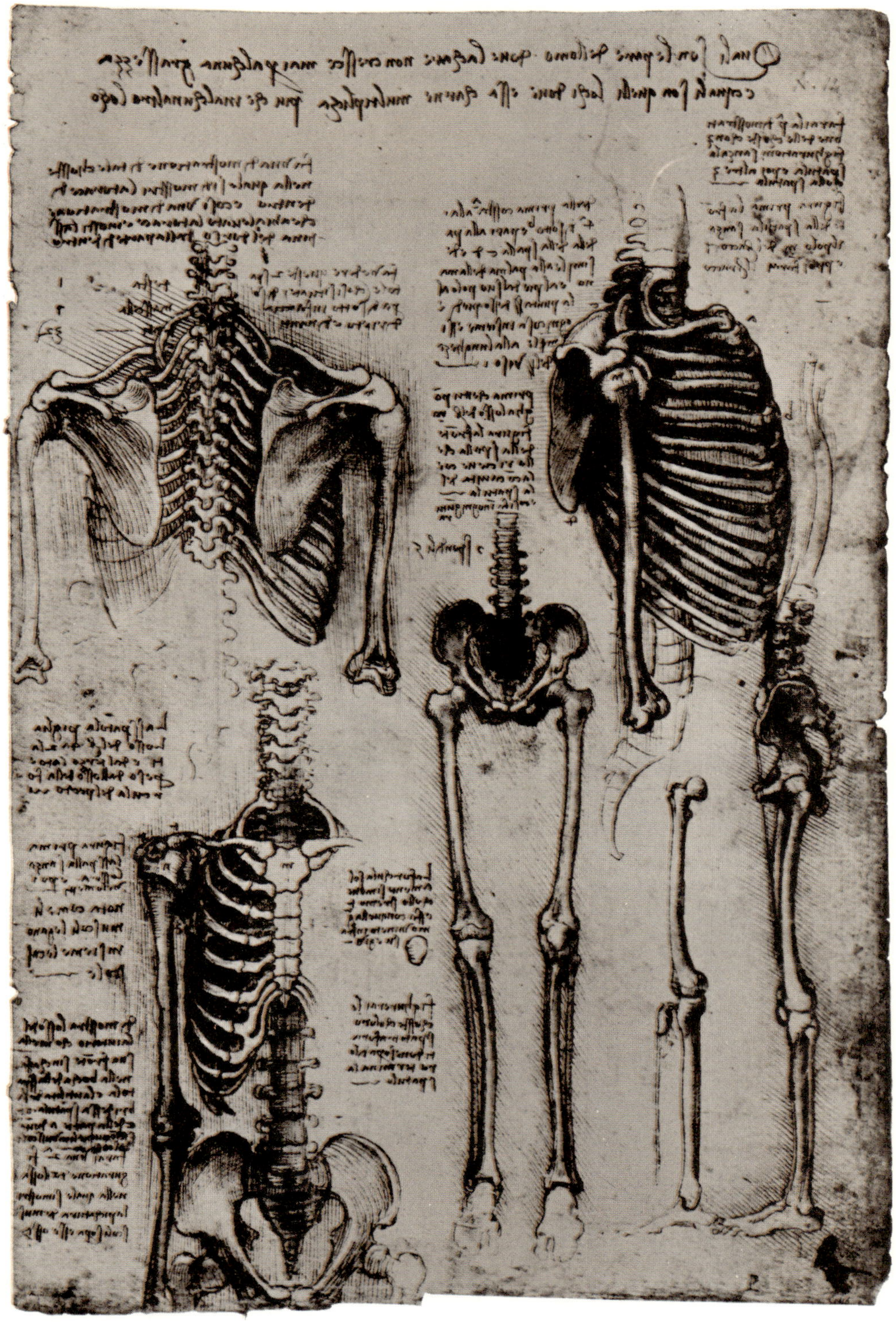

Whereas for Vesalius (1543) anatomy was to serve primarily as the basis for surgery rather than for the whole of medicine, in Leonardo's work anatomy appears as the basis for the whole study of man. His initial idea of 1489 – "This work is to begin with the conception of man" – embraces psychology, physiognomy, and the entire physiology of the senses. But at the same time he also made clear the importance of the illustrations in his work. It appears to me that in planning his textbook, Leonardo gave illustration priority over the text from the beginning. A part of his program is outlined in the notebooks that have been preserved: one sheet, which probably dates from about 1490 (the period of his first anatomical studies) outlines proposals for a systematic illustration of the skeleton and its parts; for demonstrations of myology, angiology, and neurology, each to be considered from three aspects; for studies of the surface of the body and its "measurements" or proportions; and finally for a study "of the female figure, in order to show the uterus and the menstrual vessels leading to the breasts" (Fogli B, 20^v).

LEONARDO himself testified to the degree of precedence he accorded to illustrations over text, in a note dating from 1510: "Dispel from your mind the thought that an understanding of the human body in every aspect of its structure can be given in words; for the more thoroughly you describe, the more you will confuse: it is therefore necessary to draw as well as to describe" (Fogli A, 14^v). And several years later he wrote, "I advise you not to trouble with words unless you are speaking to blind men."

LEONARDO was clearly a person who was visually oriented to an extreme degree. It is possible that this interfered with his plan to produce an anatomical textbook; for it may be that the reason the book never appeared is that he never attempted to write systematically even a simple text.

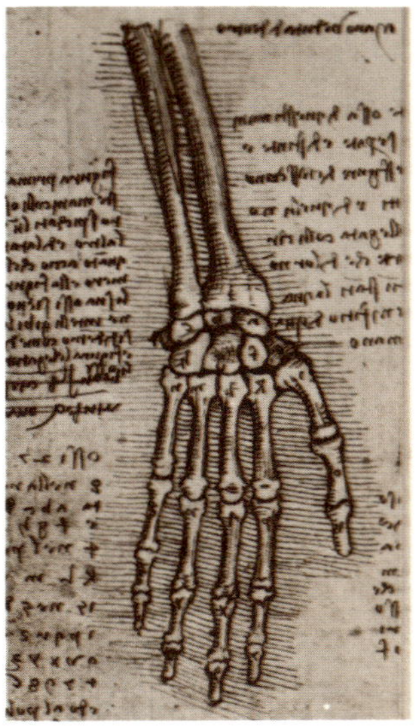

Fig. 95 Leonardo, Fogli A 10^v, 1510.

By the time he began his anatomical studies, LEONARDO had already developed great technical proficiency in drawing, so that he was quite justified in rating illustration (his own illustration!) much higher than the spoken or written word. One example of his technical proficiency can be seen in his use of undershading to achieve a three-dimensional effect – see figure 95, a drawing of the bones of the hand, which employs both undershading and white highlights. It appears to me remarkable that LEONARDO'S undershading was not more widely adopted by medical illustrators during the first half of the 16th century. It is encountered in the BERENGARIO edition of 1521 (see figure 96, from the *Commentaria super anatomia Mundini*, Bologna, 1521, page 522), but other illustrators continued to rely on more roundabout methods. The artist for VESALIUS'S *Fabrica*, for instance, generally employed a cast shadow to suggest a three-dimensional effect (see figure 97).

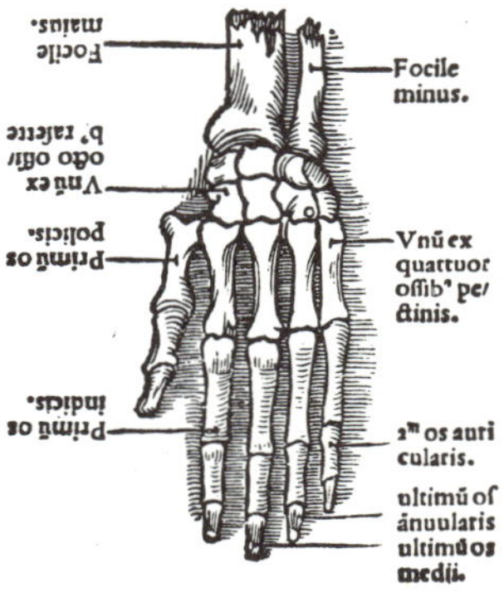

Fig. 96 Berengario da Carpi, 1521.

The vitality of LEONARDO'S anatomical illustrations is impressive. We are confronted not by a lifeless dissected figure, but – especially in the motion studies – by an anatomy which has been animated in very visual terms. It is unusual, and worth noting, that LEONARDO was able to convey this impression of life while at the same time presenting a typical anatomical figure, rather than drawing an individual anatomical example with all the accidental features that might be peculiar to this one example. Whenever LEONARDO had had the opportunity to see several examples of the same anatomical structure, he ultimately attempted a synthesis, desiring to represent what was typical rather than accidental. This problem – whether to create a typical model, or to faithfully show a real model with all its idiosyncracies – was one on which compilers of anatomies were still divided through

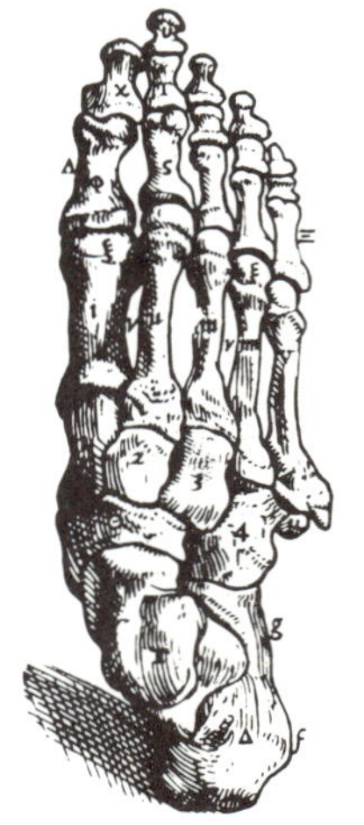

Fig. 97 Vesalius, 1543.

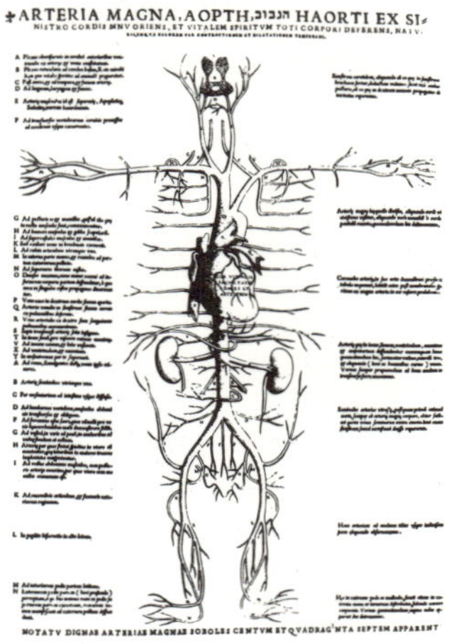

Fig. 98 Vesalius's diagram of the arteries (Tabula III) of 1538.

Fig. 99 Vesalius's vein figure in the Fabrica *of 1543.*

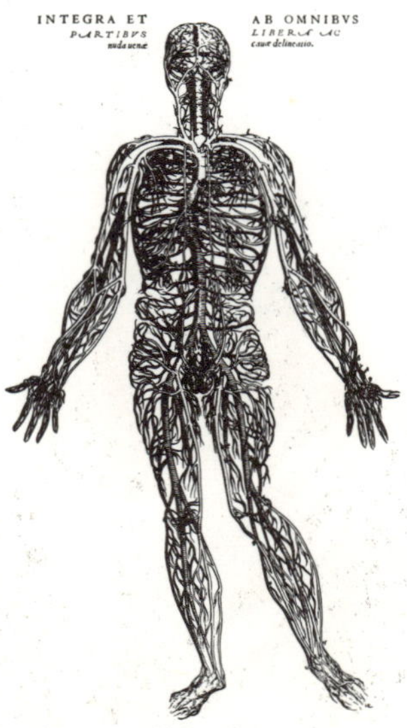

the 19th, and even into the 20th, century. The answer that seemed obvious to LEONARDO nearly five hundred years ago has thus only recently achieved general acceptance as the most reasonable solution to the problem.

In addition to the purely technical drawing skills briefly discussed above, LEONARDO also employed several technical devices of other kinds, which we shall now take up.

- *Illustrating different systems of organs in logical succession.* LEONARDO advocated that a part of the body should be systematically treated from the inside to the outside. Using the hand as an example, he explained how this was to be done: he first drew the bones, then the skeleton with the ligaments; he next added the muscles and, layer upon layer, the tendons lying partly above them; finally, he drew in the nerves, veins, and arteries, until the last illustration showed the hand covered by skin. A total of eight figures were required for this procedure. But that is not all: he also planned to show the hand of an old man, a young man, and a child; and to specify the respective length, thickness, and width of each individual part.
- *Illustrating the skeletal system.* LEONARDO wrote the following directions for illustrating the ankle: "First show all the respective bones separated from one another and arranged so that every part of each individual bone faces that side of the bone from which it has been separated, and with which it would have to be reunited if you were to replace the bones of this foot in their original positions" (Fogli A, 1r). He followed his own advice in his drawings of the top three cervical vertebrae (fig. 100) and of the clavicle and scapula (fig. 101). However, it was not until the time of JACOB HENLE (about 1850) and SPALTEHOLZ that this principle of spatial representation was firmly established in anatomical textbooks. Even today, illustrations of the bones of the wrist can be found that lack any spatial reference whatsoever and only serve to perplex the observer (in GRAY'S *Anatomy*, for example).
- *Illustrating the relations between the musculature and the skeleton.* Another of LEONARDO'S devices may have been suggested to him by the fact that the model employed for his studies was evidently extremely lean (see plate XX, on page 116, and also figures 102 and 103). LEONARDO'S drawings reduce muscles or their functional parts to cords and ultimately to a conceptual model of the motor apparatus of the shoulder joint, which shows the origin and insertion of the individual muscles and, for the person who understands how to read such a model, also demonstrates the functions of the muscles. In addition, through the reduction of its parts in this way, a region of the body becomes partly transparent; subjacent structures become visible.
- *The relation between internal organs and the surface of the body.* While in illustrations of the musculature, LEONARDO employed reduction of the superficial muscles to reveal the deeper muscles, he discovered other methods for revealing the internal organs in their topographical relationship to the body surface. He

was the first anatomist to experiment with "transparent figures." There are several illustrations with the projection of the internal organs onto the body surface. But a thigh also becomes suddenly transparent, and the femur can be observed resting on the knee-joint; otherwise there is nothing but the large vessels, the muscles having disappeared (fig. 104). The boldness of the conception has become an optical balancing act – without an intelligible transition, the eye travels up from an exterior view of the lower leg, and a vessel breaks through the barriers from the inside to the outside without our being able to perceive the point at which this actually occurs. Finally, the completely transparent torso is present, not only in a front view (fig. 90), but also from the back.

- *Cross-sections.* The frontal view with successive layers peeled away or rendered invisible is useful up to a point, but there are some relations that cannot be shown by this technique. LEONARDO found a different method – the cross-section – to show the topographical relations between the bones, muscles, and nerves. Cross-sections are already found in his earliest anatomical sketchbooks (Quaderni V, 19^{r} and 20^{r}) in the company of a systematic series of disk sections (fig. 106). Detailed cross-section drawings, however, have not come down to us.
- *Skull sections.* The special shape of the head, and its spherical structure in the region of the neurocranium, induced LEONARDO to undertake a striking combination of several of the techniques which we have already mentioned: he drew frontal sections and sagittal sections; he cut a segment out of the sphere (fig. 112); and he even separated the top of the skull from the brain and the brain from the base of the skull, to create an effective illustration that provides the additional advantage of a partial cross-section view (fig. 108).

Fig. 100 Fogli A 8^{v}, circa 1510.

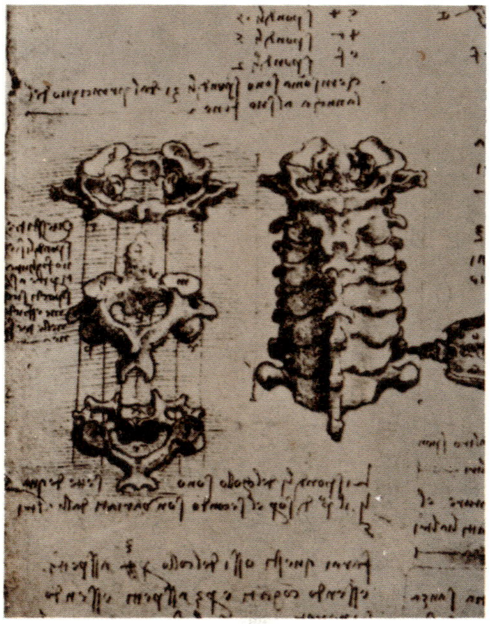

Fig. 101 Fogli A 2^{r}, circa 1510.

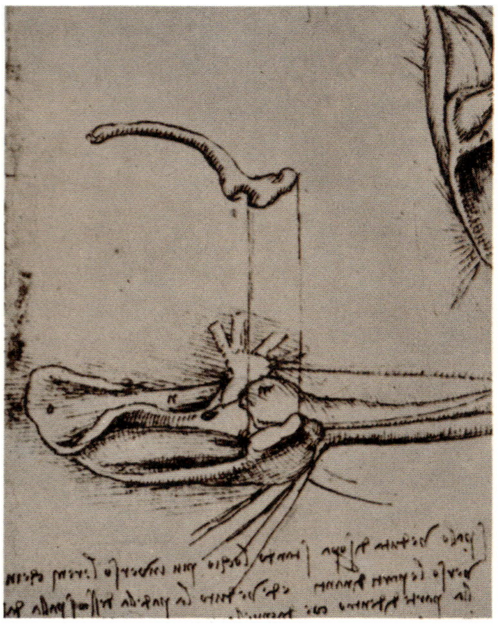

Fig. 102 Fogli A 4^{v}, circa 1510.

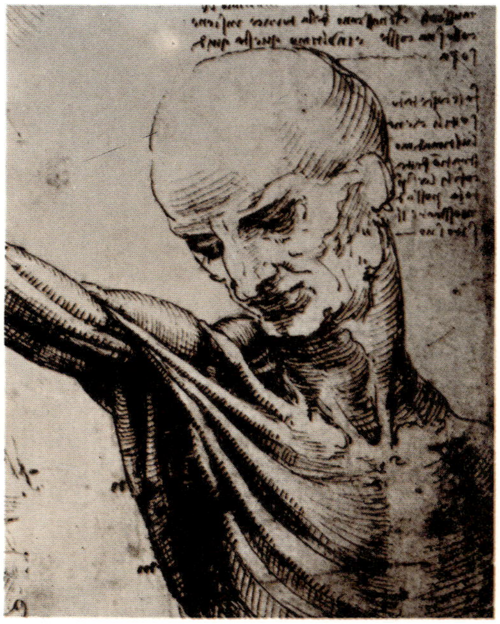

Having described LEONARDO'S ingenious solutions to some of the problems of anatomical illustration, we can now venture a guess about the sources of his technical inspiration. LEONARDO was not only an anatomist and a graphic artist, but also an engineer and an architect. It is not surprising, therefore, to suppose that he applied to one of these fields the methods used in other fields. In architecture, it had long been customary to draw a house in vertical projection combined with an oblique view. In engineering, machines had long been shown in diagrams where they were dismantled into their individual components but still spacially coordinated (see figures 107 and 111). LEONARDO merely adapted the principle used in constructional diagrams for metal cartridges in order to draw a similar diagram for the skull; the result was an anatomical illustration of a very effective kind, but a kind that had never been thought of before. The human organism is examined here by the engineer, as a mechanism which can be taken apart and analyzed. "L'homme machine" of DE LA METTRIE is anticipated in just the same way as the analytical thought of the great natural scientists of the Baroque period.

LEONARDO'S sketchbooks were not published in their entirety until the close of the 19th century, although some individual sheets were published in the 18th century. From about 1570 to 1778, the originals were kept under lock and key. Before 1570, however, they could have been inspected as the property of his heirs: and this point is of decisive importance for the question of LEONARDO'S influence upon 16th-century anatomical illustration. Of course, there were probably friends who saw the sketchbooks during LEONARDO'S lifetime; and he is supposed to have showed them to some visitors in France two years before his death. After his death in 1519, the sketchbooks, which he left in his will to his friend FRANCESCO MELZI, were brought back to Italy. According to an eyewitness account, they were

Fig. 103 Fogli A 4v, circa 1510.

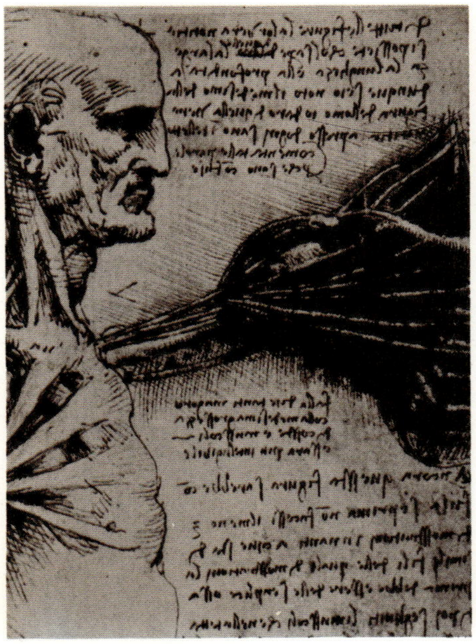

Fig. 104 Quaderni V 3v, 1505/08.

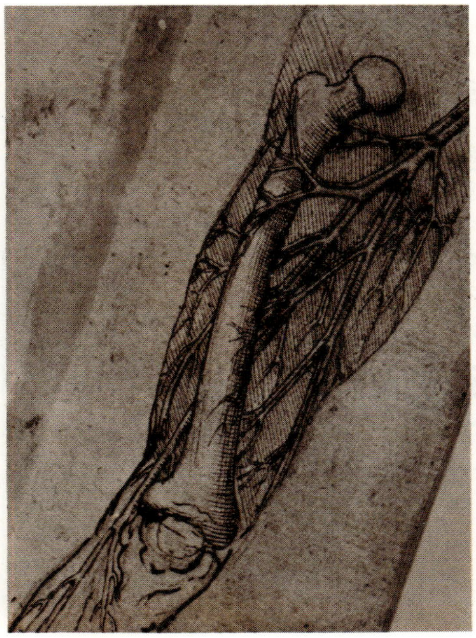

Fig. 105 Quaderni III Iv, circa 1508.

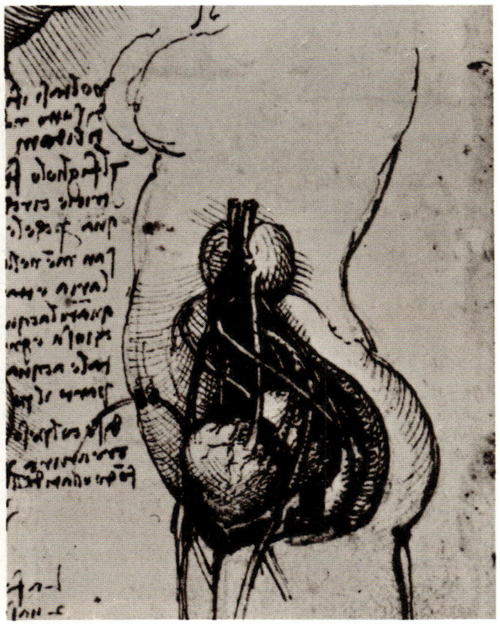

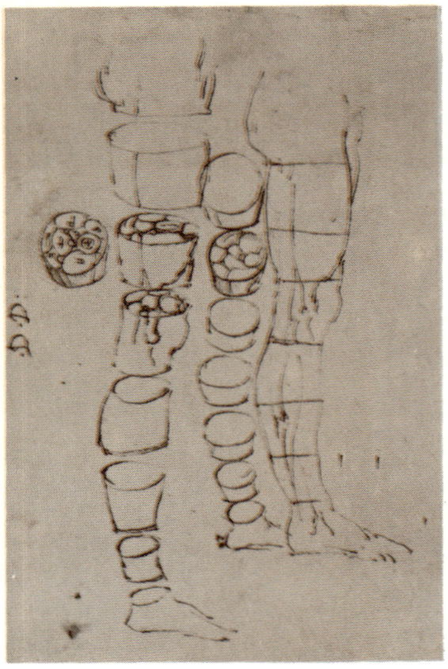

Fig. 106 Quaderni V 20ʳ, circa 1490.

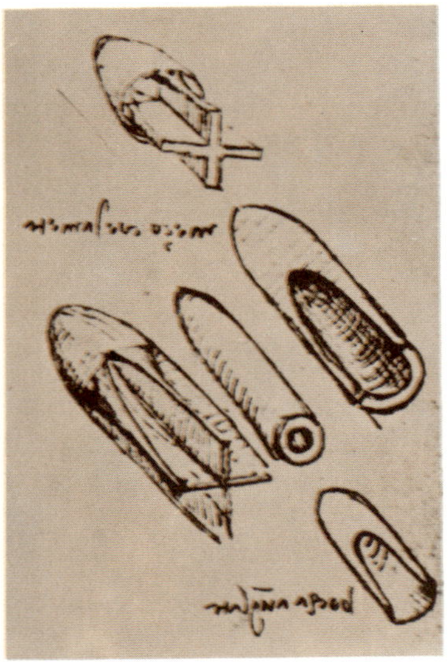

Fig. 107 Codex Arundel 54ʳ, British Museum.

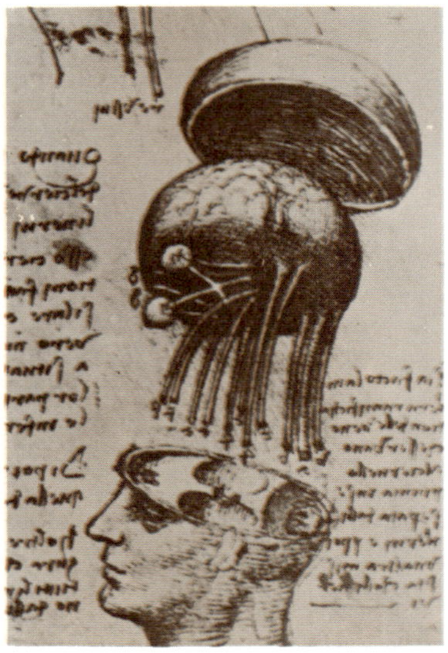

Fig. 108 Sheet Weimar recto.

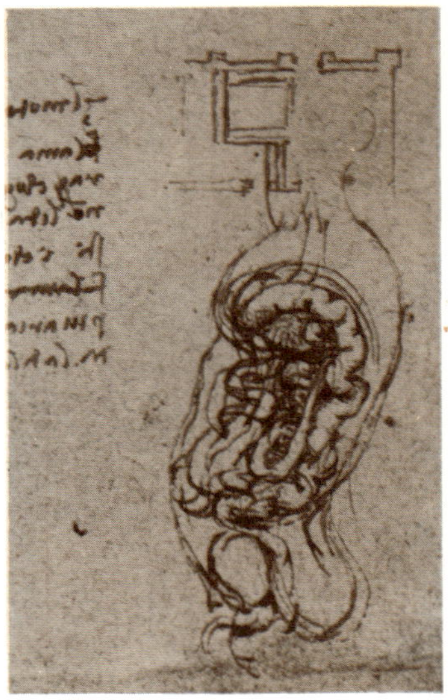

Fig. 109 Quaderni II 7ᵛ, 1513.

on view from 1537 to 1545 in MELZI'S villa at Vaprio d'Adda. Copies of individual sheets were also in circulation at that time; the Uffizi in Florence and the Galleria dell'Accademia in Venice possess fragments. A copy by DÜRER of one sketch is also known, and DÜRER may have copied others. In short, LEONARDO'S anatomical illustrations were not unknown to his contemporaries, even if they were seen by only a small circle of interested people. It is understandable, therefore, that in the first illustrated anatomical textbooks which could have profited from LEONARDO, we do detect the spirit of his anatomy. For instance, LEONARDO'S influence can be seen in a few of the woodcuts for BERENGARIO'S *Commentaria* and the *Isagogae breves*, from 1521 and 1522 (see figure 124, showing three views of the leg, and figure 96, showing the undershaded skeleton of the hand). In VESALIUS'S *Fabrica* of 1543, there are also a few places – but no more than a few – where LEONARDO'S

Fig. 110 Quaderni II 12ʳ, 1513.

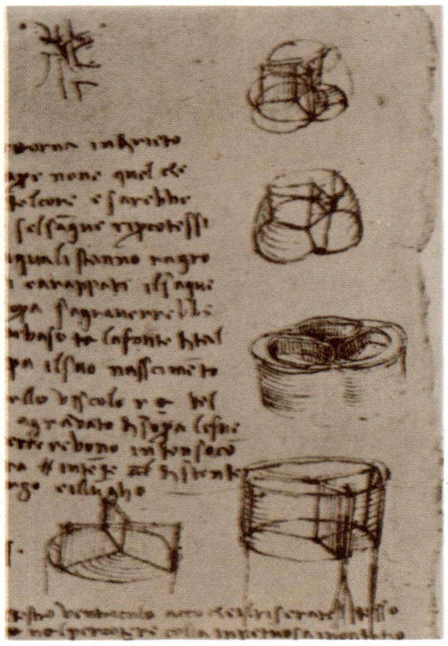

Fig. 111 MS. B 90ʳ, Institut de France, Paris.

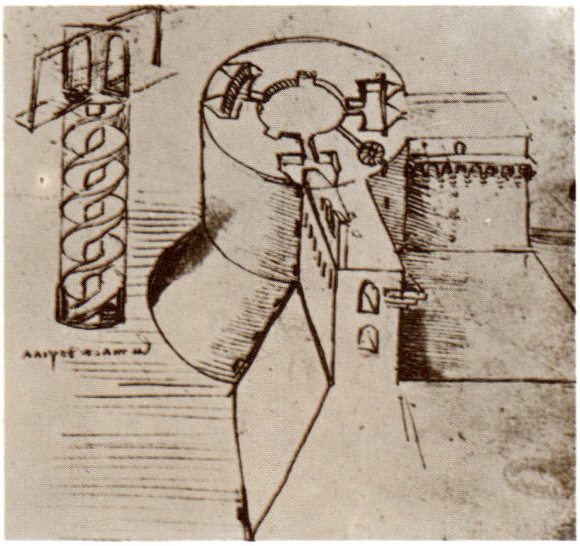

Fig. 112 Fogli B 40ʳ, circa 1500.

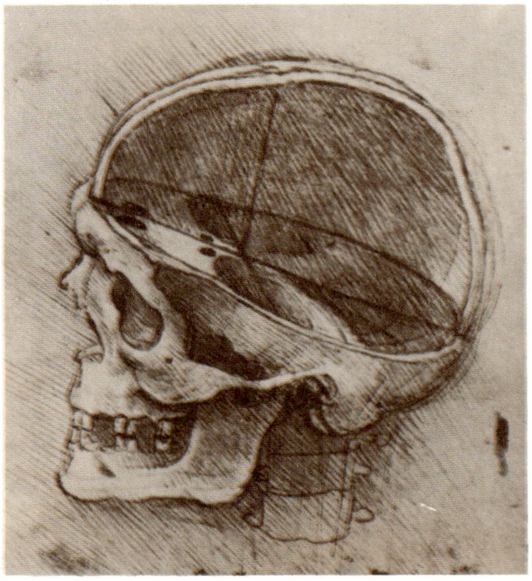

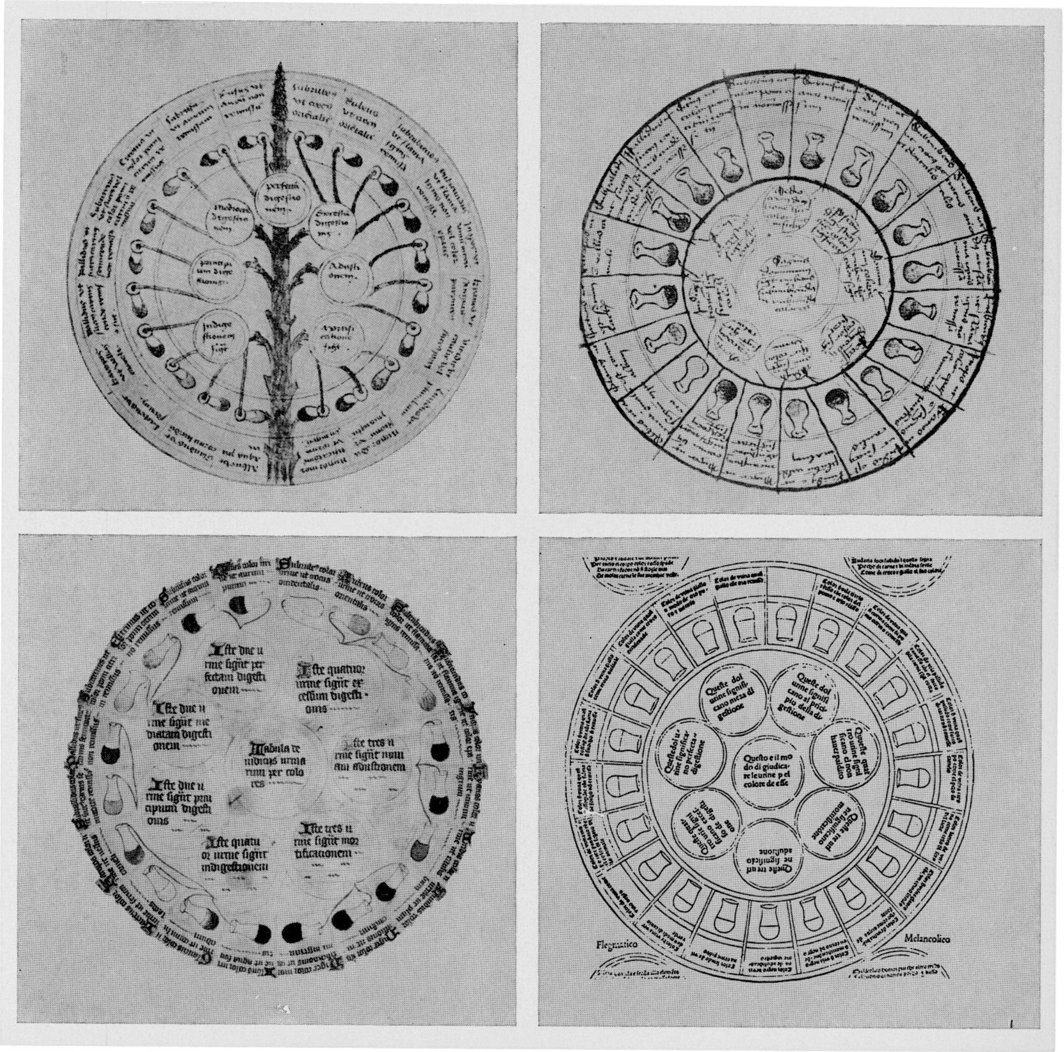

Plate XI Four examples of matula discs, pre-1500:
Genealogical type with 7 discs and 20 matulae. MS. lat. 11229, Bibl. Nat., Paris.
Scoop-wheel type with 8 discs and 20 matulae. MS. Ashmole 789, Bodleian Library, Oxford.
Spoked-wheel type with 9 discs and 20 matulae. MS. 1192, Univ. Bibl., Leipzig.
Spoked-wheel type with 8 discs and 21 matulae, from the Fasciculus medicinae, *Venice, 1491.*

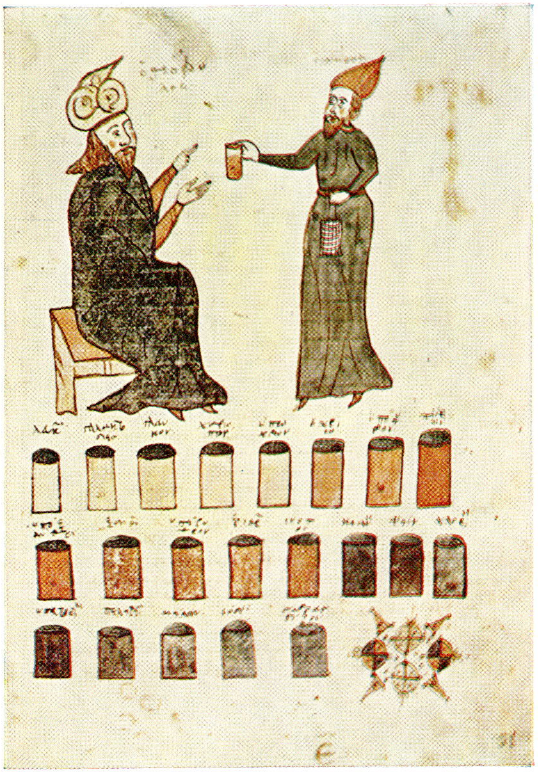

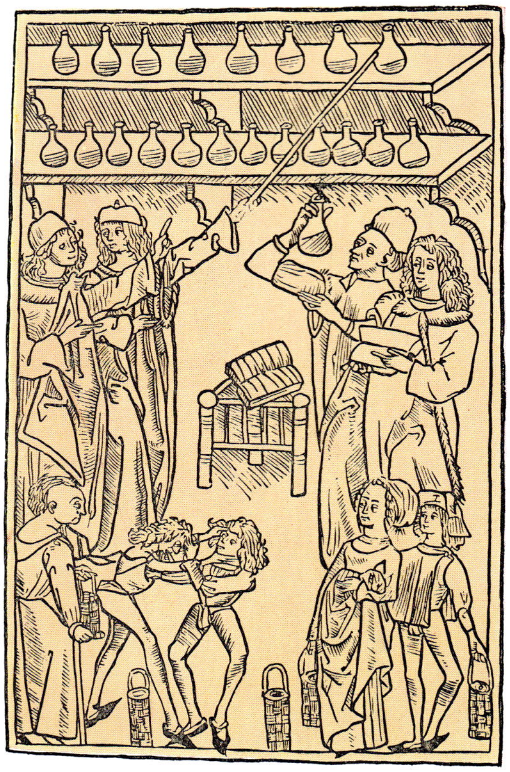

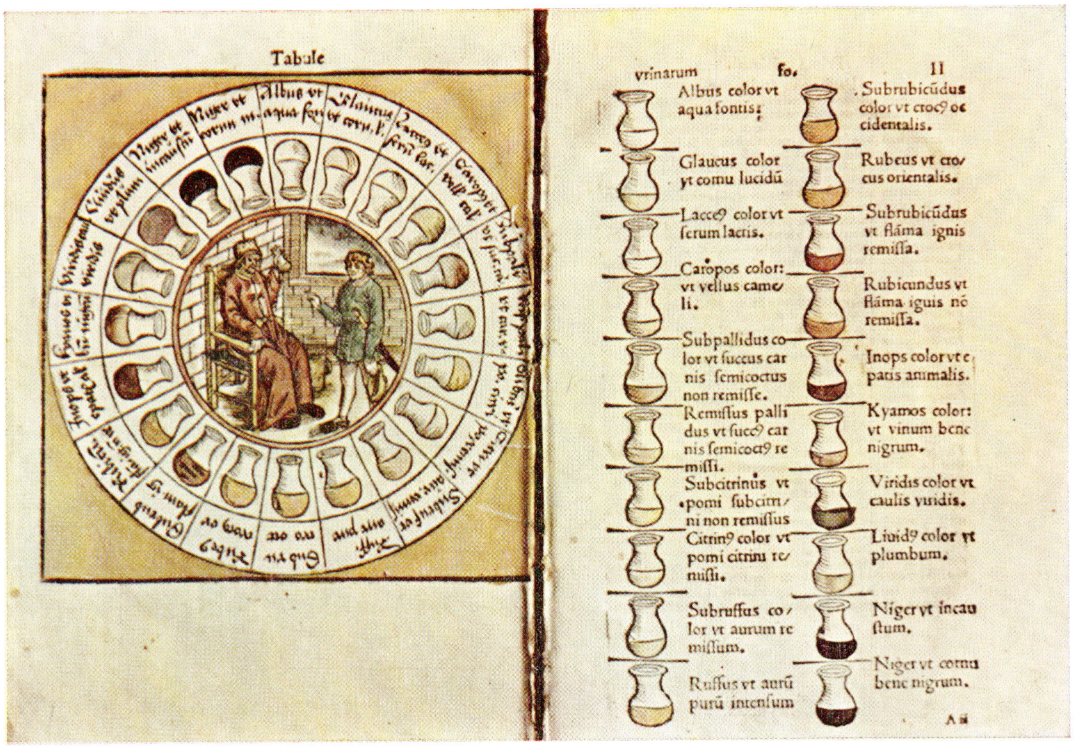

Plate XII Top left: Urine table of column type. Seated above is Theophilos Protospatharios, the author of the treatise Peri uron, *7th century A.D., Bologna, Biblioteca Universitaria, MS. 3623. Top right: Physicians examining urine. From* Hortus sanitatis, *Mainz (Meydenbach), 1491. Below: Udalricus Binder,* Epiphaniae medicorum. Speculum videndi urinas hominum, *1506. Hand-colored specimen in the Biblioteca de la Facultad de Medicina, Madrid.*

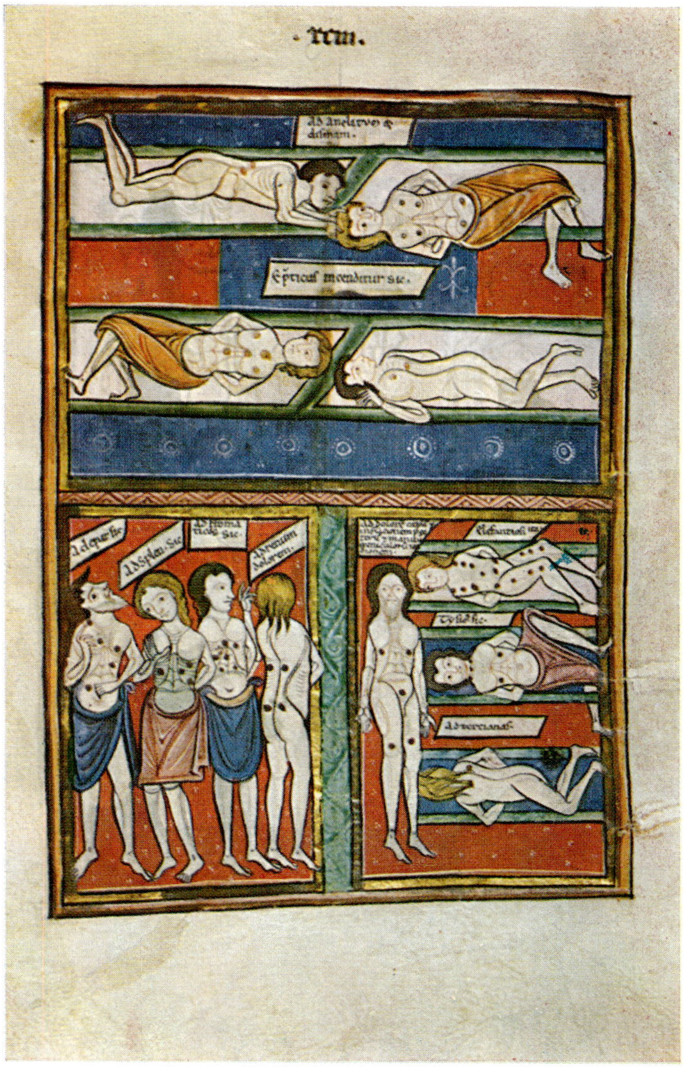

Plate XIII Fol. 92 recto of the MS. Sloane 1975, British Museum, London (see plate XIV).

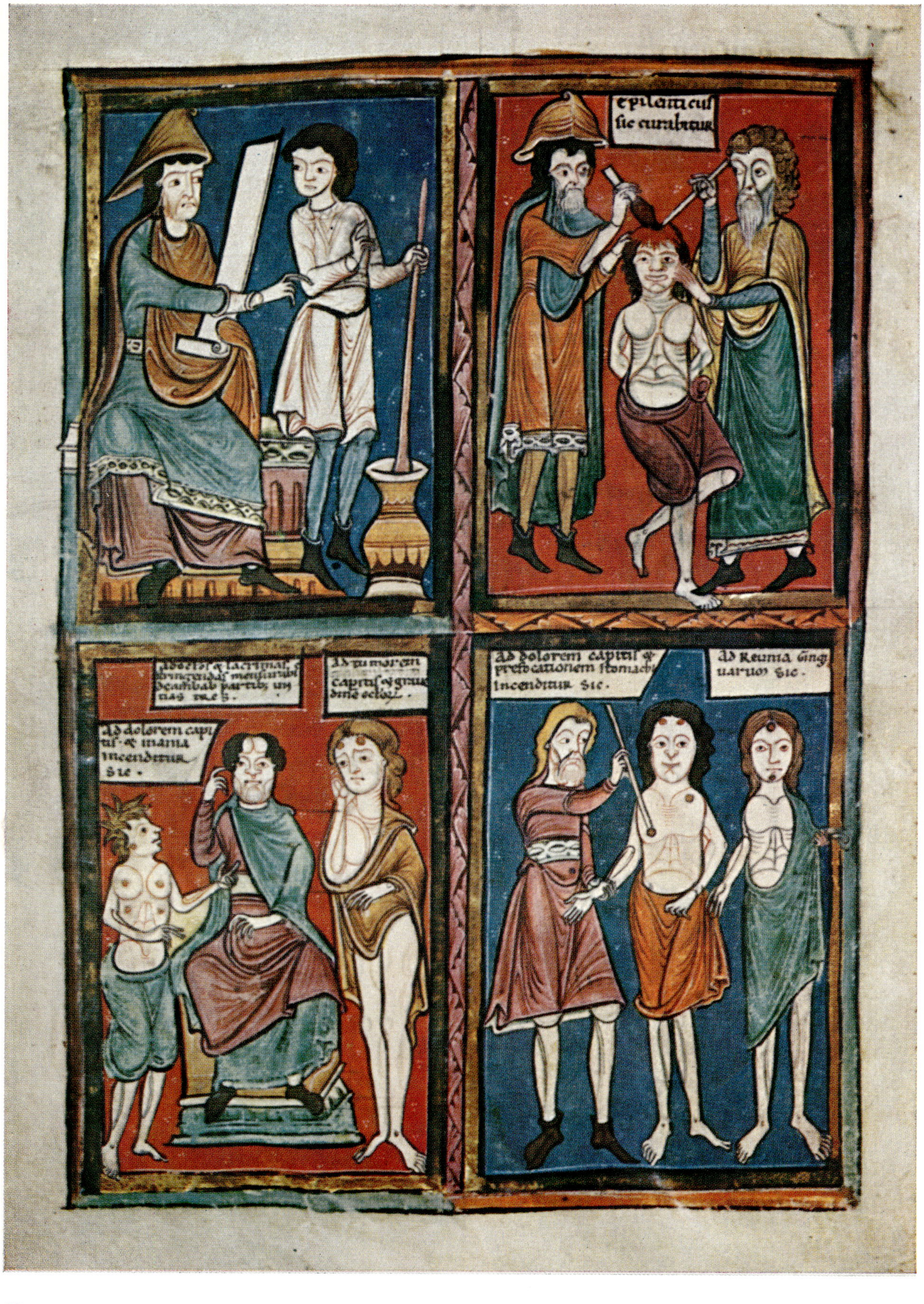

Plate XIV Fol. 91 verso of the MS. Sloane 1975, British Museum, London. The Latin codex, beginning with 'Libri IV medicinae Ypocratis Platonis Apoliensis Urbis de diversis herbis,' is a collection of excellently preserved medical scripts. It is supposed to date from the third quarter of the 12th century, and could be from the Maas Valley. The style of the miniature has been related to the school which produced the master Nicholas of Verdun. Charles Singer's suggestion of 'Anglo-Norman workmanship' (The Herbal in Antiquity, *lit. ref. p. 24) requires correction.*

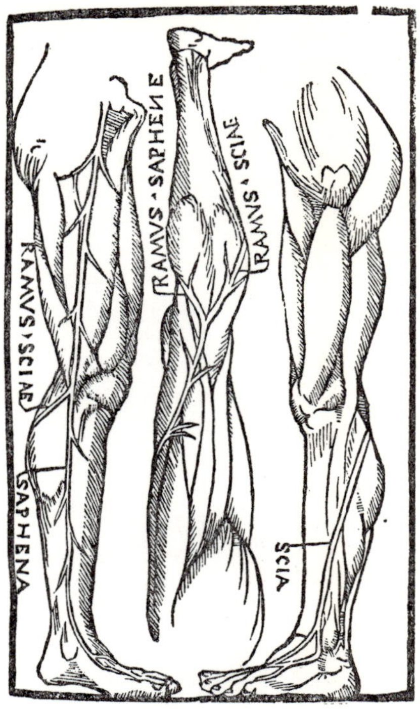

Fig. 113 Leg from three sides, from Berengario da Carpi, Isagogae breves, *Bologna, 1523. The didactic principle could well derive from Leonardo.*

influence can be surmised (compare LEONARDO'S vein figure, plate XXI, with VESALIUS'S, fig. 99).

On the other hand, after the publication of the large facsimile editions four centuries after LEONARDO'S time, a number of textbook authors adopted illustrations in LEONARDO'S manner, which was so close in spirit to the principles of 19th- and 20th-century anatomical instruction. Special mention should be made of HERMANN BRAUS, the most prominent writer of anatomies during the early decades of this century, who frankly admitted to having learned from LEONARDO; but we should also mention SPALTEHOLZ, TANDLER, BENNINGHOF, and VON LANZ-WACHSMUTH.[7] I should also add that anatomical illustrators of the 19th century – that is, prior to the facsimile editions – had already rediscovered some of LEONARDO'S methods; for instance, PIROGOFF did some angle views of figures, and HENLE contributed many ingenious sketches. All this goes to show how far LEONARDO was in advance of his time, and it explains why his anatomical sketches are still capable of fascinating anyone who studies them in detail.

[7] HERRLINGER, ROBERT: Leonardo da Vinci und Hermann Braus, in: Verhandlg. Anat. Gesch. 1950 (48 Vers. Kiel), pp. 97-99; and HERRLINGER, ROBERT: Die didaktische Originalität der anatomischen Zeichnungen Leonardos, in: Anat. Anz. *99* (1953), pp. 366-95.

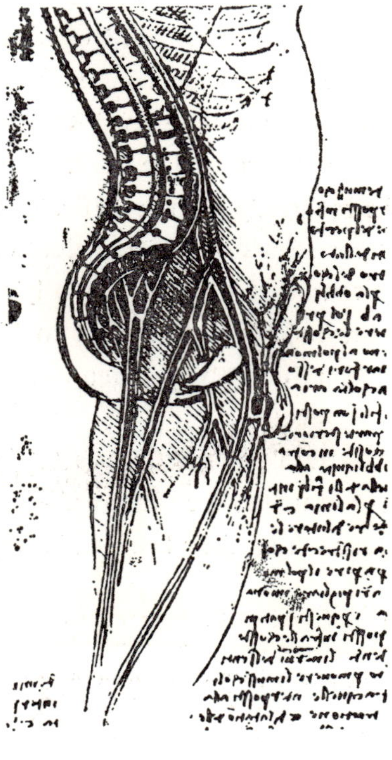

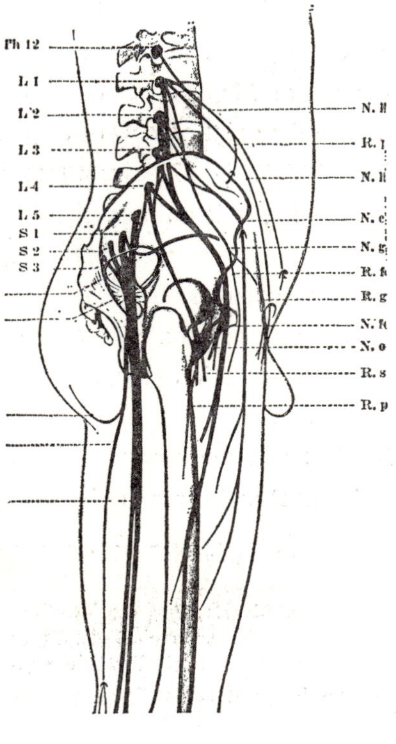

Figures 114 and 115 Lumbar and sacral plexus. Left, from Leonardo, Quaderni IV 9ʳ, circa 1500. Right, from Von Lanz-Wachsmuth, Praktische Anatomie *I/4, fig. 38 (detail), 1938.*

Berengario, Dryander, and Canano

The general opinion that the illustrations of VESALIUS'S *Fabrica* are remarkably innovative is, as we have already indicated, not wholly true. We certainly do not intend to underestimate the importance of VESALIUS and his designer, but it has been known to historians since CHOULANT that there were predecessors to the *Fabrica* with regard to graphic art work. There are a number of innovations in the illustrations contained in the work of BERENGARIO DA CARPI (after 1521) and JOHANNES DRYANDER (after 1537), which VESALIUS only needed to adopt and develop. VESALIUS certainly had an advantage over these predecessors in having a larger page-size for his illustrations, as well as in having an extremely skillful designer, but we need not confuse an artistically impressive result with artistic originality.

JACOPO BERENGARIO (actually BARIGAZZI) DA CARPI was a surgeon and anatomist who taught in Bologna from 1502 to 1527. He wrote two anatomical textbooks: the *Commentaria super Anatomia Mundini,* 1521, and the *Isagogae breves,* 1522. The *Commentaria* is quite extensive, compared to the original text of MONDINO DE' LUIZZI of 1316. Drawings of the viscera, with the exception of the female reproductive organs (fig. 120), are missing. The skeletons and the muscle figures are drawn against landscape backgrounds (figs. 122, 123) in a way that we shall later observe in ESTIENNE and VESALIUS. The full figures are shown performing specific actions: a skeleton is holding a skull in each hand, thereby demonstrating three different and well-conceived views of the cranium – a trick which is repeated in VESALIUS'S *Epitome* in the second plate of the muscle figure and dissected skull (figs. 123, 124). The figures demonstrating the abdominal muscles hold back the dissected flaps of skin themselves (figs. 116-118); this type of presentation, when it appears more than one century later in CASSERIO and his successors, is usually considered to be an example of Mannerism. The series of illustrations relating to the female organs is, from the point of view of the didactic principle, the same as the second KETHAM situs of 1493 (fig. 89), except that the woman no longer is portrayed in a stilted and unnatural archaic attitude (fig. 120). ESTIENNE follows directly from here (fig. 121). BERENGARIO'S figure demonstrating the opened uterus stands with the left foot on two book volumes and points with the right hand toward a dissected uterus lying upon a pedestal. Later, VESALIUS hangs a diaphragm on the wall next to his eviscerated muscle figure, and ESTIENNE lays the stomach on a tree stump next to the full figure.

The fact that the representation of detail in BERENGARIO'S illustrations is totally inadequate[1] and that the illustrations – as far as our examples are concerned – are not accompanied by descriptive text in no way detracts from their being eminently

[1] See ROTH, MORITZ: Andreas Vesalius Bruxellensis, Berlin, 1892, pp. 49 ff. ROTH quite correctly observes that the anatomical details drawn into BERENGARIO'S full figures are descended from scholastic diagrams. Such illustrations are sheer graphic hybrids, naturally with a dominant modern component.

116

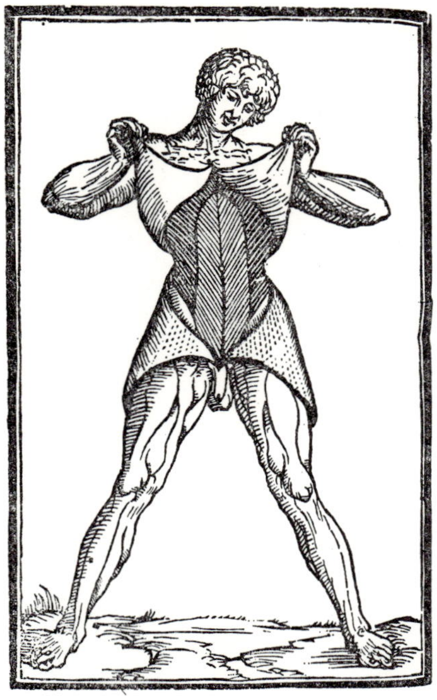

117

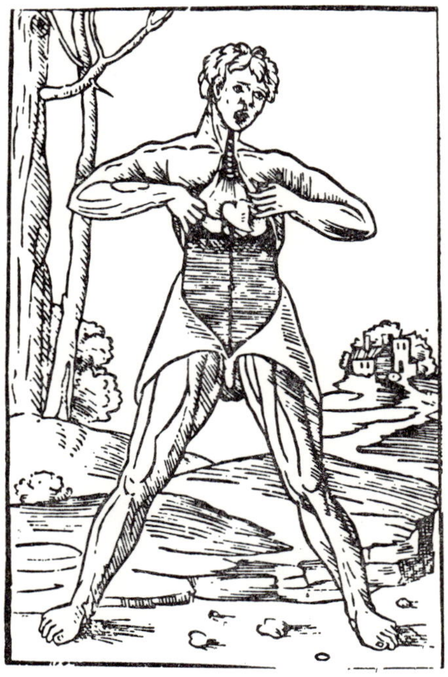

118

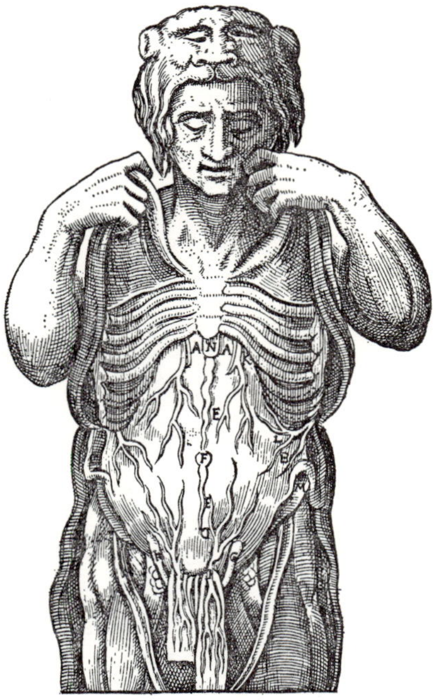

119

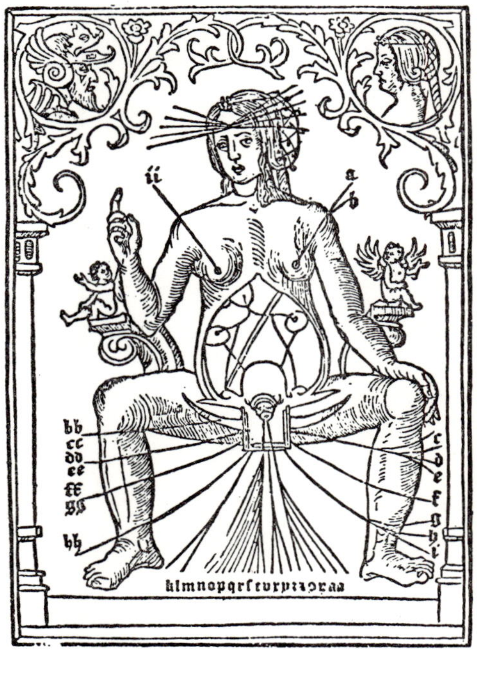

120

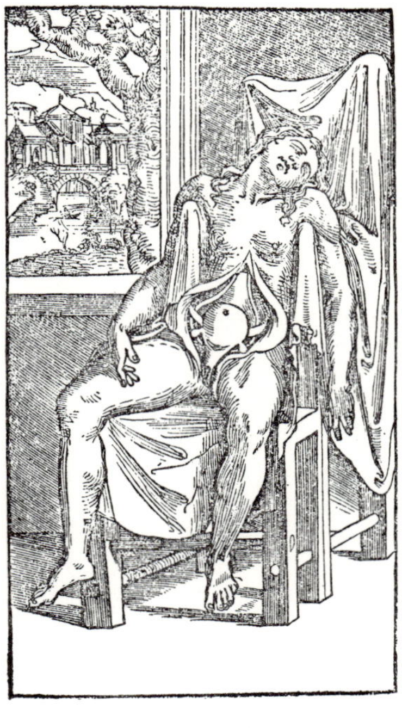

121

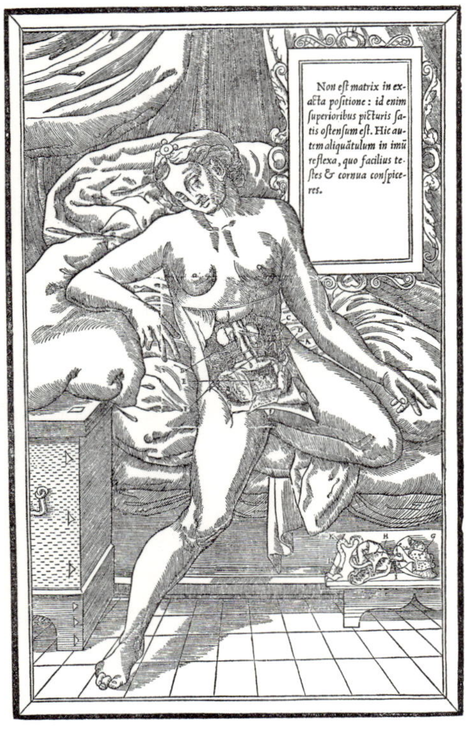

Figures 116 to 118 Figures holding back dissected flaps of skin. Left, from Berengario, Commentaria, *1521, and* Isagogae, *1523. Center, from Mondino, French edition, Paris, 1532. Right, from Valverde,* Anatomie, *Antwerp, 1568.*
Figures 119 to 121 The female reproductive organs, from Ketham to Estienne. Left, from Ketham, Antwerp edition of 1512. Center, from Berengario, Isagogae, *Bologna, 1523. Right, from Estienne,* De dissectione, *Paris, 1545.*

122

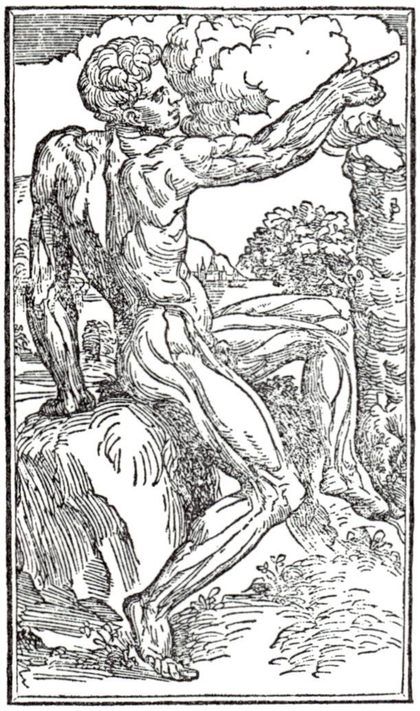

123

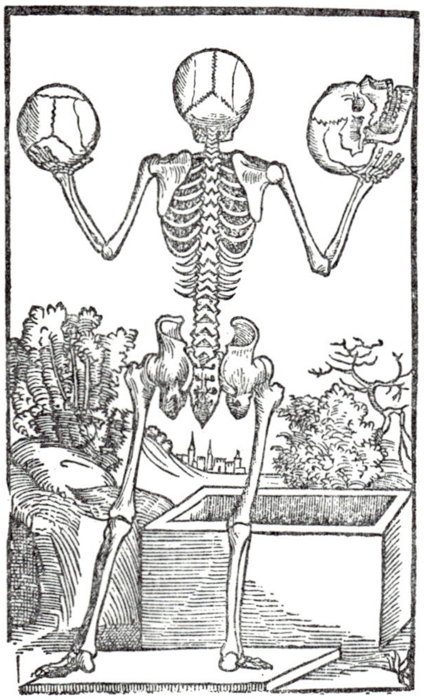

124

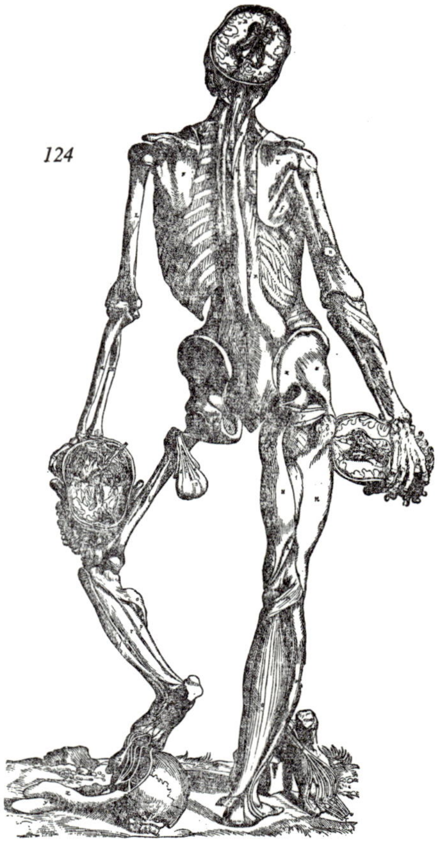

125

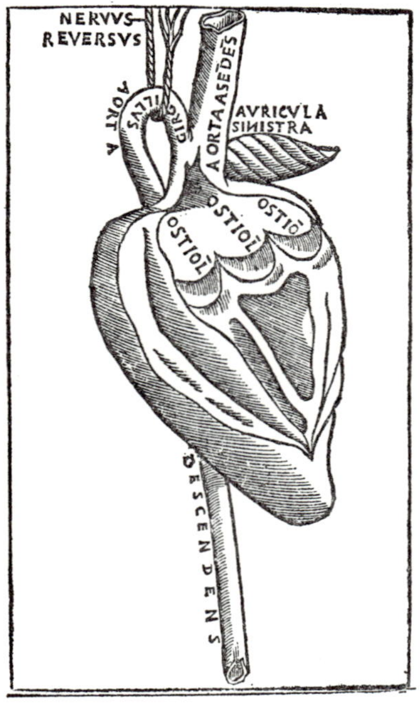

126

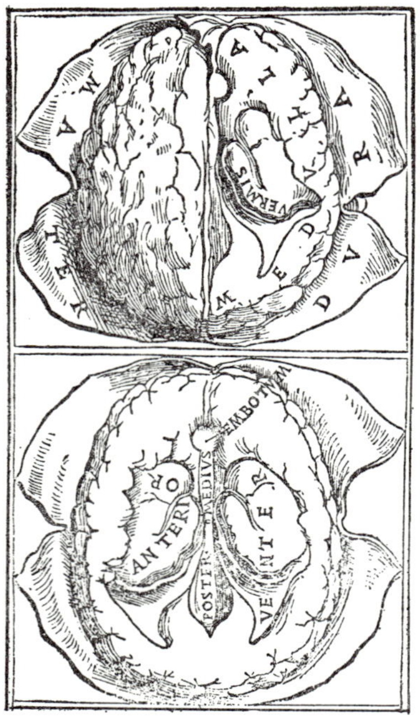

127

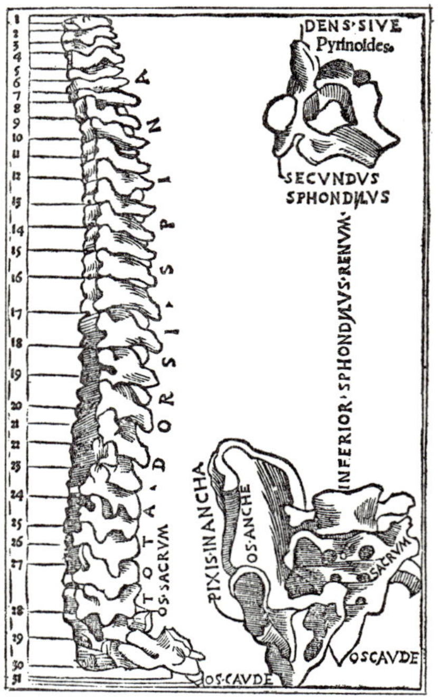

Fig. 122 Muscle figure from Berengario, Isagogae, *1523, 'in hac figura videntur musculi exteriores, laterales et partim posteriores.'*
Figures 123 and 124 Skeletons with skulls in each hand. Left, from Berengario, Isagogae, *1523. Right, from Vesalius,* Epitome, *Basel, 1543.*
Figures 125 to 127 Illustrations showing the influence of Leonardo da Vinci, from Berengario da Carpi, Isagogae breves, *Bologna, 1523.*

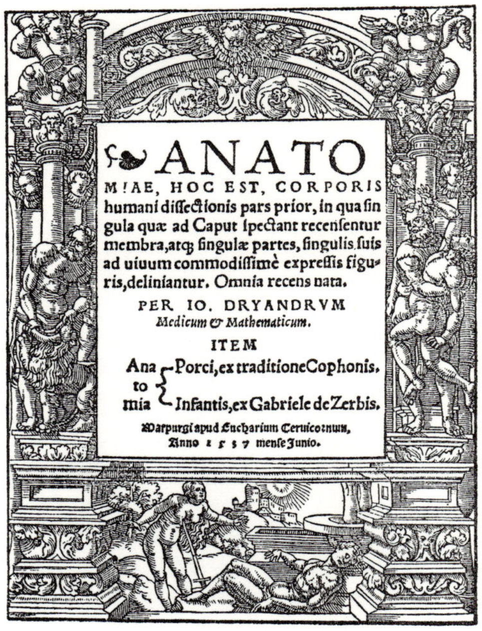

ANATO
MIAE, HOC EST, CORPORIS
humani dissectionis pars prior, in qua sin
gula quæ ad Caput spectant recensentur
membra, atq; singulæ partes, singulis suis
ad uiuum commodissimè expressis figu-
ris, deliniantur. Omnia recens nata.
PER IO. DRYANDRVM
Medicum & Mathematicum.
ITEM
Ana- Porci, ex traditione Cophonis.
to-
mia Infantis, ex Gabriele de Zerbis.
Marpurgi apud Eucharium Ceruicornum,
Anno 1537 mense Junio.

Fig. 128 Title page of Dryander's Anatomiae . . . pars prior, *Marburg (E. Cervicornus), 1537.*

Fig 129 Skull with hourglass, from Dryander's Anatomia capitis humani, *1536.*

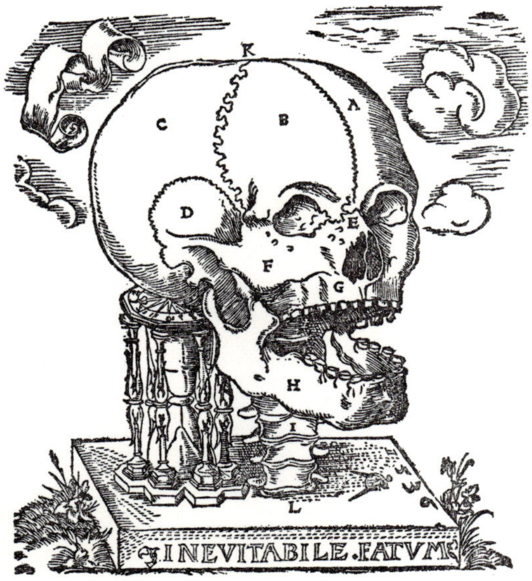

representative of their type. They would only require enlargement and descriptions to become extremely useful. Several other of BERENGARIO'S illustrations, including the vein figures (fig. 113), seem to incorporate techniques learned from LEONARDO.[2] Several illustrations of the heart also show the influence of LEONARDO (an example is shown in figure 125), as does a double illustration of the brain, which is crude but surprisingly modern in principle (fig. 126), and a no less Leonardesque drawing of the spinal column (fig. 127).

JOHANN EICHMANN, who adopted the more elegant name of DRYANDER, was a professor and author of a small *Anatomia* published by the Marburg printer EUCHARIUS CERVICORNUS in 1537. Although the name of the artist who illustrated the book is not known, he employed a monogram showing an open pair of compasses above the letter G, frequently with the initials G V B inscribed above, or with V B only. G V B has recently been identified as a member of the Basel school of woodcut designers.[3]

The full title of the book (see figure 128) indicates that this is Part I of a publishing project of which Part II never appeared. Nevertheless, the illustrator of the book took a very promising step in a new direction, toward the systematic presentation of a dissection series – that is, a group of illustrations showing the successive stages of an anatomical dissection. Remarkably enough, he began with the skull rather than with the large body cavities, the skeleton, or the musculature.[4] Each of the woodcuts, as a rule, fills a whole page of the quarto volume; the illustrations are consequently of adequate size. In some, the dissected head lies upon a table, frequently with instruments in the foreground; in others, the skulls are mounted upon an ornamented socle, or a diagram of the exposed skull is shown as part of a living head (see figures 129-33). A thorax is treated rather like a statue of Hermes (fig. 134); an anatomical preparation of the heart with the great vessels rests on the diaphragm as though this were a round socle; and an illustration of the lungs which, in contrast to most of the other illustrations, is quite primitive, is shown against a landscape containing clouds and birds (fig. 135). The parts drawn from life are provided with cast shadows; the explanation is facilitated by means of letters inscribed into the figure; and occasionally indication lines are also used. Many of these features reappear in VESALIUS, as does the *memento mori* theme invoked here by the hourglass and by plaques bearing the inscription *"Inevitabile fatum"* ("inevitable fate").

Several features in the DRYANDER illustrations are scarcely conceivable without

2 Further observations on prototypes can be found in ROTH, *loc. cit.*

3 See NAGLER, G. K.: Die Monogrammisten II, Munich, 1860, No. 2619. His work is still treated as anonymous here. HANS KOGLER connected it with the woodcutter GEORG (JÖRG) THOMAS of Basel, in the supplementary volume to the Swiss Künstler-Lexicon (Vol. IV), Frauenfeld, 1917. The pair of compasses – the symbol of the apostle Thomas – could refer to the family name of THOMAS.

4 The eleven plates relating to the anatomy of the head were brought out by the same publisher one year earlier, in 1536, under the title *Anatomia capitis humani.*

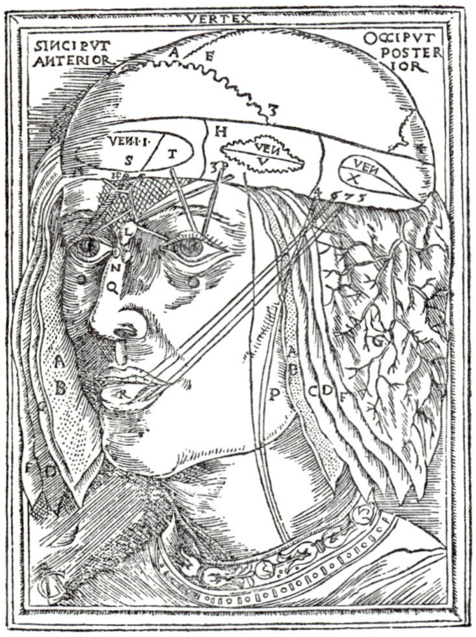

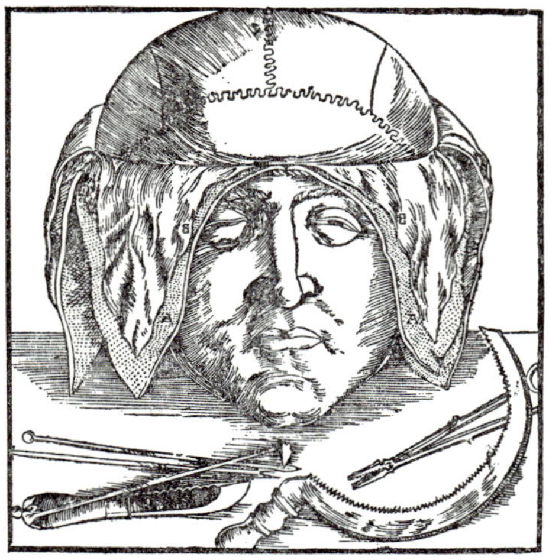

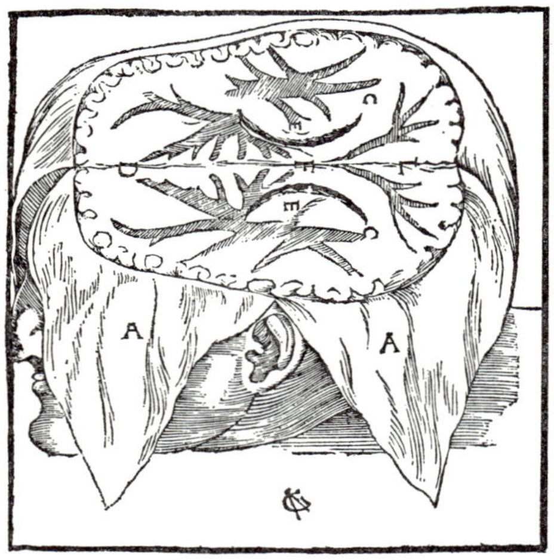

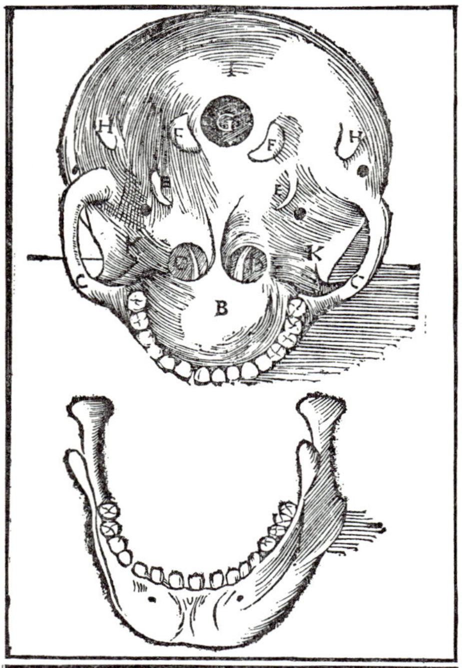

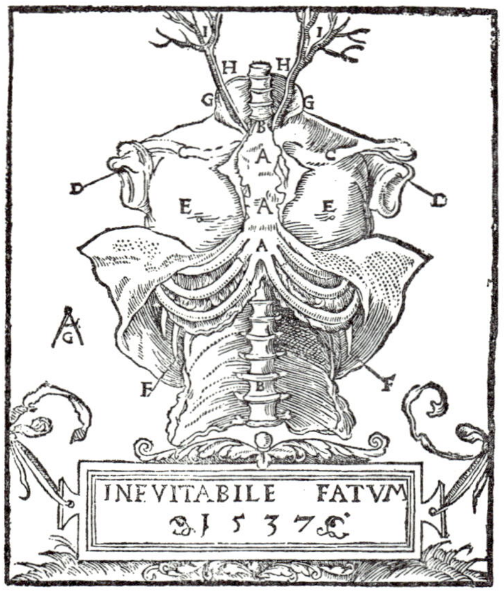

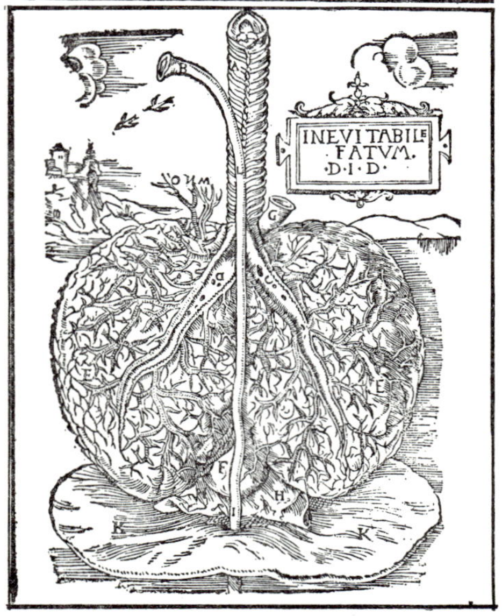

Figures 130 to 135 Six illustrations from Dryander, Anatomiae, *1537.*

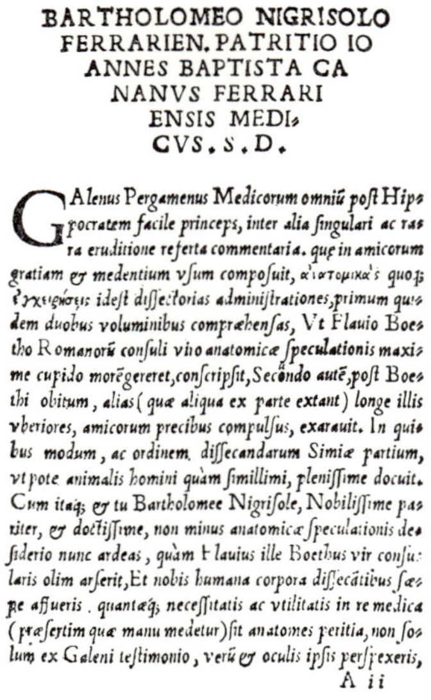
BARTHOLOMEO NIGRISOLO
FERRARIEN. PATRITIO IO
ANNES BAPTISTA CA
NANVS FERRARI
ENSIS MEDI-
CVS. S. D.

GAlenus Pergamenus Medicorum omniũ post Hip-
pocratem facile princeps, inter alia singulari ac ra-
ra eruditione referta commentaria. quę in amicorum
gratiam & medentium vsum composuit, [illegible] quoq;
[illegible] idest dissectorias administrationes, primum qui-
dem duobus voluminibus compræhensas, Vt Flauio Boe-
tho Romanorũ consuli viro anatomicæ speculationis maxi-
me cupido morẽgereret, conscripsit, Secundo autẽ, post Boe-
thi obitum, alias (quæ aliqua ex parte extant) longe illis
vberiores, amicorum precibus compulsus, exarauit. In qui-
bus modum, ac ordinem dissecandarum Simiæ partium,
vt pote animalis homini quàm simillimi, plenissime docuit.
Cum itaq; & tu Bartholomee Nigrisole, Nobilissime pa-
triter, & doctissime, non minus anatomicæ speculationis de-
siderio nunc ardeas, quàm Flauius ille Boethus vir consu-
laris olim arserit, Et nobis humana corpora dissecãtibus sæ-
pe affueris. quantæq; necessitatis ac vtilitatis in re medica
(præsertim quæ manu medetur) sit anatomes peritia, non so-
lum ex Galeni testimonio, verũ & oculis ipsis perspexeris,
A ii

Fig. 136 Preface to G. B. Canano's Musculorum humani corporis picturata dissectio, *Ferrara, 1543.*

the influence of BERENGARIO and PHRYES; the scholastic woodcuts in PEYLIGK, HUNDT, and REISCH must also be classified as forerunners of these illustrations;[5] and SIGRID BRAUNFELS-ESCHE is of the opinion that "one can not fail to recognize LEONARDO'S influence upon them."[6]

CHARLES SINGER finally goes so far as to maintain that the best of DRYANDER'S illustrations were obviously "stolen from Vesalius, who was then at work preparing his masterpiece"; he refers to the figure of the heart with the vascular roots, trachea, and esophagus, among other examples. In view of everything we know of the early history of the *Fabrica*, this is impossible, but CUSHING is certainly correct in asserting, without treating SINGER'S argument in detail, that "There was nothing to which Vesalius could object in all this."[7] The situation could well be quite the reverse. There are several illustrations in Books VI and VII of VESALIUS'S *Fabrica* which could be regarded essentially as improvements – indeed, necessary improvements – of the corresponding woodcuts in DRYANDER, but which are exactly similar in conception (see p. 112). DRYANDER and his publisher EGENOLPH did not actually steal from VESALIUS until 1541, when they made use of his "Tabulae sex," and only this can have provoked the displeasure of VESALIUS (p. 121).

GIOVANNI BATTISTA CANANO of Ferrara (1515-1579) deserves attention from historians of medical illustration for several reasons. In the year 1541 he published a slim quarto volume of twenty sheets with twenty-seven illustrations; it opens with the title *Musculorum humani corporis picturata dissectio* and concludes with the words *Libri primi finis* ("end of Book One"). It was intended to comprise seven books, all devoted to myology; it would have become, therefore, the first anatomical textbook to be devoted exclusively to one of the great organ systems.

The first – and only – book to appear treats the muscles of the upper limbs. What induced CANANO to suddenly stop work, and even withdraw the remaining copies from sale, has been frequently discussed by medical historians. The current hypothesis, which goes back to ZAFFARINI (1809),[8] that CANANO resigned after seeing the illustrations of VESALIUS, has recently been questioned by L. MÜNSTER.[9]

As far as we know today, CANANO'S illustrations are the first copperplate engravings to be used in medical illustration. Their failure as publications, which coincided with the triumphal success of VESALIUS'S *Fabrica*, spoiled the first chance for gravure printing to become established in the field. The designer, GIROLAMO DA CARPI (1501-1556), was an important painter, but the engraver – and even more, the printers – did not satisfactorily solve the technical problems which arose at the start.

5 TURNER, EDOUARD: Les planches anatomiques de J. Dryander et de G. H. Ryff. Gaz. Hebd. Méd. Chir., 2e sér. *13*, 1876, pp. 785 ff., 817 ff.

6 Leonardo da Vinci. Das anatomische Werk, Ars docta VIII, Basel, 1954, p. 64.

7 CUSHING, HARVEY: A Bio-Bibliography of Andreas Vesalius, New York, 1943, p. 29.

8 ZAFFARINI, NICCOLO: Scoperte anatomiche di G. B. Canani, Ferrara, 1809.

9 MÜNSTER, LADISLAO: Giovanni Battista Canano und seine Muskelanatomie, 1541, Med. Mon. schr., Munich, *19*, 1965, pp. 266-71.

Unsuitable printing ink also contributed to this failure. The few preserved specimens – there are twelve altogether, of which two are at the Bibliotheca Ariostea in Ferrara, and two at the Bibliotheca Pinali in Padua – contain perforations in the illustrations and in the text. The paper was too thin and practically useless for printing purposes.

The graphic achievement of GIROLAMO DA CARPI also leaves much to be desired. He, or perhaps only the engraver, failed to clearly represent the differences in texture between bone and muscle. The chiaroscuro used by GIROLAMO[10] is a painter's technique that marks him as a follower of LEONARDO (through CORREGGIO, PARMIGIANINO, and the DOSSI brothers), but it is out of place in these anatomical illustrations, or at least premature, due to inadequate transposition onto the copperplate. Only the highlights on the tendons, which are technically easier to achieve in an engraving than in a woodcut, justify the attempt and have the power to convince the observer (see plate XXIIa).

It is unproductive to speculate on the line of development that medical illustration and the teaching of anatomy would have taken if CANANO had not abandoned his work, but it must be said that the didactic mode of representation used in his illustrations was really quite new. He drew only one, or very few muscles, in each illustration, and he included the corresponding movement of the finger and the hand.[11] This teaching approach remained unique for a long time in the history of medical illustration.

[10] This matter is discussed in LORIS PREMUDA: Storia dell' Iconografia anatomica, Milano, 1956, pp. 134-36.
[11] This was first remarked upon by L. MÜNSTER, *loc. cit.*

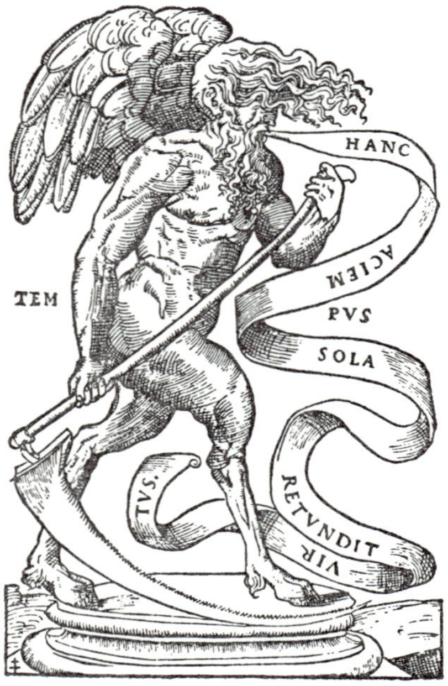

Fig. 137 Title-page colophon from Estienne, La dissection des parties du corps humain, *Paris, 1546.*

Charles Estienne and Estienne de la Rivière

The ugliest anatomical work that we know... wholly devoid of grace or beauty.[1]
Ces planches ne sont pas sans quelque beauté.[2]
Affermare che le tavole . . . siano belle e piacciano non ci pare possible.[3]
La partie iconographique de ce livre conserve un certain charme . . . cette série de gracieux corps féminins . . .[4]
In part, the drawings are neither elegant nor anatomically correct . . . the human body, too, is often drawn in strange and offensive positions.[5]
One's first reaction to the book is entirely favourable.[6]

Illustrations that were done four hundred years ago must be rather unusual, to provoke such varied reactions from modern critics. And, indeed, this work does immediately either attract or repel the reader. The illustrations in question are contained in CHARLES ESTIENNE and ESTIENNE DE LA RIVIÈRE'S *De dissectione partium corporis humani libri III*, which was published in Paris in 1545.
Going against traditional custom, the names of the two authors (in Latin) were actually given in the title of the book, which continues: . . . *a* CAROLO STEPHANO, *doctore medico, editi. Una cum figuris, et incisionum declarationibus, a* STEPHANO RIVERIO CHIRURGO *compositis.* This unusual wording was the result of a lawsuit tried in the Paris courts. By a court decision, ESTIENNE DE LA RIVIÈRE forced his reluctant former friend and colleague to include his name in the title. As the foreword clearly explains, this court case delayed the publication of the book for six years, from 1539 to 1545. In the meantime, of course, VESALIUS had stolen a march on them.
This book is quite a spectacle, in the full sense of the word; and it is an exciting spectacle, appealing even to the personal taste of the observer, as our quotations have shown. Despite the fact that the book may appear at first to occupy a minor place in the history of medical illustration, a closer study will reveal that both CHARLES ESTIENNE and ESTIENNE DE LA RIVIÈRE are more important links in the historical chain of events than has previously been admitted.

De dissectione partium corporis humani has always stood "in the shadow of Vesalius," as G. RATH has pertinently observed.[7] This statement applies not only to the text but also to the illustrations (in which RATH was less interested). The illustrations are entirely pre-Vesalian, despite the opinion of such experts as MORITZ ROTH[8] and

Fig. 138 Estienne, De dissectione, *p. 262 (detail).*

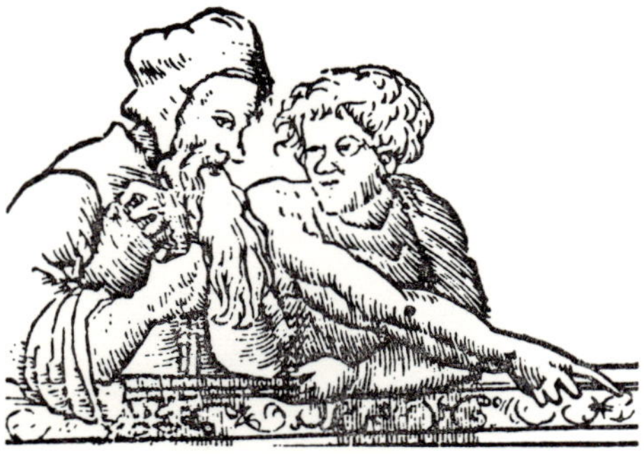

[1] SINGER, CHARLES and C. RABIN: A Prelude to Modern Science, Cambridge, England, 1946, p. xix.
[2] HAHN, ANDRÉ, PAULE DUMAITRE and JANINE SAMION-CONTET: Histoire de la Médecine et du livre médical, Paris, 1962, p. 129.
[3] PREMUDA, LORIS: Storia dell' Iconografia anatomica, Milan, 1957, p. 104.
[4] HUARD, PIERRE and MIRKO DRAZEN GRMEK: L'oeuvre de Charles Estienne et l'école anatomique parisienne, Paris, 1965.
[5] CHOULANT, LUDWIG: Geschichte und Bibliographie der anatomischen Abbildung, Leipzig, 1852, p. 37.
[6] KELLETT, C. E.: Two Anatomies, in: Medical History, London, *VIII*, 1964, p. 343.
[7] RATH, GERNOT: Charles Estienne, Anatom im Schatten Vesals, in: Südhoff's Arch. Gesch. Med. Naturw. *39*, 1955, pp. 35-43.
[8] ROTH, MORITZ: Andreas Vesalius Bruxellensis, Berlin, 1892, pp. 209-12.

HARVEY CUSHING,[9] who could not free themselves from the idea that the authors must have stolen ideas from VESALIUS. This is far from being the case – on the contrary, there is reason to believe that VESALIUS became acquainted with their work during his stay in Paris, and himself gained essential inspiration from it. VESALIUS was in Paris from September, 1533,[10] until the outbreak of the war between Francis I and Charles V in the summer of 1536.[11] During these years, the first woodcuts for the *De dissectione* – perhaps even the majority of them – must have been completed.

The *De dissectione* is a handy folio volume containing approximately four hundred pages.[12] A facsimile edition has recently been published,[13] but it is less accessible than the French edition referred to below. The originals of 1545 and 1546 are examples of the best Parisian printing of that period. The printing only barely fails to match that of Venice and Basel, which we shall treat in detail later. The general layout is bold and clean; the type, in italics, is clear and easy to read. The main sections begin with large initials, and the chapters with small initials of the same purely ornamental type; an oversize initial "A" is employed at the beginning of each of the three "Books."[14] The lines are numbered by fives on one side, and the outer margin contains notes. The first two books contain full-page illustrations; the legends are printed on separate pages where necessary. From page 318 on of the third book, small illustrations are distributed throughout the text. All the illustrations are woodcuts, and a number of them reveal the unmistakable style of one artist. There are three different artists' signatures, however, and this fact has puzzled historians for more than a century.[15] On the title page, the observer is immediately confronted with a cross of Lorraine, which also appears on several plates, but evidently only in the older ones. The symbol was often used in the 16th century and has long been connected with the workshop of GEOFFROY TORY. Several plates also bear the monogram of the designer JOLLAT – it is unquestionably his monogram, for he occasionally uses it as the first letter when writing his name in full.[16] The monogram appears in all three books, and particularly on those illustrations which C. E. KELLETT[17] has recently connected with PERINO DEL VAGA (1501-1547), a pupil of

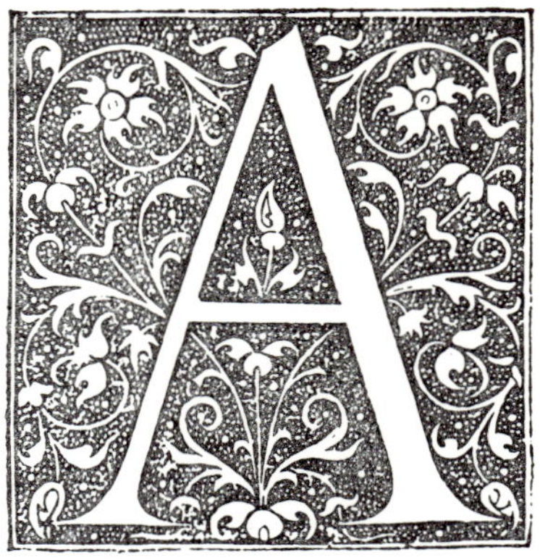
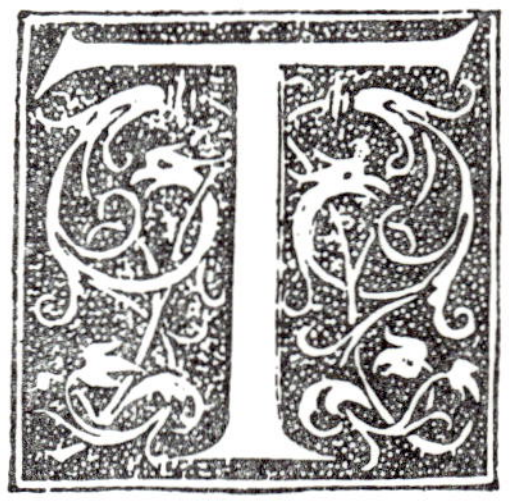
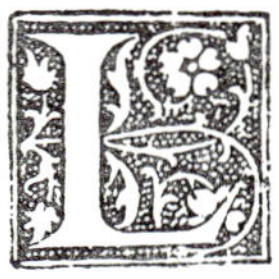

Figures 139 to 142 Initials of the workshop of Simon de Colines ('lettres fleuries'), from Estienne, De dissectione, *1545. They were used as early as 1526 and pass as the work of Geoffroy Tory.*

9 CUSHING, HARVEY: A Bio-Bibliography of Andreas Vesalius, New York, 1943, pp. 33-39.
10 O'MALLEY, C. D.: Andreas Vesalius of Brussels, 1514-1564; Berkeley and Los Angeles, 1964, pp. 35-61.
11 ROTH, M., *op. cit.*, p. 73, footnote 2.
12 The Latin edition of 1545, XXIV + 379 pp. The French edition of 1546, XVI + 406 pp.
13 With an introduction by P. HUARD and M. D. GRMEK (see p. 87, footnote 4), Paris, Au Cercle du Livre Précieux, 1965.
14 For these embellished capital letters (figs. 139-142), which are dated 1526, see BERNARD, AUGUSTE: Geoffrey Tory, peintre et graveur, premier imprimeur royal, Paris, Tross, 1865; reprint Nieuwkoop, de Graaf, 1963.
15 Relevant details can be found in NAGLER.
16 Art historians offer two JOLLAT'S: one generally well-known and one – perhaps completely hypothetical - "Mercure" JOLLAT, a designation derived from our monogram, which is also the symbol for Mercury. See NAGLER, *loc. cit.*
17 KELLETT, C. E.: Perino del Vaga et les illustrations pour l'anatomie d'Estienne, in: Aesculape, Paris, *37*, No. 4, 1955, pp. 74-89.

RAPHAEL. These illustrations will be discussed in greater detail later. In contrast, the third signature occurs only once, on the first plate of the book. It is a monogram "S.R." inscribed on a small tablet suspended from the branch of a tree in the background landscape. These initials were interpreted by CHOULANT as belonging to "Stephanus Riverius" (ESTIENNE DE LA RIVIÈRE). It is noteworthy that there are a whole series of plates in the *De dissectione* which, although they bear no artist's signature, do contain blank tablets in one corner.

The illustrations to the *De dissectione* are far more ambitious in scope than those found in earlier texts. Osteology, for example, is treated in four full-figure illustrations, just as LEONARDO himself had planned. Myology is illustrated in the same way; but in this case only with anterior and posterior views, each accompanied by a corresponding skeleton. At this point, by the way, a problem of chronology arises, for both skeletons (figs. 147-148) are of later date than the corresponding muscle figures. The peripheral nervous system is also accorded two full-figure illustrations. These illustrations, rather astonishingly, combine nerves with a skeleton – the nerve branches coil like worms around the long cylindrical bones and the skeleton of the trunk, to produce two extremely macabre figures (fig. 149) which stand alone in the middle of a landscape. The vascular system, too, is demonstrated

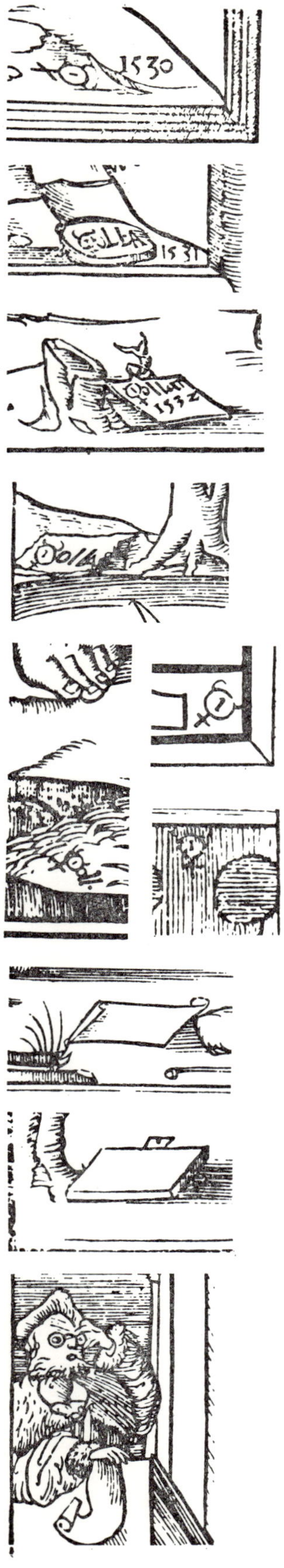

Fig. 143 (Left hand margin) The upper four signatures of Jollat are from Books I and II, the three middle signatures from Books I, II and III. The two empty signature plates are both from Book II, and the man with the blank scroll from Book III.

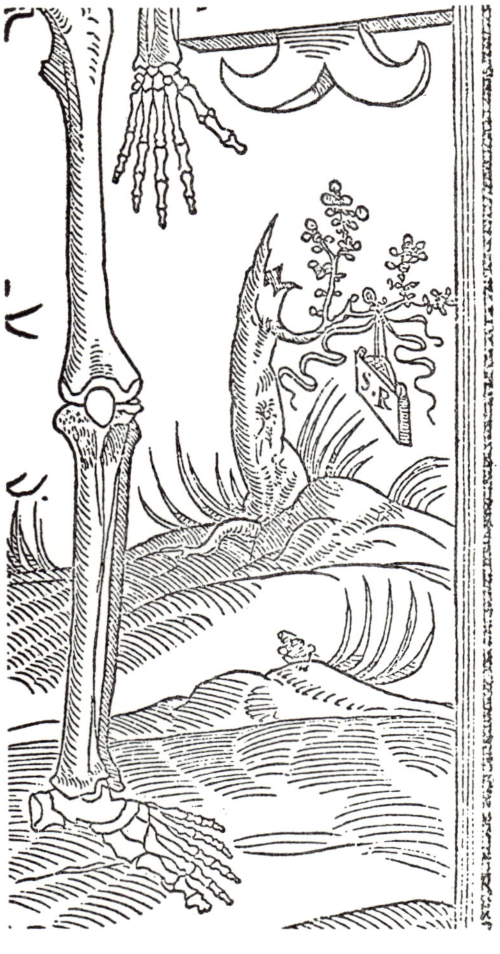

Fig. 144 Monogram 'S. R.' on the first plate of **Book I.**

in two figures; but the attempt to accomodate the great veins and great arteries in on anterior view of the extremities, is, quite apart from the crude technical errors, a failure (fig. 150). Three full-figure illustrations of the surface musculature derive in turn from another world: they are remarkably inflexible, as though they were of leather. Their detail was certainly not drawn from life; and there is no form of explanation. Two of these figures are dated 1532 and signed by JOLLAT. The last two illustrations in Book I show far less artistic accomplishment. The figures, which seem to be drawn from life, are provided with traditional, clumsy inscriptions. They are the oldest in the entire book, dated 1530 and 1531, and – to the astonishment of the modern observer who notices the difference in quality – they are also signed by JOLLAT (fig. 152).

The illustrations in Book I give us a chance to study JOLLAT'S successive attempts at solving the problem of presenting clear, instructive anatomical drawings. He made a sincere effort with the inscriptions, trying out everything known within the tradition that extended from KETHAM and the venesection figures to GERSSDORFF and PHRYES. His pronounced feeling for stylization led him to attach indication lines to his muscle figures like geometrically arranged needles (fig. 146), after he had evidently become dissatisfied with the confusion prevailing in the corresponding skeletons. The four osteological figures at the beginning of Book I are still clearly influenced by the KETHAM type of illustration with inscriptions inserted in the margins (fig. 147). A unique example of anatomical inscription, however, is found in JOLLAT'S attempt to incorporate the borders into the substance of the illustration in the form of two thin, hollow walls with holes along their edges, from which the threadlike indication lines emerge (fig. 145). Quite casually, the artist allows his skeleton to extend his hand into the border of the picture. Had JOLLAT not added his signature to so many of the illustrations, no one would imagine that they are all the work of the same designer.[18] Throughout the book, however, the attentive observer can note an abundance of masterly details revealing the sense of humor of the artist (figs. 153-155).

There are several other typical features to be found in these earlier illustrations which reappear as leitmotifs throughout the rest of the book: for instance, the board hanging from the top margin and bearing the explanatory text,[19] or the pedestal ornamented with a mask (figs. 147 and 154). These are not to be taken as JOLLAT'S "signature," however, for they belong to the standard repertoire shared by most European illustrators of the period.

Book II treats the internal organs of the abdomen, thorax, and skull; and it is much more uniform than the first book. The artist now seems to have found his style; these illustrations were probably produced during a period of persistent work

[18] The designer generally signed his name, but the person who actually executed the woodcuts did not.

[19] The motif also appears, bearing the book title, in the frontispiece of LINACRE'S 1530 edition of GALEN. The cross of Lorraine proves the identity of the artist, or at least of the workshop (fig. 298).

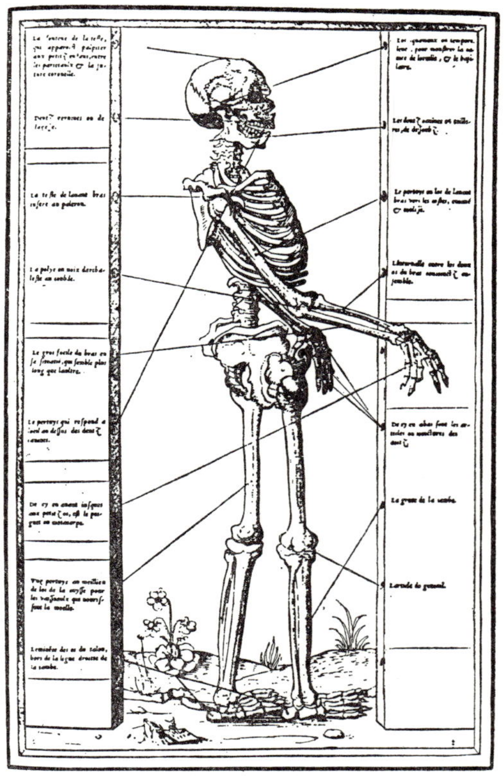

Fig. 145 Third plate of Book I.

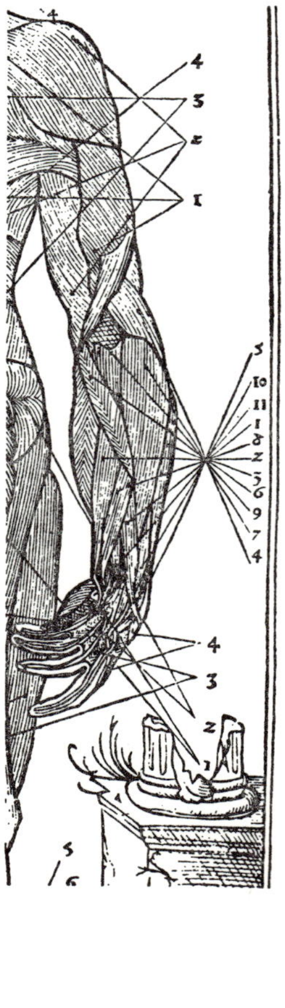

Fig. 146 Page 113 from Estienne, La dissection *(detail).*

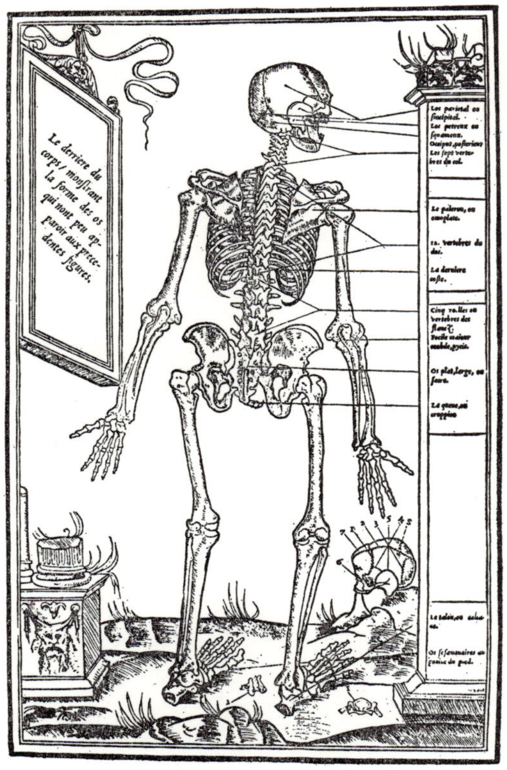

Fig. 147

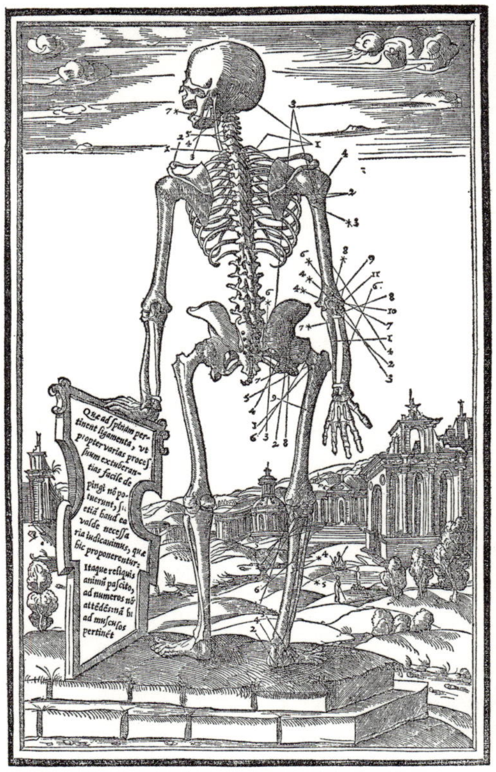

Fig. 148

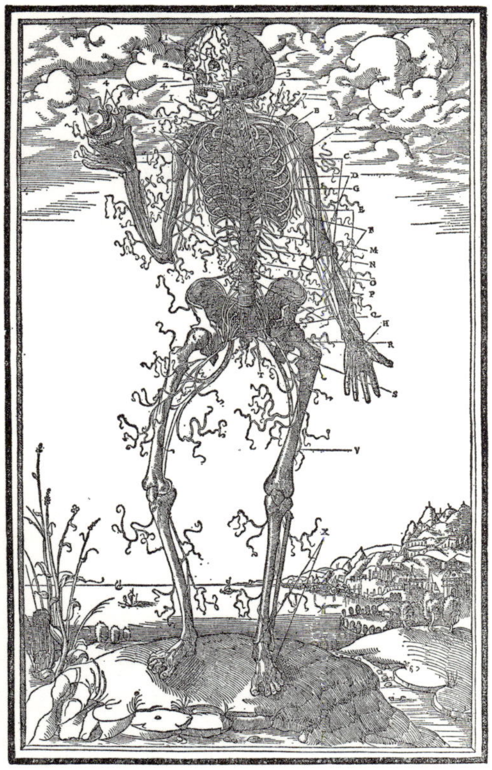

Fig. 149

Figures 147 to 152 *The first five illustrations from Book I. Figure 152 ends Book I.*

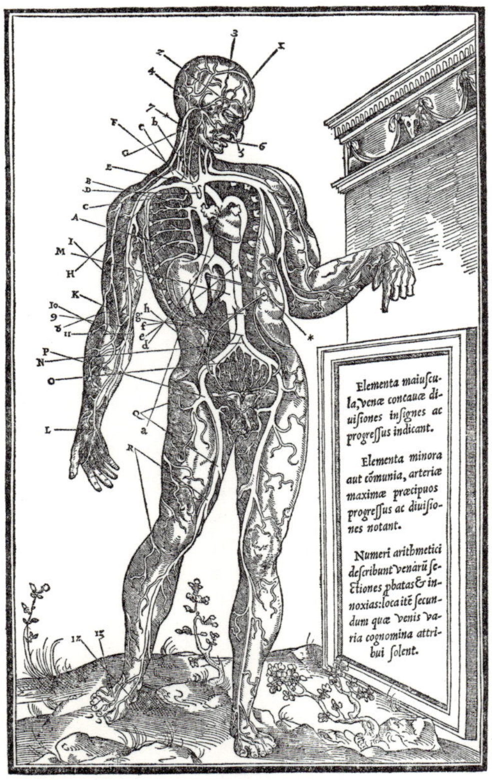

Fig. 150

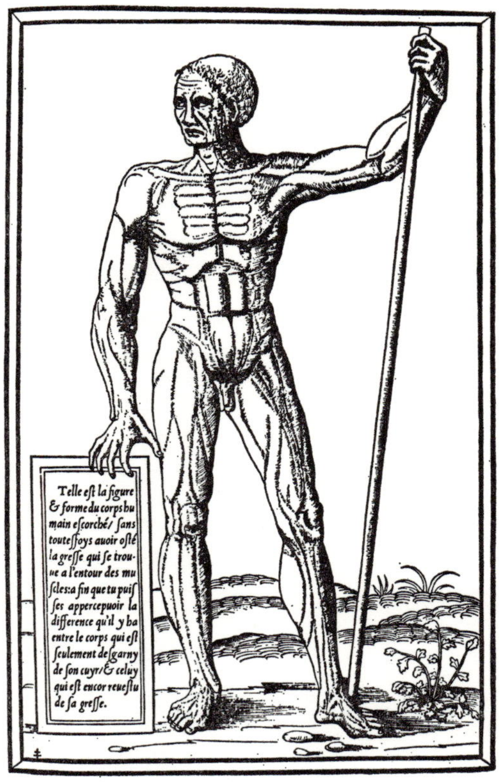

Fig. 151

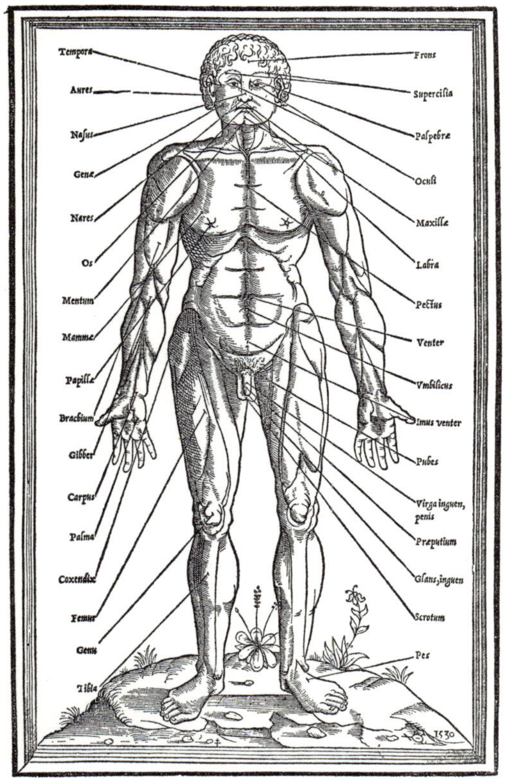

Fig. 152

immediately following the execution of the three muscle figures for Book I, and were therefore probably cut in 1534 or shortly afterwards. JOLLAT'S signature also appears on two occasions.[20] Yet we are faced here (from page 168 onwards) with a new problem, which must be regarded as unsolved: with two exceptions,[21] all the illustrations contain one or two corrective inserts of the type already encountered in BRUNSCHWIG'S *Cirurgia* (see pages 50 and 51). If the intention was to create "new" illustrations with a minimum of trouble, then we are presented with a riddle; for nowhere does the same full-figure illustration occur twice with inserts. There must, therefore, have been a special illustration for each anatomical subject from the beginning. What is the actual purpose of the inserts? The most plausible theory is that all the anatomical illustrations were revised to correct errors and inadequacies.[22] This is supported by the fact that there are plates without inserts. But since most of the illustrations are quite unobtrusive with respect to their anatomical content, it is difficult to imagine what actually required correction. The spirit which prompted such corrections of details in the first place is certainly still the same as it was in BRUNSCHWIG'S case. The representation of a medical subject – in BRUNSCHWIG, a wound on various parts of the body; in the *De dissectione,* mostly a visceral situs – still traditionally required a picture of the whole human body. In such figures, the human body was really only a kind of scenic setting for the specific theme, or a logical artistic surrounding. This has nothing to do with the quality of the illustration. The type of medical illustration that showed only a specific part of the body was abandoned, even though only for a short time, with the abandoning of the scholastic tradition characterized by diagrammatic and semi-diagrammatic illustrations. But the idea was already recovered, at least in part, by the end of the *De dissectione,* where the forms of the larger muscles are represented individually.

The approach used in Book II was so far ahead of its time that it bears a great similarity to the approach that was used in J. SOBOTTA'S atlas of descriptive anatomy, which appeared in 1904 and was regarded then – and for several decades following – as strikingly "modern." Just as SOBOTTA'S atlas does, Book II of the *De dissectione* contains series of illustrations of an abdominal situs (figs. 158-167) and of a thoracic situs, each demonstrating the successive stages of dissection from the skin to the evisceration of the body cavities; the *De dissectione* series comprise twelve pictures and eight pictures, respectively. The topography of the soft parts of the neck, illustrated in three pictures, is the weakest part of Book II; whereas the eight pictures of the skull, despite their small size, are surprisingly good compared with those of PHRYES, which are of approximately the same size and appeared fifteen years earlier (see page 61). Anyone wishing to compare the skull figures with those

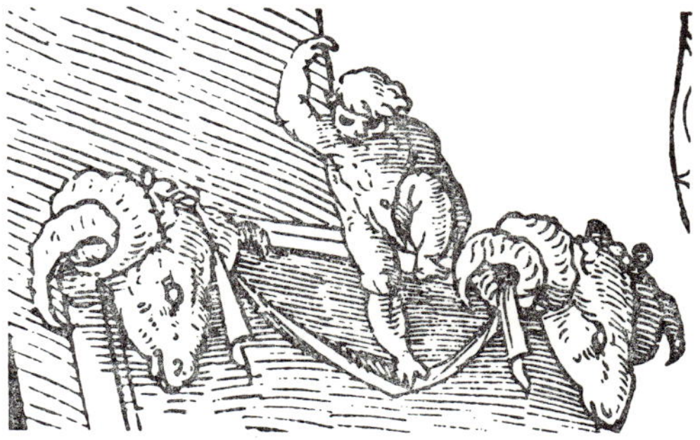

Fig. 153 Detail from La dissection, *p. 136.*

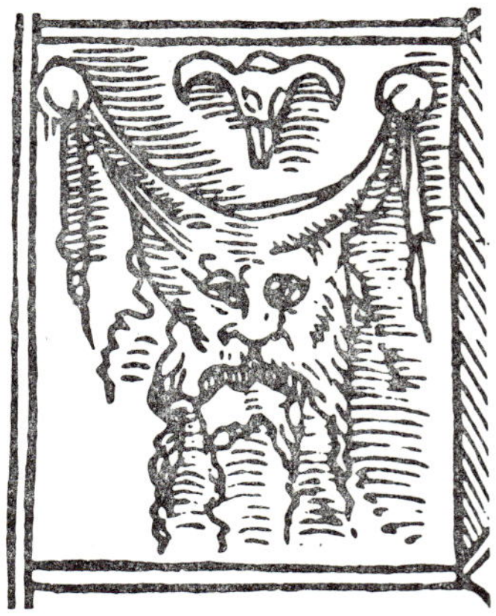

Fig. 154 Detail from p. 12 (from our fig. 147).

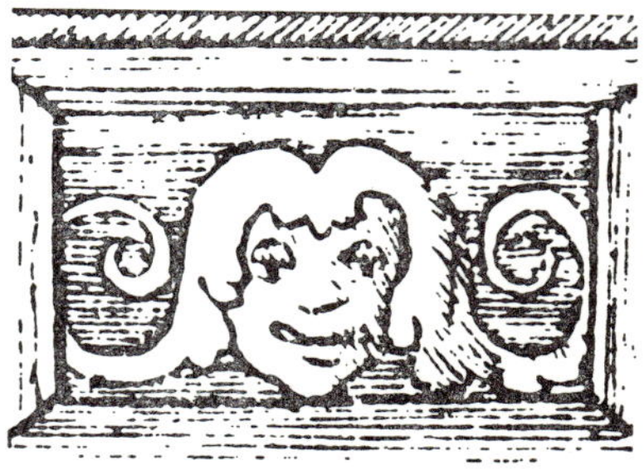

Fig. 155 Detail from p. 300.

20 French edition, pp. 210, 255.
21 French edition, pp. 265, 271.
22 The opinion sometimes expressed that the woodblocks were not cut for anatomical purposes, but were transformed into anatomical illustrations by means of the inserts, is based upon inadequate study of the originals.

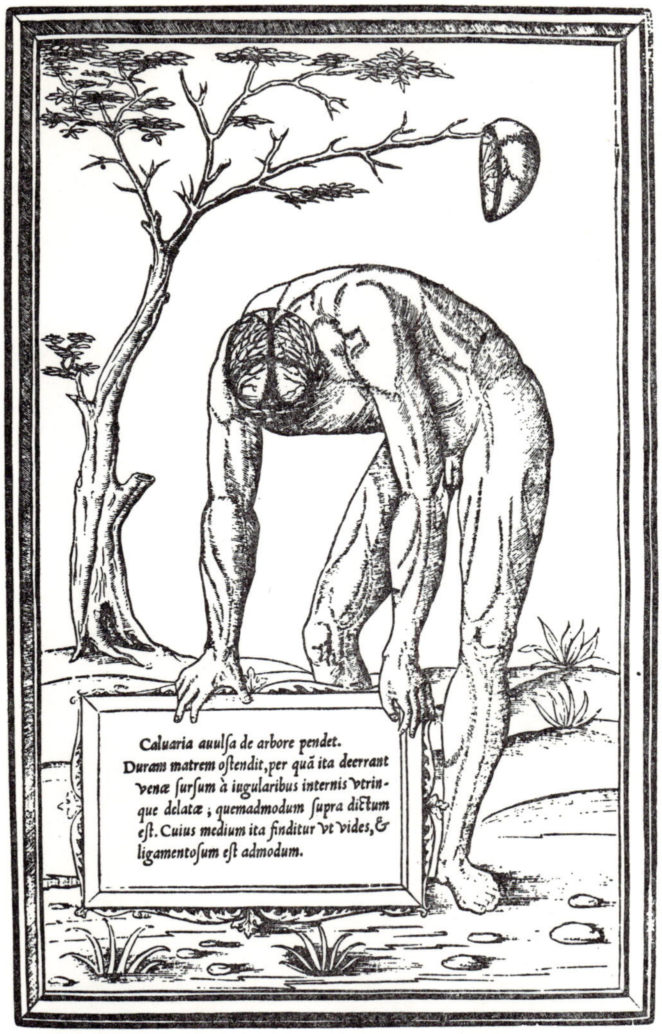

Fig. 156

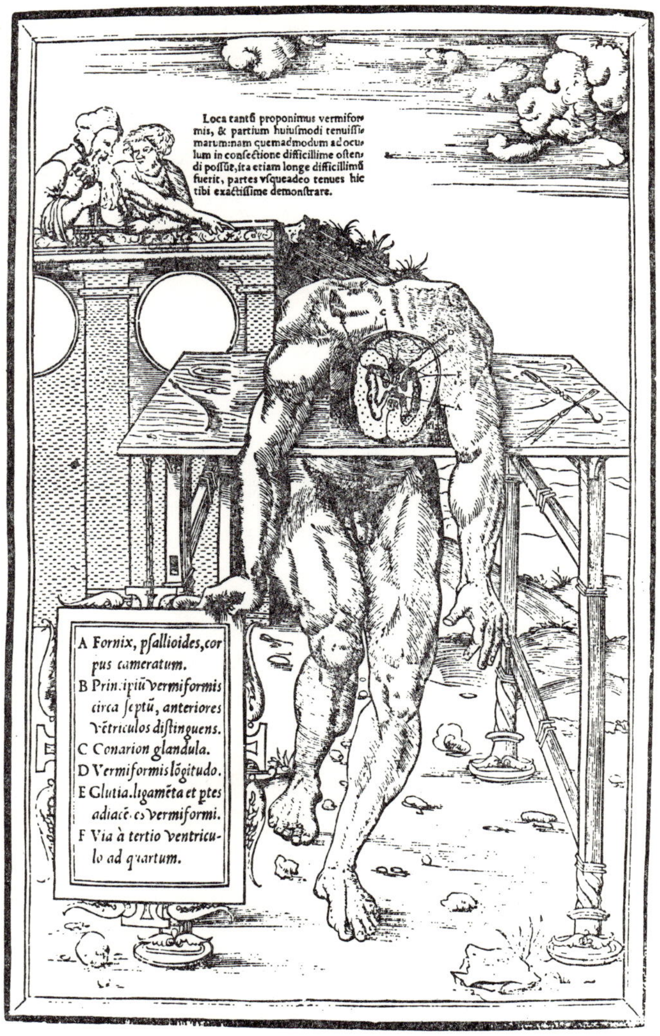

Fig. 157

Figures 156 and 157 Charles Estienne and Estienne de la Rivière, La dissection des parties du corps humain, *Paris, 1546. The left illustration is from one block, whereas the one on the right has a small insert. Left, Book II, p. 256; right, Book II, p. 262.*

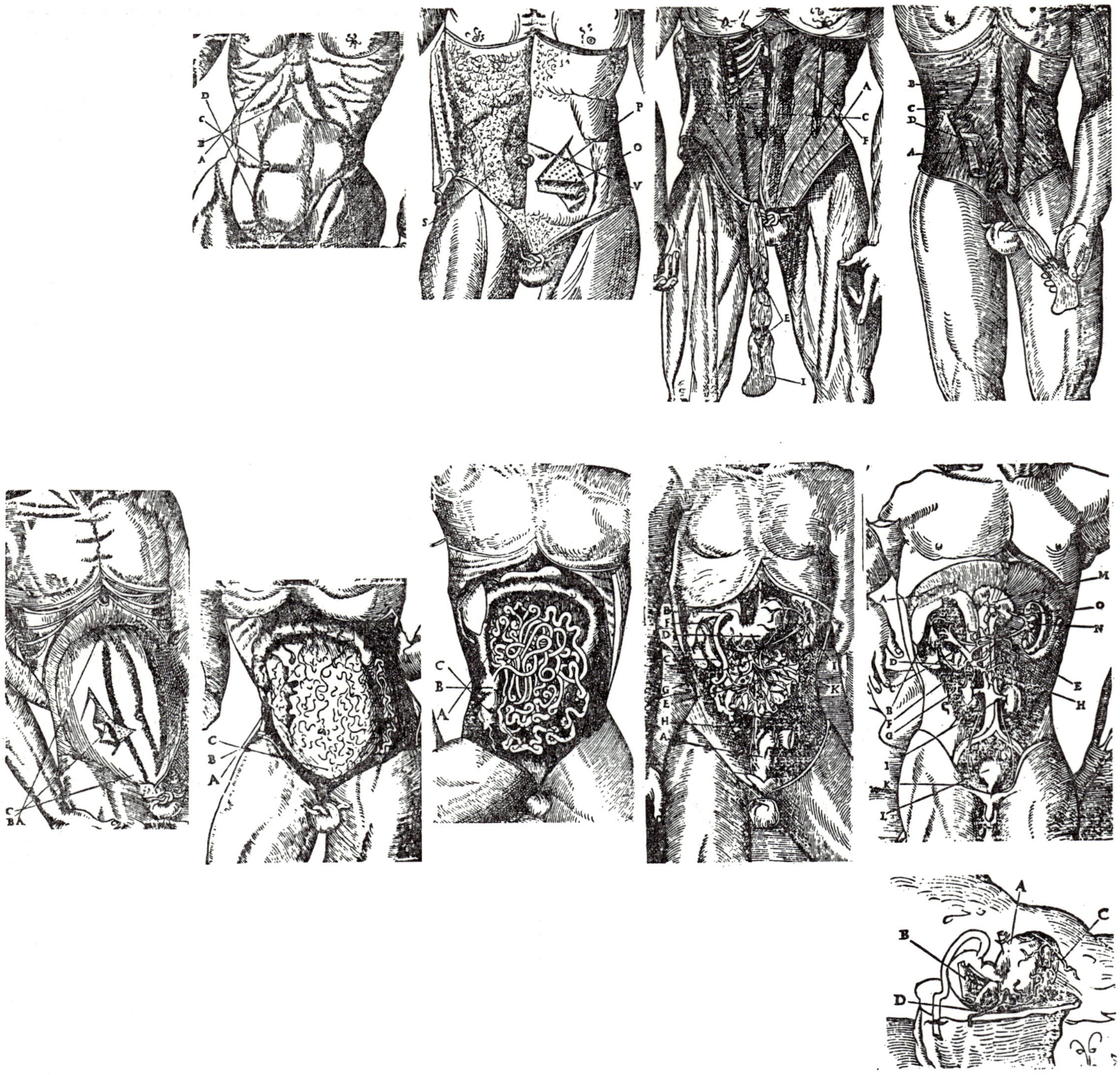

Figures 158 to 167 Estienne, Book II: Dissection of the abdominal viscera in a consecutive series of illustrations. The inserts have been taken form the full-figure illustrations and arranged in sequence. Compare the corresponding series in the Fabrica *of Vesalius (p. 111).*

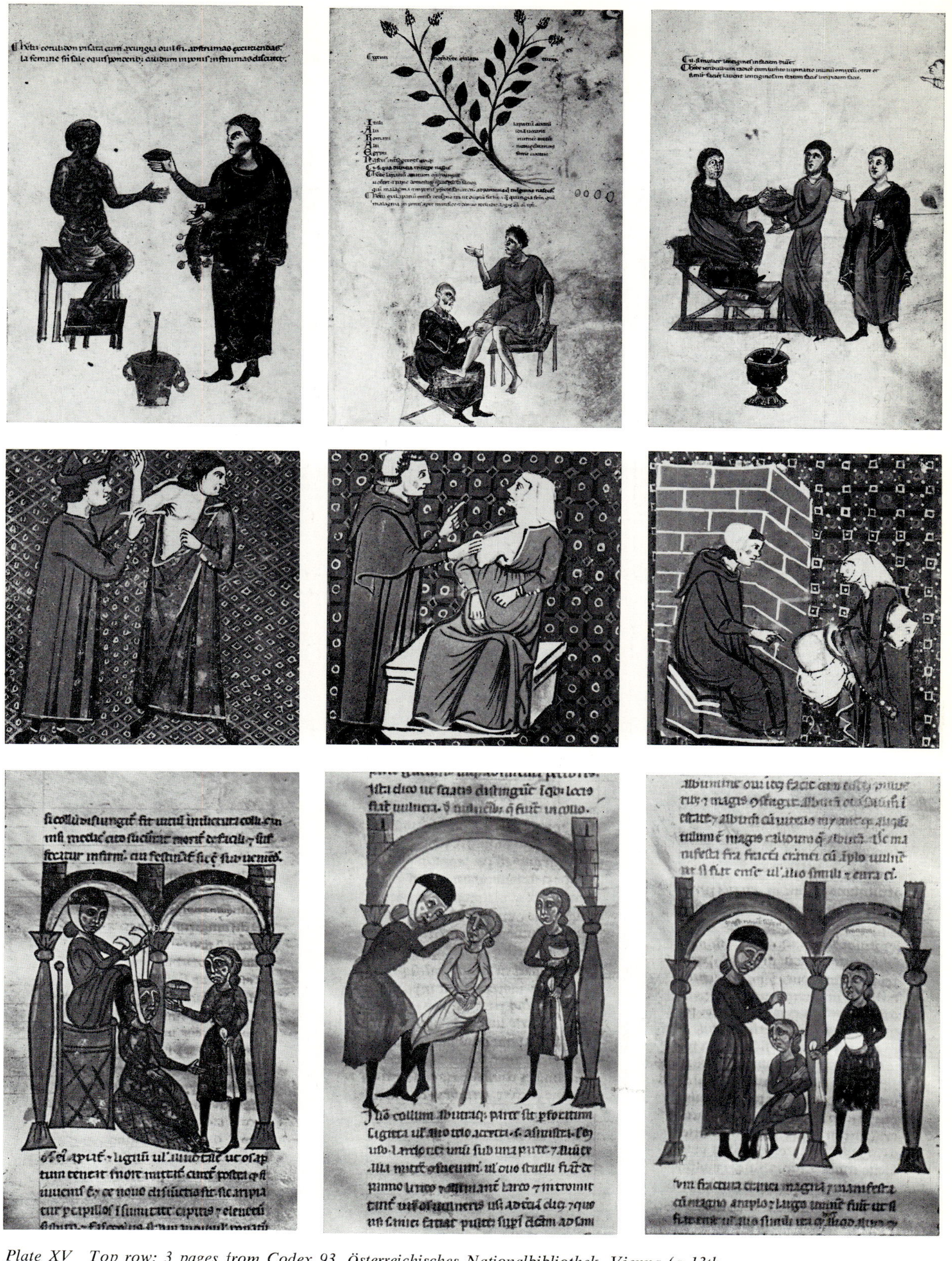

Plate XV Top row: 3 pages from Codex 93, Österreichisches Nationalbibliothek, Vienna (a 13th-century copy of a late-classical original dating from about the 6th century). At the bottom of the center illustration is a pen and ink drawing (cf. fig. 33). Middle row: 3 miniatures from the Cod. Voss. 3, the University Library, Leyden (Teodorico de Cervia, Chirurgia*), each measuring approximately 8 x 8 cm and dating from circa 1375. Bottom row: 3 miniatures from the Cod. 1382, Biblioteca Casanatense, Rome (Chirurgie of Rolandus Parmensis), circa 1300.*

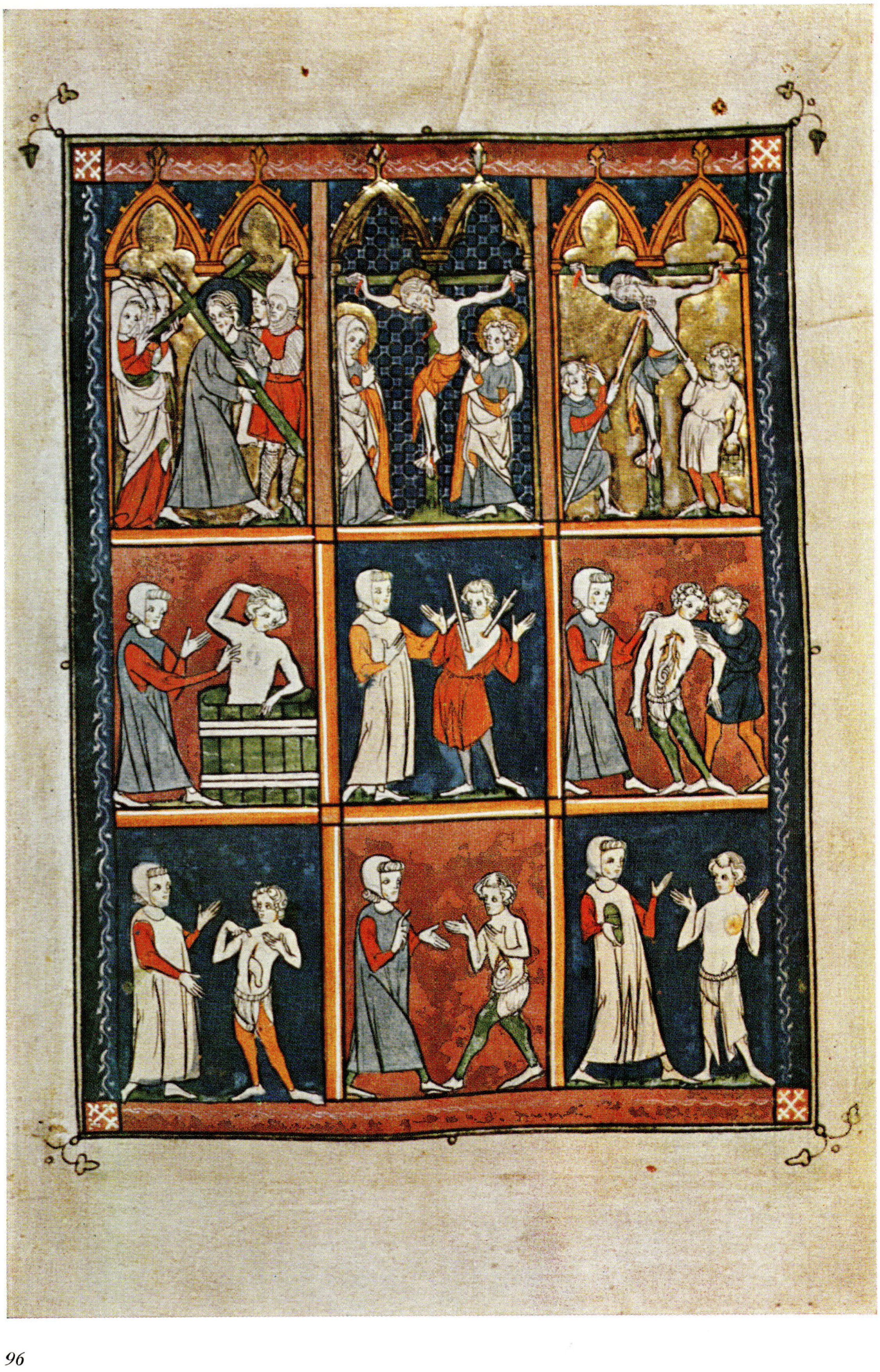

Plate XVI A page (fol. 7r) from the magnificent MS. Sloane 1977 in the British Museum. Gothic miniature painting of the French school, 13th century. (See p. 34.)

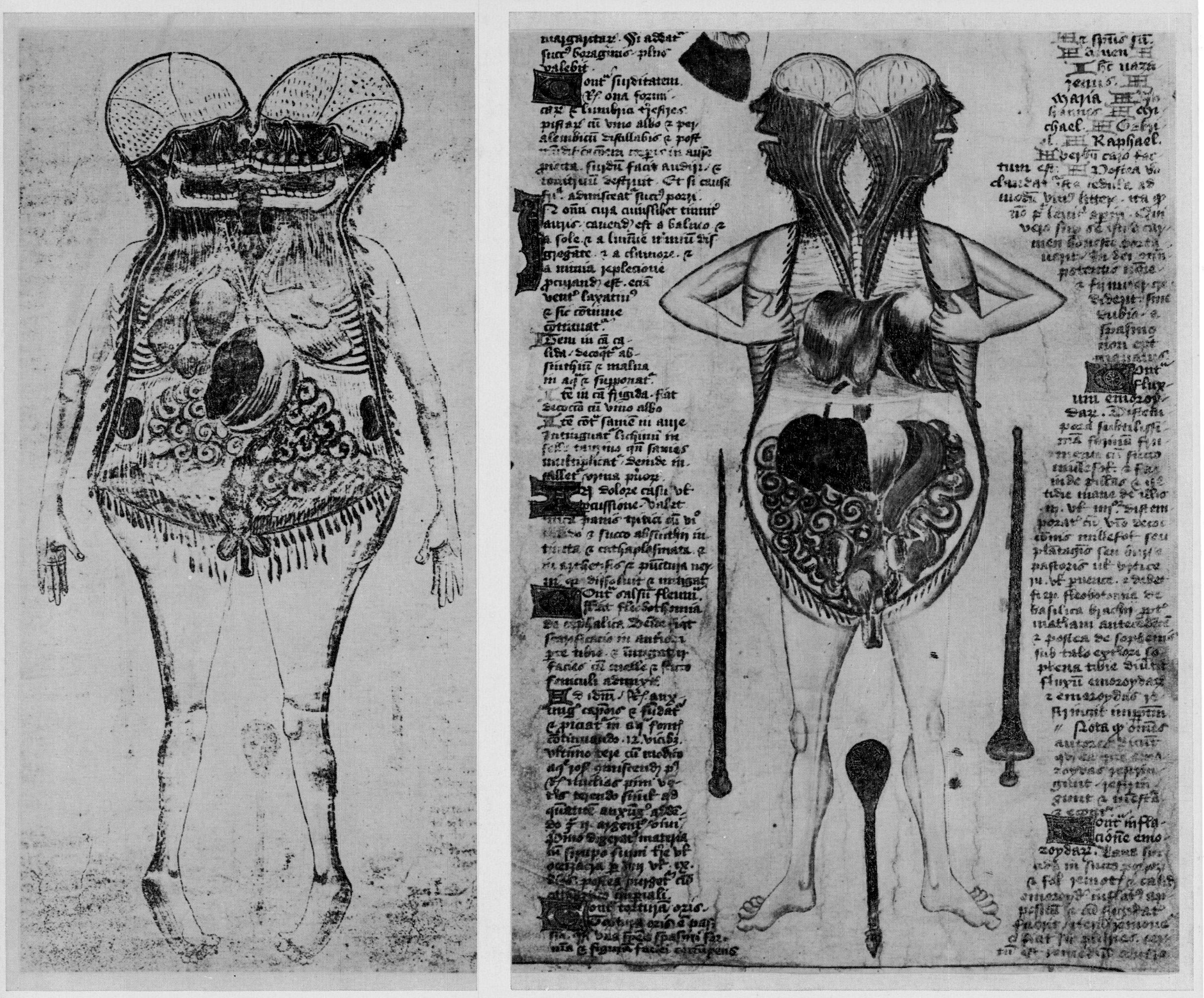

Plate XVII Medio-longitudinal dissection of a human corpse. Ventral and dorsal exposure, respectively, Kungliga Biblioteket, Stockholm, MS. X 118 (John Arderne), circa 1412. The whole manuscript is reproduced in monochrome and translated in De Arte Physicali et de Cirurgia of Master John Arderne, Surgeon of Newark, *translation by Sir D'Arcy Power (Wellcome Historical Medical Museum, Research Studies in Medical History No. 1), London (Bayle and Danielsson), 1922.*

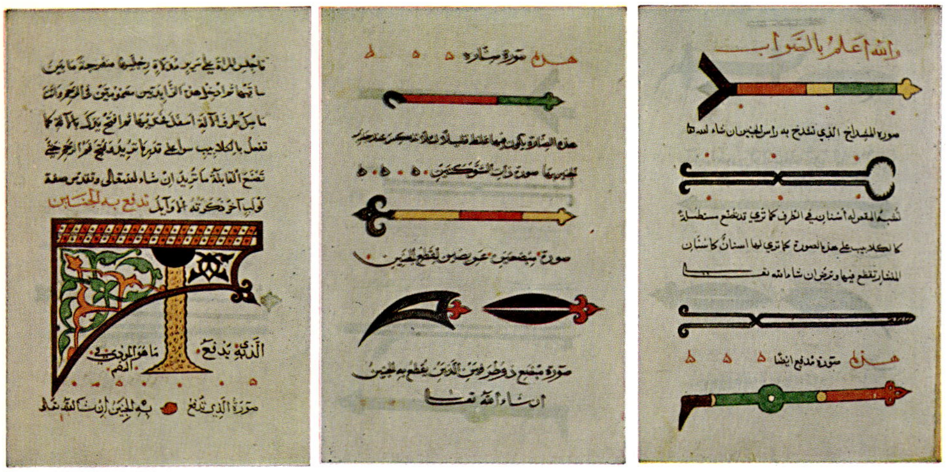

Plate XVIII a Three pages from the Cod. arab. 91, Tübingen, former Preuss. Staatsbibliothek, Berlin. Illustrations from Schipperges, Schmerzbekämpfung in der arabischen Chirurgie.

Plate XVIIIb Resetting the spine, according to Abulcasis. Miniature from Codex S, n. 2641, Österr. Nationalbibliothek, Vienna. What actually occurred when Gibbus was 'reset' remains a mystery.

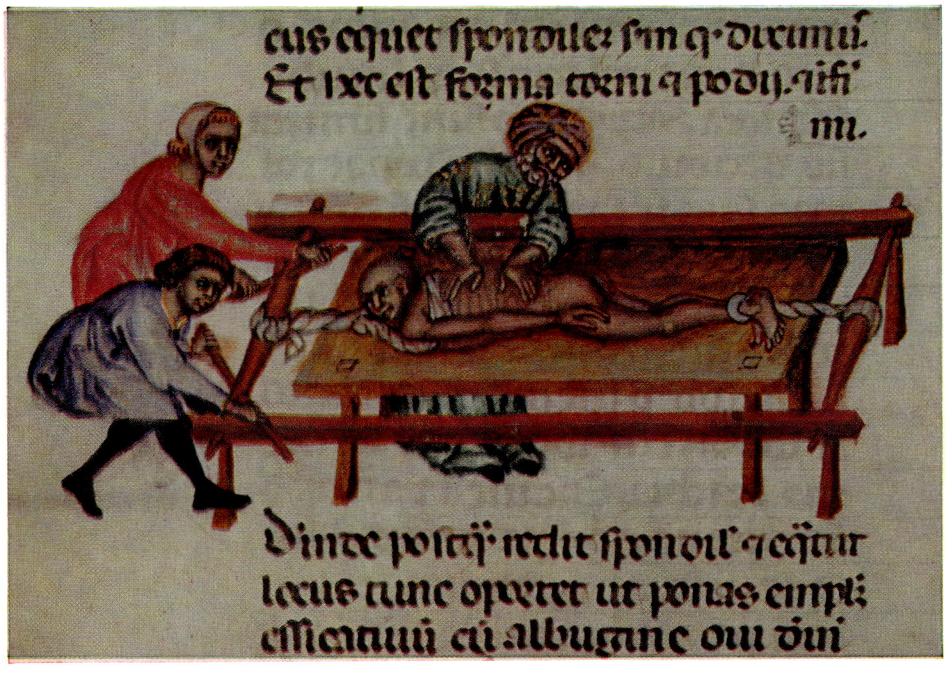

Figures 168 to 179 Estienne, Book II: Dissection of the brain demonstrated in a sequence of illustrations.

in DRYANDER should not forget that they are about five years older; however, the achievement of DRYANDER'S artist, who had progressed beyond the full-figure illustration, becomes obvious through comparison with the *De dissectione.* With the exception of the inserts, we are inclined to attribute all the woodcuts in Book II to JOLLAT. The tentativeness of JOLLAT'S first step from the medieval to the modern approach is demonstrated by his interiors with a chair and a view through a small window; or by the architectural framework in the "Bathsheba scene" (page 299 in the French edition); but most of all by the confused perspective in several plates in the first book, where the "vanishing lines" do not converge at a single point in the distance but go off in random directions. JOLLAT might be said to have skipped over the Renaissance entirely, and can be counted as an example of an early, and typical, Mannerist, with one foot still in the late Gothic period.

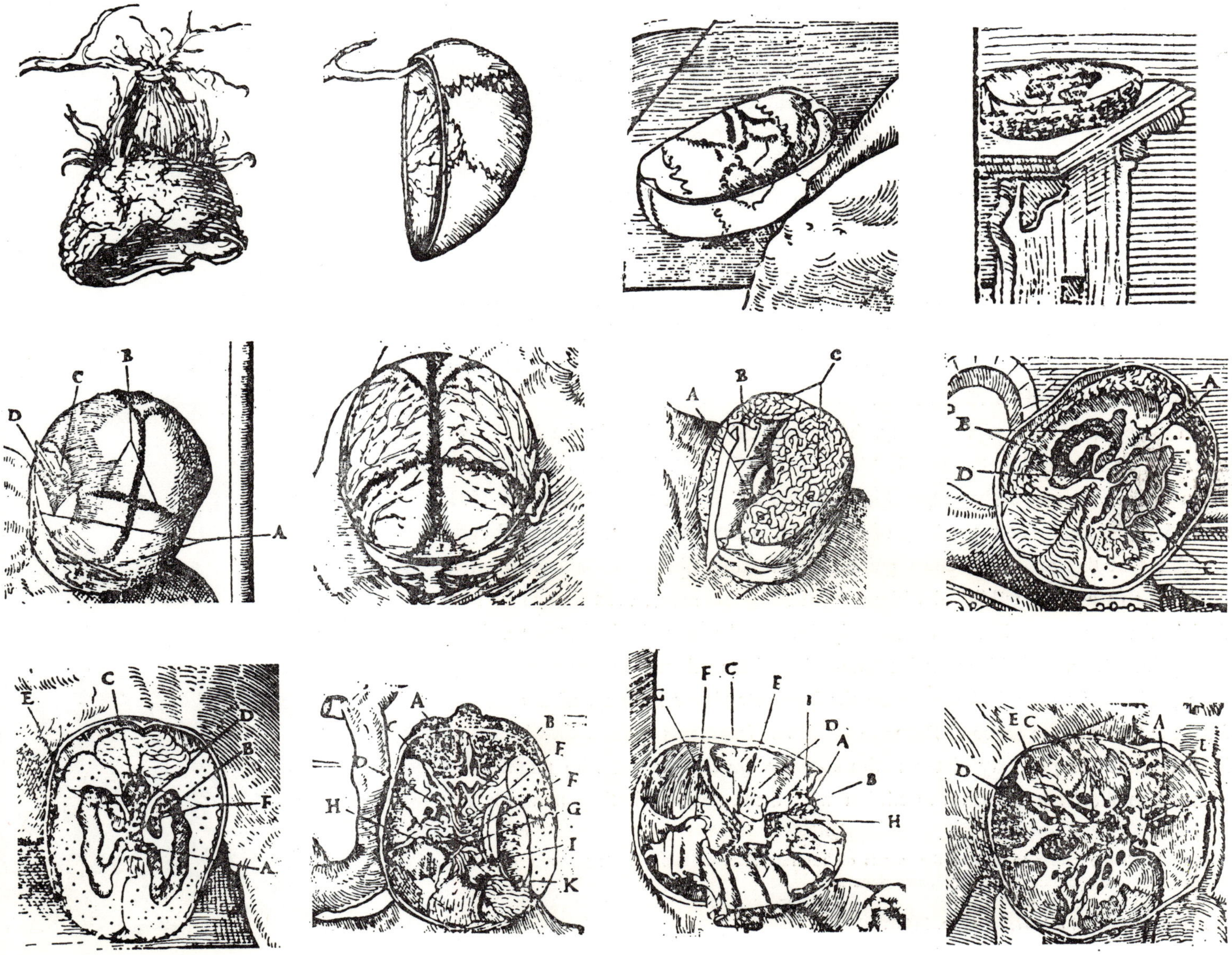

It cannot be doubted that the artist who produced the woodcuts in Book II made use of older models. Kellett has convincingly proved that Berengario's illustrations served as model for the gynecological series. There is no direct prototype for the male figures of Book II, which however have been connected with Rosso de' Rossi and his circle. The sources of this series should be sought in a sketchbook rather than in printed graphic art. Is it not possible – to take a typical example – that Michelangelo's "David" served as the model for the visceral figure on page 202 of the French edition? As we have already indicated, the adaptation of Perino del Vaga's "Amours des Dieux," which also only partially served as a model, is to be attributed to Jollat. The proof for this is contained in the plate on page 303 of the French edition (page 279 of the Latin edition) where Jollat's signature is found in the left-hand border of the picture, in the shadow beneath the trunk. Even more legible is a second specimen on page 290 of the French edition, which is inscribed in the right-hand corner of a bench (fig. 143).

The inserts can scarcely have been made by the same artist who did the original woodcuts. They are of lower quality, and some are so poor as to be practically unintelligible. Jollat never produced such inexpert crosshatching as occurs throughout Book II.[23] Whether we can ascribe the inserts to Estienne de la Rivière and – like the actual anatomical illustrations from books II and III – also regard them as the main part of the surgeon's co-authorship, must be left undecided for the moment.[24] Taken as a whole, the inserts represent a bold step into the future for the history of anatomical and obstetrical illustration; their immediate failure was caused merely by the deficient artwork. However, putting artistic value aside, the inserts are not drawn from life, but rather represent partially diagrammatic simplifications. Consequently, they detract from the full-figure illustrations, which are in the naturalistic tradition of mural and canvas painting.

From the point of view of art history, the anatomical illustrations in the *De dissectione* can be described as thoroughly Mannerist. The connection with the Fontainebleau School is not merely geographical. Rosso de' Rossi worked between 1531 and 1540 principally at the gallery of Francis I in Fontainebleau. Is it at all conceivable that this artist, the court painter of the king, himself collaborated on a book which was then published without mentioning his name, even though he had died in the meantime? Kellett[25] recently developed a hypothesis that not only is daring, but also reveals his extensive knowledge of the subject: Rosso may already have performed anatomical studies on the human cadaver in Italy, after escaping from the terror of the Sacco di Roma in 1527. The fragments of these drawings may have become the property of the authors of the *De dissectione*, who might have planned to illustrate a Mondino edition with them, for which they naturally re-

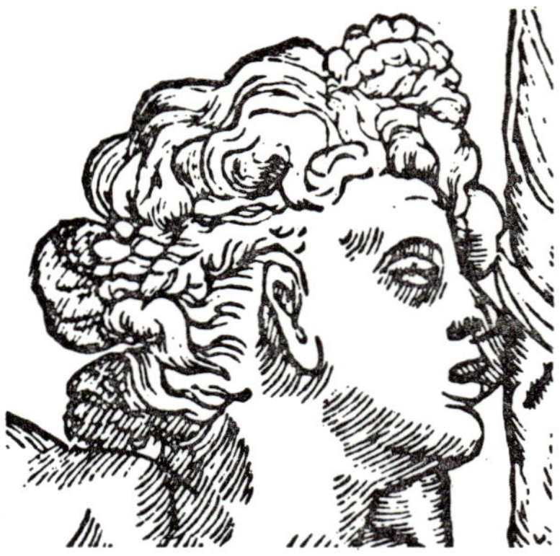

Fig. 180

Figures 180 to 182 Three heads from Estienne: center, from Book I; bottom, from Book II; top, from Book III.

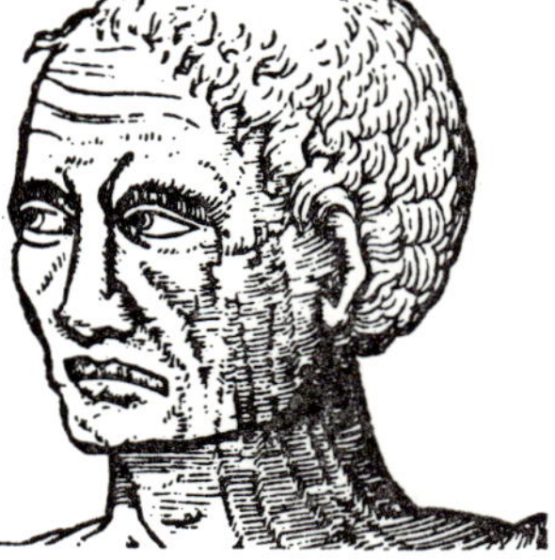

Fig. 181

Fig. 182

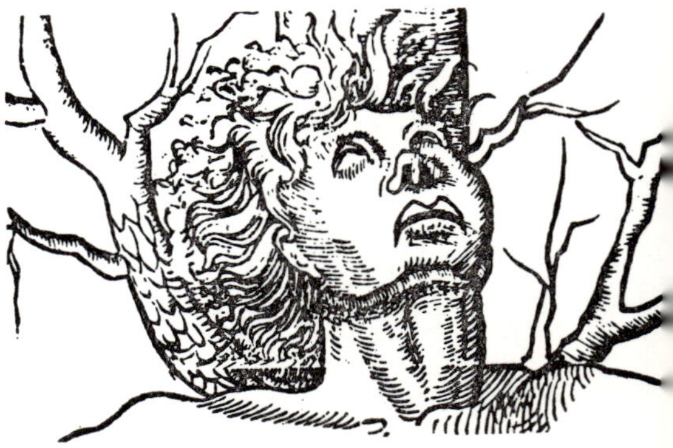

[23] I would choose rather to ascribe the inserts on several plates of Book III (e.g., those on pages 290 and 305) to the master with the Mercury signature.
[24] See Premuda, *op. cit.*, p. 105.
[25] Kellett, Med. Hist. *VIII*, 1964, pp. 344 ff.

quired redrawing. Estienne de la Rivière, who had become associated with the project as surgeon, could have prepared a cadaver for the skeleton illustrations according to the method of water maceration which several years later was depicted on the initial "C" in Vesalius's *Fabrica.*[26] But in Paris, events were precipitated by the rediscovery of Galen, who then took the place of Mondino, because the Galen edition by Winther von Andernach (to which we would also add his anatomy of the female organs) set new standards. De la Rivière, according to this theory, was then the moving force in replacing the inadequate situs illustrations with better ones, which was only possible by employing inserts or by starting anew. This would be the reason for the choice of these inserts, which disturb the observer and have encouraged speculation on the part of all subsequent historians.

This theory of Kellett's is attractive, but the historical support is too scanty for it to be accepted as more than a working hypothesis. All the same, a better hypothesis has yet to be offered. Kellett's most interesting assumption is that the "new" Galen of the humanists stands between Berengario and Vesalius. The first, and only, illustrated text dedicated to Galen is the *De dissectione.* Since it combines the spirit of Winther von Andernach with that of the Mannerists of Fontainebleau, the result had to be a hybrid.

The lawsuit over this book occurred in Paris while Vesalius was there. It is wholly possible that he left the city with the idea that there must be a better solution to the current problem of anatomical illustration.

[26] Herrlinger, R.: Die Initialen in Vesals "Fabrica," in: Index Gesch. Med. Naturw. Technik *1,* 1953, pp. 4-5.

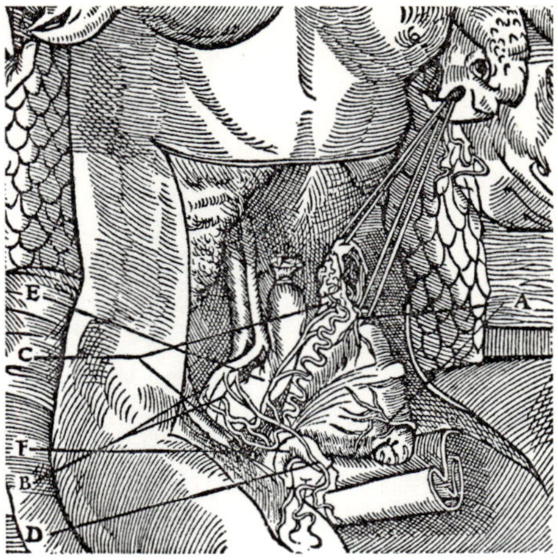

Fig. 183 An insert from Book III. For better demonstration, the uterus is suspended from a chair arm which has the unusual shape of a parrot's head.

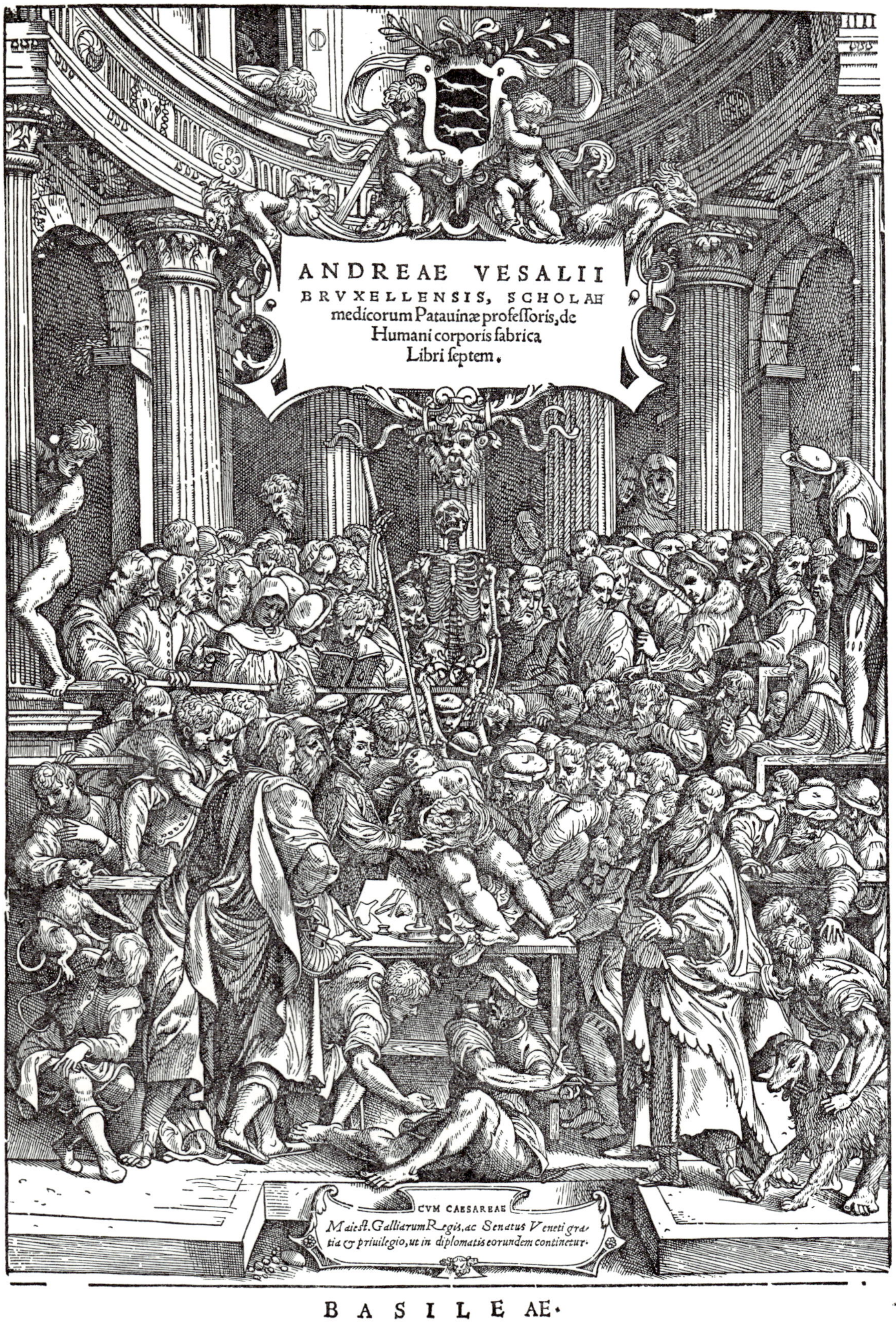

Fig. 184 Title-page woodcut for the Fabrica *of Vesalius, Basel, 1543 (reduced 3 : 5). Attributed to Jan Stevenszoon van Calcar.*

Vesalius

VESALIUS'S *De Humani corporis fabrica libri septem*, published in 1543 by JOHANNES OPORINUS in Basel, is both a classic work in the field of medicine and a classic example of the art of printing. There is no other medical text that has been accorded so high a rank in both fields at once.

At the time he wrote the *Fabrica*, ANDREAS VESALIUS was a lecturer in surgery[1] at the University of Padua. He had arrived in Padua in 1537, after having lived in Paris from 1533 to 1536.[2] VESALIUS was twenty-eight years old when the book appeared.

The *Fabrica* is a large folio volume of 663 pages, illustrated with more than two hundred woodcuts. The imposing layout and the spectacular illustrations immediately impress anyone who opens the text; even the title-page woodcut is a masterly work of art which must have caused a sensation when it first appeared (fig. 184). In this woodcut, whose artist still remains anonymous,[3] VESALIUS is shown giving an anatomy lecture like those which he frequently delivered before students and professors in Padua and Bologna. Not only is he demonstrating from the cadaver, but he himself is the prosector. The idea of picturing an anatomical lecture was not new[4] – such scenes had already been shown, although in an abstract and symbolical way, in late medieval illustrations (fig. 86); and a woodcut in a naturalistic style showing a demonstration from the cadaver had been recently published in Paris, in 1531. This latter illustration, which was also a piece of title-page art,[5] shows a surgeon standing at the cadaver and disputing with a doctor of medicine – a dramatic scene about which unfortunately we have no further particulars. Even in this scene, there is a break from the traditional procedure of demonstrating dissection; in contrast to earlier illustrations in KETHAM (1493), in the *Mondino* editions of POLLICH (1495), or in BERENGARIO (1521), the professor is no longer shown lecturing from a chair while a prosector and a demonstrator work on the cadaver.

VESALIUS'S title page possesses greater merit than the 1531 illustration not only as a work of art, but also as a practical indication of the contents of the book.[6] Rather than depicting an academic dispute, it shows the teacher of anatomy demon-

1 On the title page he is called, quite rightly, *Scholae medicorum Patauinae professoris.*

2 Further biographical information can be found in O'MALLEY, C. D.: Andreas Vesalius of Brussels, 1514-1564; Berkeley and Los Angeles, 1964.

3 A monogram, the letter "I" over a letter "O," is inscribed at the top edge of the picture. WILLY WIEGAND, who is especially qualified in this field, would like to interpret this monogram as standing for "Io(annes Stephanus van Calcar)." The hypothesis conforms to an older theory of ROTH and SPIELMANN, who regard the two heads looking down from the gallery as representing the young Fleming JAN STEVENSZOON VAN CALCAR and the old TITIAN. The degree to which the composition conforms to the taste of the contemporary Venetian school of painting is revealed by TINTORETTO'S "St. Mark Rescuing a Slave" (1548) in the Accademia.

4 See SINGER, CH. and C. RABIN: A Prelude to Modern Science, Publication of the Wellcome Historical Medical Museum I, Cambridge, 1946.

5 CLAUDII GALENI: Pergameni De anatomicis administrationibus libri IX, JOANNE GUINTERIO ANDERNACO Medico interprete. Parisiis apud SIMONEM COLINAEUM 1531. The artist could be identical with the master of the *De dissectione*. The cross of Lorraine suggests at least the same workshop, perhaps that of JOLLAT or TORY (see pp. 88-89).

6 O'MALLEY, *op. cit.*, pp. 139 ff. The minute description offered here probably overinterprets.

strating the abdominal situs of a female cadaver to his audience. The actual lecture-room is a wooden construction in the form of a theater, overflowing with a motley public. The illustrator presents the scene in part realistically, in a manner comparable to a modern eyewitness report, but he is nevertheless still partially indebted to the traditional way of depicting a theatrical scene (see figure 186), as W. ARTELT demonstrated in 1950.[7] Many details were probably worked into the scene in accordance with the special wishes of VESALIUS. The author himself is shown facing the observer, while his hands are unmistakably engaged in demonstration

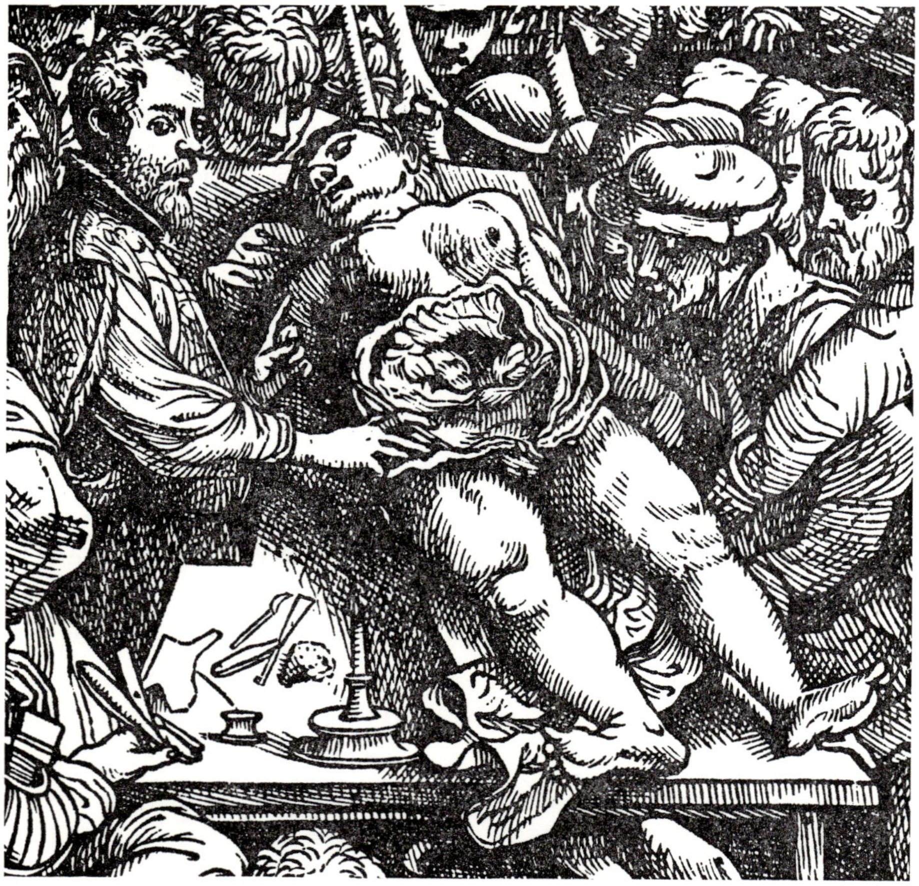

Fig. 185 Andreas Vesalius giving a public lecture in anatomy. Detail from fig. 184, greatly enlarged.

(see the detail from the title page, given in figure 185). In this way the reader is prepared for the subject matter of the book, expecting a description of the human body that will be based on the author's observations. In the foreword, by the way, VESALIUS specifically mentions the use of the hands, which he says has been "completely neglected" by physicians since the time of the Romans. "Because physicians left the manual work to others and thus lost their practical acquaintance with anatomy," medicine itself had declined from its former splendor.

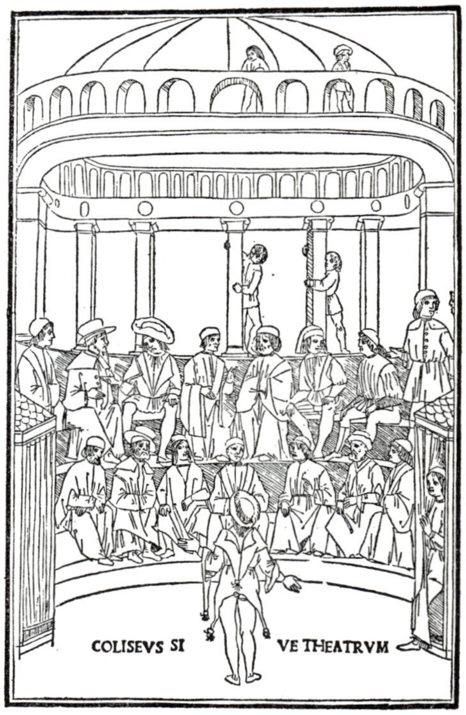

Fig. 186 Terentius, Comoediae cum V commentis, *Venice, 1497.*

Fig. 187 Portrait of Vesalius on fol. 6ᵛ, opposite the beginning of the text of the Fabrica *of 1543. Unknown artist.*

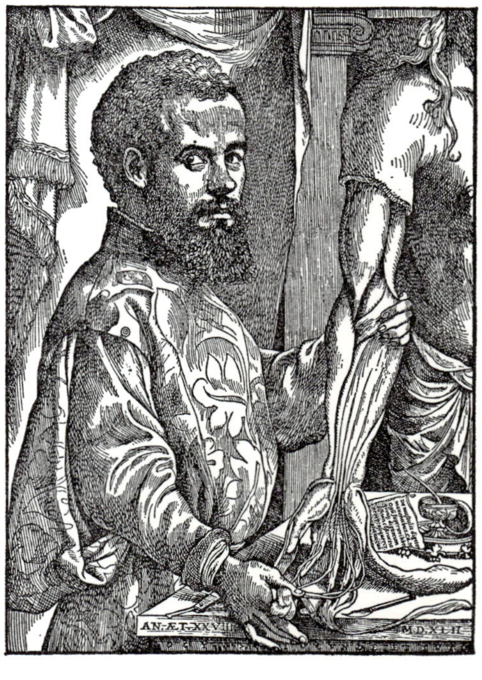

[7] ARTELT, WALTER: Das Titelbild zur "Fabrica" Vesals und seine kunstgeschichtlichen Voraussetzungen, in: Centaurus, Copenhagen, *1*, 1950/51, p. 66.

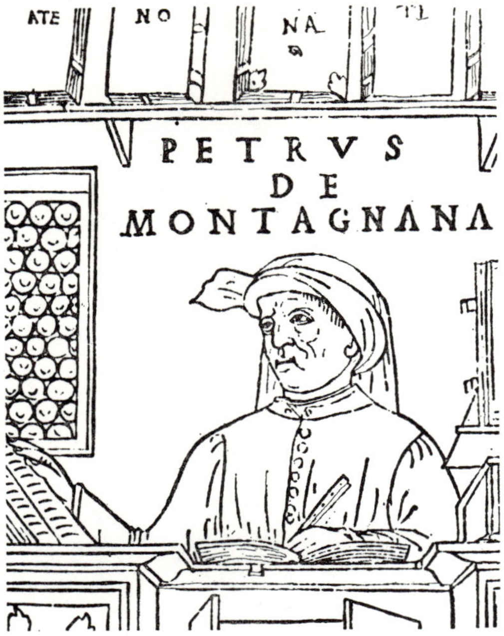

Fig. 188 Portrait of Petrus de Montagnana (1405-1460), on fol. Ir of the Fasciculus medicinae, *Venice, 1493 (detail). There is a title-page woodcut for Aesop's* Fables, *Venice, 1491, by the same unknown master.*

Fig. 189 Sketch after Tintoretto's 'St. Mark rescuing a slave,' Accademia, Venice. The stylistic similarity to Vesalius' frontispiece extends to numerous details (see fig. 184).

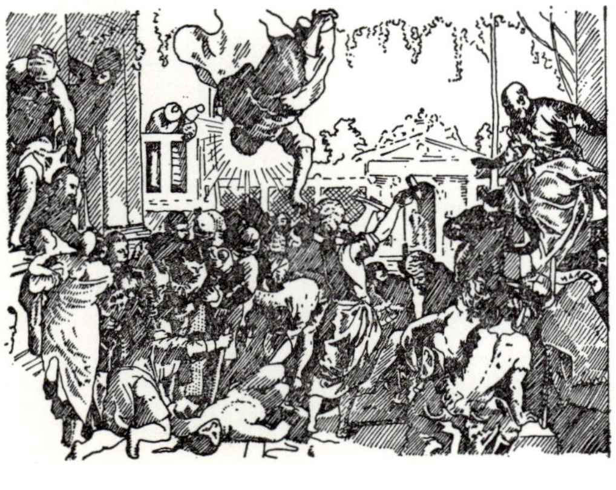

This book was intended to provide a text for those who had attended VESALIUS'S dissection classes, a text which would permit them "to demonstrate anatomy to others with little difficulty." But a person who had no cadaver as a demonstration object would find the text "even more useful," because "every small part of the human body is represented in adequate detail to show its number, position, form, size, composition, connection with other parts, purpose, function, and very much more than we are accustomed to investigating in the dissection of the parts; in addition, instructions are given for the correct dissection of dead and living bodies. Moreover, the text contains illustrations of all the parts, which are so inserted into the book that the eye of whoever is occupied with the works of nature is simultaneously presented with a dissected body." VESALIUS did not exaggerate. Never before had such a textbook been attempted.

The portrait of the author, which appears on the page facing the beginning of the text, is more traditional in conception than the great title-page woodcut. The portrait, as an artistic genre, had reached its height one century before VESALIUS in the works of JAN VAN EYCK and his followers. These Flemish artists, whose work has never been surpassed so far as lifelike representation is concerned, led the whole of Europe in the field of portraiture. It is surely not a coincidence that VESALIUS, who grew up in Brussels and Louvain – the centers of Flemish art – should have commissioned such a portrait of himself for his book.[8] When we look at the portrait of our anatomist[9] (fig. 187), we are confronted with a very self-confident young man. He has a round head, a trimmed beard, a turned-up nose, and a small mole above the right eyebrow. His dark eyes fix the observer with a challenging stare. However, the scene containing the portrait is not fully realistic in the modern sense of the word. In spite of the fleshy appearance of the dissected arm that the anatomist is holding, the arm belongs to an unrealistically conceived body, a cadaver seemingly in a standing position. Here we have a medieval symbol which corresponds in some respects to the illustrations in the *Anathomia* by GUIDO DA VIGEVANO DE PAPIA (see p. 40), where the corpse also appears to stand next to the dissector. Actually, rather than representing a real cadaver, the corpse is primarily symbolic. The text lying on the table also seems symbolic; it is written in a code so complicated that historians have been unable to decipher its meaning. The quality of the woodcut has been repeatedly commended, but the engraver does not possess that same mastery of line, in the surface-hatching and shadow-hatching, as the master of the title page and the full-figure anatomical illustrations.

8 The oldest portrait of an author in a medical work is that of PETRUS DE MONTAGNANA in the *Fasciculus medicinae* of 1493. A portrait of the author on the title page was by no means unusual by 1543. KRISTELLER compiled a small catalogue of such portraits: PAUL KRISTELLER, Kupferstich und Holzschnitt in vier Jahrhunderten, Berlin (Cassirer), 1922, pp. 285-86.

9 For further information on portraits of VESALIUS, see recent studies by PAZZINI, ADALBERTO: Uno sconosciuto ritratto di Andrea Vesalio, Rome, 1966, and GUERRA, FRANCESCO: Juan de Valverde de Hamusco, in: Clio Medica *3*, 1968, Vol. I.

The first page of the text (plate XXIIIa), with its magnificent capital letter "O", reveals the art of the printer, who produced a masterpiece in this work. The best printers of Basel, Paris, and Venice produced little to compare with it. The heading of Book I displays some of the typefaces to be used in the book: a Roman type, which was also employed by the VON FROBEN in Basel and by others; and a cursive type, which is used in the *Fabrica* for the legends of the illustrations and to a lesser extent for the marginal notes. The second edition of 1555 – to mention this in advance – used a new typeface, the celebrated Parisian script design copied by CLAUDE GARAMOND from the classical Roman type of the Renaissance. It is characterized by a horizontal stroke in the "e" and by a pointed "A". The "A" of the older Roman types, including that of the 1543 edition of the *Fabrica*, had a small stroke over the point. In the 1543 edition, marginal notes are placed in the outside margins of the first four pages, but thereafter they appear also in the inside margins; the notes in the outer margins refer to the contents of the text, and those in the inner margins are cross-references to the illustrations (see plate XXIIIb). The cross-references continue through all seven books – no mean achievement, and probably the work of the author himself.

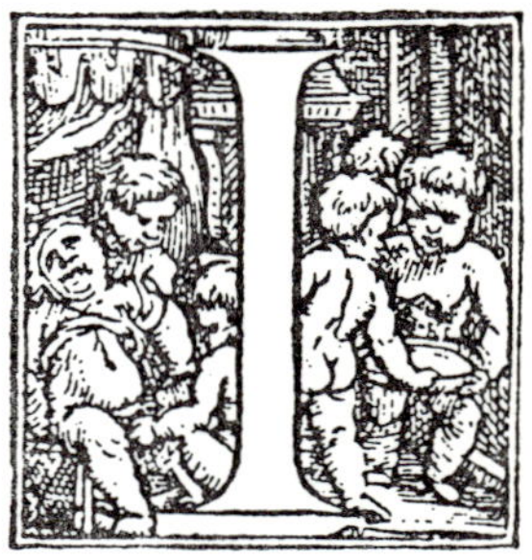

Each of the seven "books," and each of the two hundred and eight chapters, begins with an ornamented capital letter. The scenes shown in these capital-letter illustrations were undoubtedly also conceived by the author: they depict the art of dissection (legitimate and illegitimate procurement of corpses, techniques of dissection, vivisection), surgery (blood-letting, catheterization, fontanelle cautery, theory of fractures), and obstetrics. An "L" from HANS HOLBEIN'S alphabet shows a symbolic child in the act of defecating – the sole "internal" motif. For the second edition of 1555, new and somewhat larger initials were cut, preserving the original motifs, but on the whole they are of slightly poorer quality.[10] H. S. FRANCIS has been shown that the production of new initials for the second edition was a necessary consequence of the adoption of another, larger typeface.[11]

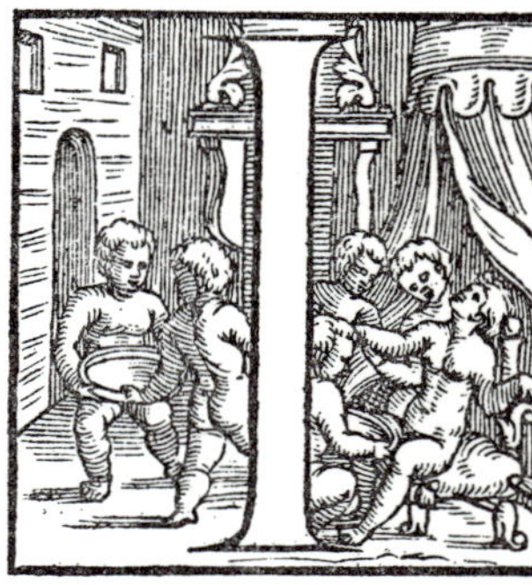

Figures 190 and 191 The initial 'I' in the 1543 edition (above) and the 1555 edition (below).

The two great editions of the *Fabrica* were published in Basel by JOHANNES OPORINUS (HANS HERBST). The reason why VESALIUS did not have his book printed in Venice has often been discussed.[12] It is certain that he had been connected with the Basel publishers before, and that he had worked for several years as an author for the partnership of PLATER, RUCH/LAZIUS, WINTER, and HERBST/OPORINUS, which had emerged as the successor of ANDREAS CRATANDER. When the *Fabrica* was ready for typesetting, OPORINUS was the sole owner of the publishing house, which under

[10] HERRLINGER, ROBERT: Die Initialen in der "Fabrica" des Andreas Vesalius, in: Acta Medicae Historiae Patavina, Padova, *X*, 1963-64, pp. 97-117.

[11] FRANCIS, H. S.: The woodcut initials of the Fabrica, in: Bull. Med. Libr. Assoc. *31*, 1943, pp. 228-39.

[12] ROTH, *op. cit.*, p. 129; CUSHING, *op. cit.* p. 75; but also IVINS, WILLIAM M. JR.: What about the Fabrica of Vesalius? in: Three Vesalian Essays, pp. 78 ff.; O'MALLEY, 1964, *op. cit.*, p. 133. For details on the publisher Oporinus, see FISCH, MAX H.: The printer of Vesalius's Fabrica, in: Bull. Med. Libr. Assoc. *31*, 1943, pp. 240-59, and ROSTENBERG, LEONA: Johann Oporin, Printer, Publisher, and Scholar, 1507-68; in: Library Quarterly *14*, 1944, pp. 207-13.

his expert management had already become famous throughout Europe. He took special care to read the proofs himself, which must have particularly recommended him to a perfectionist like VESALIUS. Moreover, OPORINUS was sympathetic toward the modern developments of his time, and he risked several sensational publications, such as a Latin edition of the Koran during the wars against the Turks – an affront to public opinion – which shortly afterwards led to his imprisonment. The *Fabrica* was also a potentially explosive work, with its new teaching methods and its taunts against prevailing dogma. It has been repeatedly surmised that VESALIUS trusted the Venetian authorities less than he did the council of the city of Basel. Nevertheless, it appears not only that the illustrations were designed in Italy, but that the woodcuts were also executed there. Unless appearances deceive, then, all the praise expressed by twentieth-century admirers of the engravings in the *Fabrica* should actually be conferred on the Venetians rather than on artists in Basel.[13]

It is the illustrations that have contributed primarily to the fame of the *Fabrica* in our century. The text has probably only been read by a few specialists, who, naturally, have mainly concentrated on specific chapters. Text and illustrations, however, comprise a unit, and should properly be discussed together.

The *Fabrica* is amply illustrated, but it is not an anatomical atlas. While he was writing his textbook, VESALIUS had already become aware of the demand for such an atlas, and in 1543 OPORINUS brought out the *Epitome* – published in German, this book for students was also intended for surgeons, and apparently it sold very well. It was conceived independently of the *Fabrica* to a large extent, not least in respect of the illustrations, and it was soon translated into other languages: into English in 1553, Dutch in 1569, and French in 1569.[14]

Fig. 192 Vesalius, 1538, Table III of the Tabulae Sex: *Arterial system showing heart, kidneys and brain plexus.*

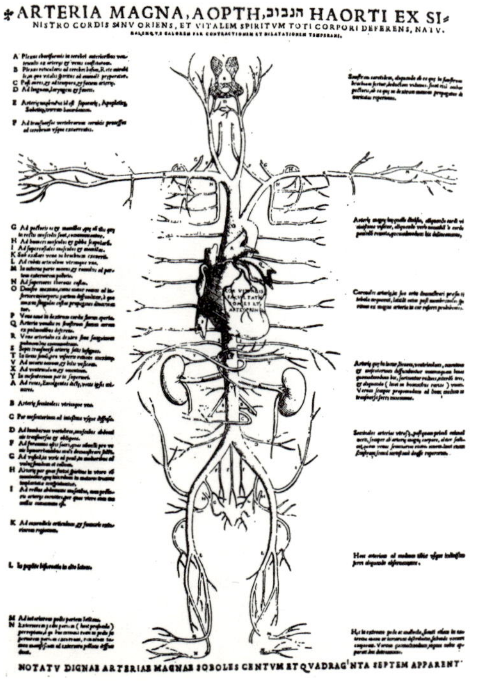

The precursor of both the *Fabrica* and the *Epitome* was the *Tabulae sex* of 1538, which consisted of six single sheets with anatomical illustrations. The six *Tabulae anatomicae*, as VESALIUS called them, contained illustrations arranged in two groups of three. The first group was made up of Table I, showing semi-schematic representations of the portal vein system with the reproductive organs next to it; Table II, showing the entire venous system; and Table III, showing the arterial system. The second group, Tables IV-VI, showed the skeleton from the front, in profile from the right, and from the back. Since CHOULANT, these sheets have been among the favorites of students of VESALIUS,[15] but only two complete sets have been

13 WIEGAND, WILLY: Marginal Notes by the Printer of the Icones, in: Three Vesalian Essays to Accompany the Icones Anatomicae of 1934, The History of Medicine Series, ed. Library New York Acad. Med. No. 11, New York, Macmillan, 1952.

14 The English surgeons initially received the Latin text of the *Epitome* together with illustrations by GEMINUS (see p. 121).

15 Facsimile editions: London, 1874, ed. SIR WILLIAM STIRLING-MAXWELL; Leipzig, 1920, ed. M. HOLL and K. SÜDHOFF; New York/Munich, 1934, ed. New York Academy of Medicine and Univ. Lib. Munich, as appendix to the *Icones anatomicae* of the Bremer Presse, and in SINGER, CHARLES and C. RABIN: A Prelude to Modern Science. Being a Discussion of the History, Sources and Circumstances of the *Tabulae anatomicae sex* of Vesalius, Cambridge, 1946. These works provide the illustrations for SANDERS, J. B. de C. M. and CHARLES D. O'MALLEY: The Illustrations from the Works of Andreas Vesalius of Brussels, Cleveland/New York, 1950.

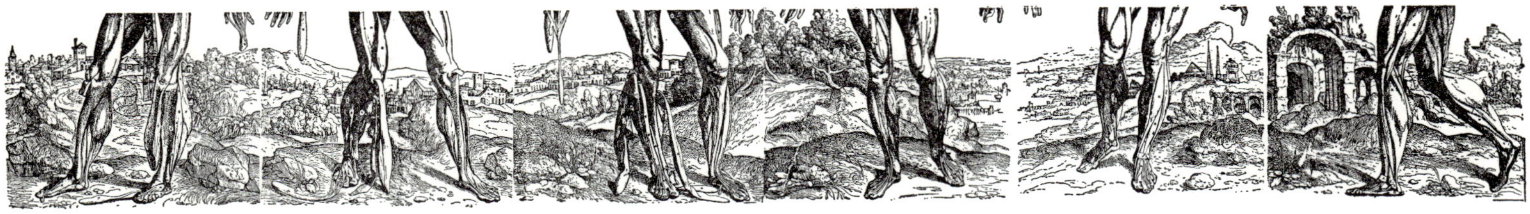

discovered. Modern historical research has been misled by VESALIUS'S own boasting into considerably overrating them. Compared with those in ESTIENNE'S *De dissectione*, the skeletons are to be preferred in some respects, but in several details they are inferior. The *De dissectione* skeletons of 1532 are definitely of lower quality, but later examples, which were printed in 1539, were not necessarily copied after those in the *Tabulae anatomicae* of 1538. In any case, the muscle figures in the *De dissectione*, dated 1532, represent the same stage of stylistic development as VESALIUS'S skeletons of 1538.

The woodcuts in the *Fabrica* vary considerably in size and importance. The book explores the whole range of possibilities open to medical illustration, and in this respect it is far superior to the *De dissectione*. This is VESALIUS'S own achievement. Among the large woodcuts, each occupying a whole page, are the full-figure illustrations for osteology and myology. The most brilliant graphic art work in the *Fabrica* is contained in these plates. The fourteen muscle figures form a series of closely related illustrations which are linked by a continuous background motif, a magnificent panorama which has been indentified as a landscape view of the Colli Euganei region near Padua (figs. 193-194).[16] Even in this respect, however, the *Fabrica* is not without precedent. In Book I of the *De dissectione*, there were several plates with background landscapes of remarkably high quality (figs. 149, 195). The tradition itself is even older, and can be traced in a direct line through BERENGARIO (1521) back to the scholastic title-page woodcut in the *Mondino* edition of POLLICH (see p. 63), and thence to the incunabula and to medieval illustrations.

Criticism of the muscle figures and skeletons in the *Fabrica* has, for obvious reasons, fastened upon an elementary problem of anatomical illustration.[17] The series consists largely of figures of "living" cadavers, which, depending on the critic's point of view, can be interpreted either as an absurdity or as a deliberate artifice. Portrayals of "living" skeletons and muscle figures had been in use since LEONARDO DA VINCI (see p. 70), and all the illustrations of the surface musculature belong to this category. IVINS, in a logical analysis based upon his own experience, has explained that such illustrations are works of art, and that only very competent artists are capable of creating convincing solutions to the problems posed by illus-

Fig. 195 Background from Estienne, La dissection, *1546. Detail from fig. 149.*

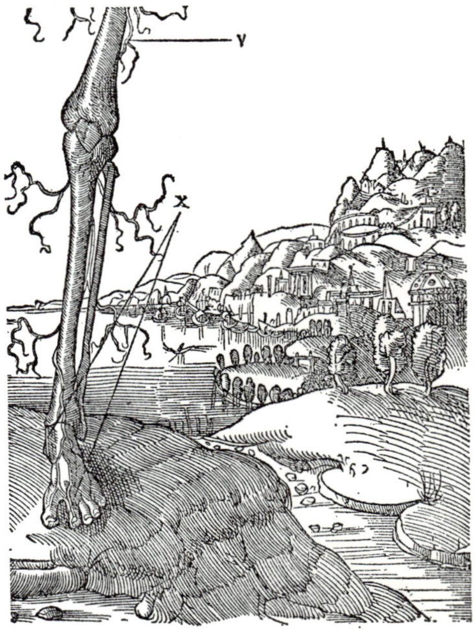

16 WIEGAND, *op. cit.*, pp. 40 ff., but previously by E. JACKSCHATH: Mitt. Gesch. Med. Naturw. *2*, 1903, p. 282 and Janus *9*, 1904, p. 238; CUSHING, *op. cit.*, p. 87.

17 IVINS, pp. 87 ff.; ROTH, *op. cit.*, pp. 155 ff.; SAUNDERS and O'MALLEY, *op. cit.*, p. 25; JACKSCHATH, *op. cit.*; IVINS.

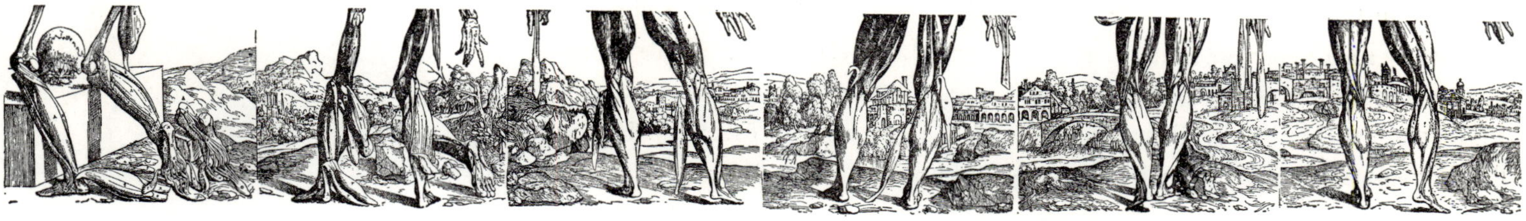

Figures 193 and 194

tration of this type.[18] Whether JAN STEVENSZOON VAN CALCAR was such an artist, or whether TITIAN himself sketched the poses and only the anatomical details can be ascribed to JAN STEVENSZOON (or some other pupil of TITIAN), cannot be determined on the basis of our present knowledge. But there is still no reason for denying VESALIUS credit for having conceived the complete program of illustration.

The full-figure illustrations in Books I and II are by no means the most original feature of the *Fabrica,* though they may be the most spectacular. It should not be forgotten that most of the illustration plates for the *De dissectione* had already been printed when VESALIUS was in Paris. The first two muscle figures of the *Fabrica,* which, as he himself explains, were drawn for purely artistic purposes, belong to the same type as the muscle figures of the *De dissectione.* A direct comparison with the Parisian work, however, clearly shows that VESALIUS took anatomical illustration a decisive step further. The authors of the *De dissectione* had used full-figure drawings of the human body for almost all of their anatomical illustrations and, since this

[18] See comments by the anatomist C. ELZE who – together with VESALIUS – speaks of the "homo absolutus," by which he means that only the anatomist can know him. ELZE, CURT: Vesals Anatomie, in: Zschr. Anat. Entwick. Gesch. *124*, 1964, p. 240, and especially the relevant footnote 34.

Figures 196 to 198 Three muscle figures, dorsal view. Left and center figures from Estienne, the center one dated '1532'; righthand figure from Vesalius's Fabrica *of 1543.*

Fig. 196

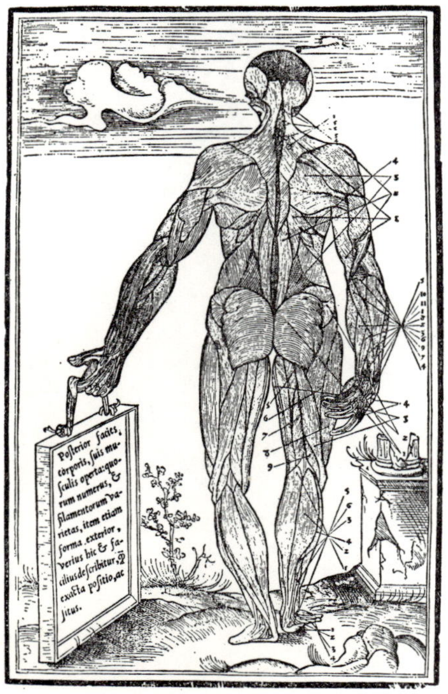

Fig. 197

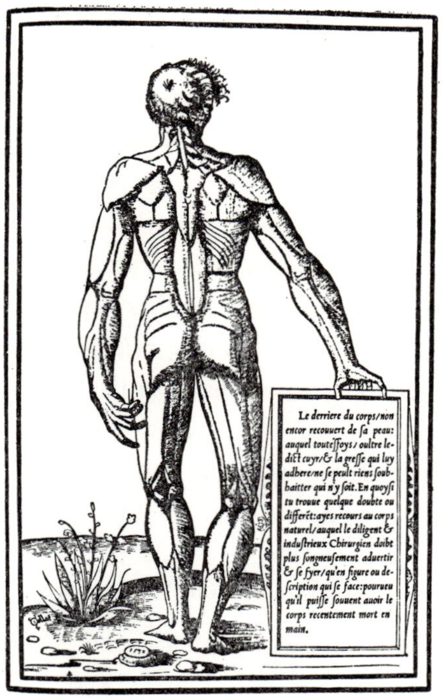

Fig. 198

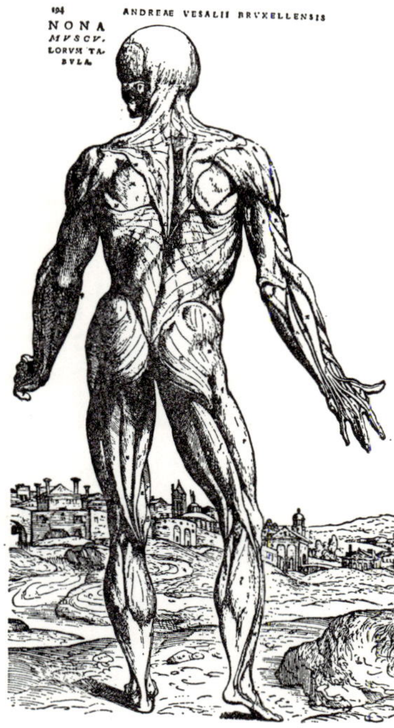

kind of illustration is almost useless for showing details, had failed[19] to illustrate adequately such important features as the viscera (Book II) and the female reproductive organs (Book III). VESALIUS, however, included illustrations of details within the text from the very start of the *Fabrica*, beginning with osteology. He did this in two ways: (a) by arranging groups of illustrations of details together at the beginning of each chapter, with extensive legends, and (b) by repeating single details throughout the text where for pedagogical reasons, repetitions were necessary.[20] In addition to full-figure illustrations and illustrations of details – all drawn from nature – we also find a third kind of illustration: schematic or semi-schematic diagrams, which are also built into the text (figs. 200, 201).

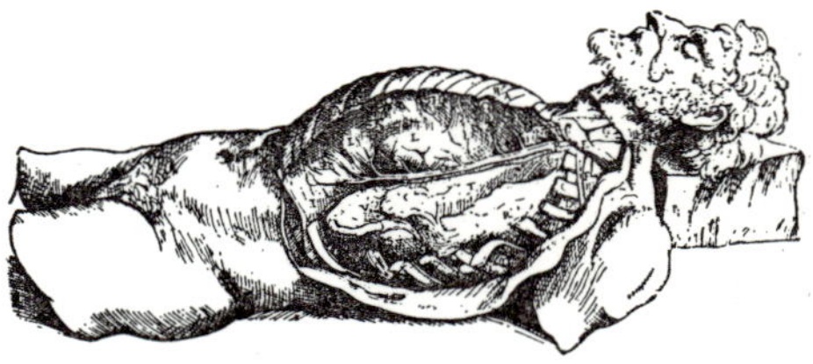

Fig. 199 Torso of a corpse from Vesalius's Fabrica, *Book VI, fig. I.*

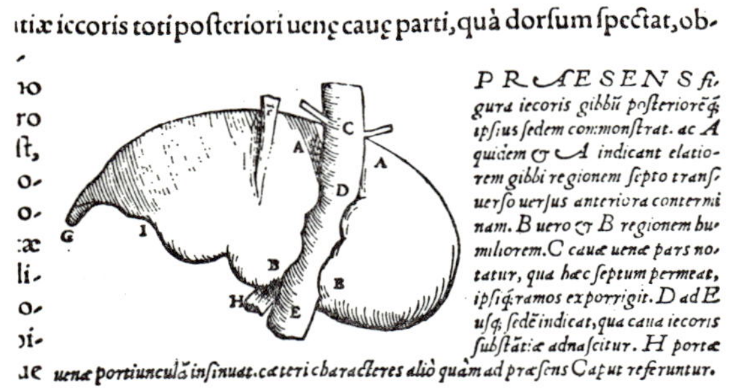

ıtiæ iecoris toti posteriori uenę cauę parti, quà dorsum spectat, ob-

PRÆSENS figura iecoris gibbū posterioreq́; ipsius sedem commonstrat. ac A quidem & A indicant elatiorem gibbi regionem septo transuerso uersus anteriora conterminam. B uero & B regionem humiliorem. C cauæ uenæ pars notatur, qua hæc septum permeat, ipsiq́; ramos exporrigit. D ad E usq; sedē indicat, qua caua iecoris substātiæ adnascitur. H portæ uenæ portiunculā insinuat. cæteri characteres aliò quàm ad præsens Caput referuntur.

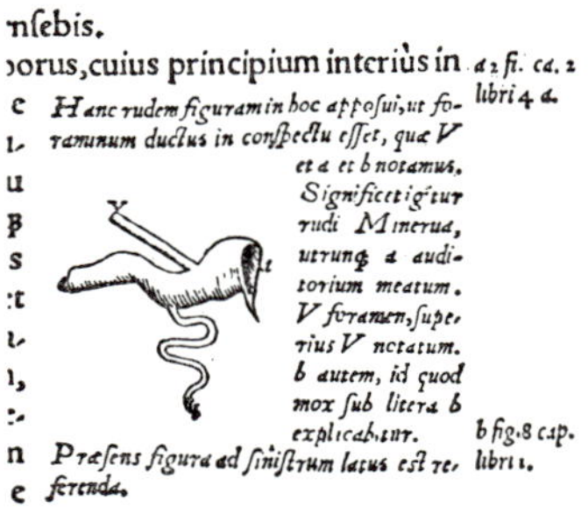

nſebis.

ɔorus, cuius principium interiùs in

Hanc rudem figuram in hoc apposui, ut foraminum ductus in conspectu esset, quæ V et a et b notamus. Significet igitur rudi Minerua, utrunq; a auditorium meatum. V foramen, superius V notatum. b autem, id quod mox sub litera b explicabitur.

Præsens figura ad sinistrum latus est referenda.

a 2 fi. ca. 2 libri 4 a.

b fig. 8 cap. libri 1.

Figures 200 and 201

VESALIUS used a novel method for representing the viscera: as though he were familiar with the Parisian attempt to solve this problem and had perceived its faults, he used torsos to set off his situs figures (figs. 203–210), thus dispensing with the complete body. However, these partial figures are not all drawn in the style of classical torsos. Several are artistically unsatisfying, the impression of an autopsy on the corpse being dominant. In fact, the two figures demonstrating the thoracic situs dispense altogether with the illusion of a living body and show what is clearly a cadaver on the dissecting table (fig. 199). (In JUAN VALVERDE'S adaptation, published in Rome in 1560, VESALIUS'S two thoracic situs figures were combined into a macabre double figure, in which one cadaver is exploring the opened thorax of the other in the manner of a demonstrating anatomist; see figure 202.) The drawings of the anatomy of the heart (figs. 212, 213) represent the extracted organ in the most diverse stages of anatomical dissection. We are familiar with one earlier illustration of the dissection of extracted organs in the one existing plate prepared by HANS WÄCHTLIN for JOHANNES SCHOTT (1517), reprinted in the *Spiegel der Artzny* of LORENZ PHRYES (fig. 82).

In VESALIUS'S work, the detail illustration finally supersedes the traditional full-figure illustration. VESALIUS was certainly not the first anatomist to illustrate

Fig. 202 Valverde (see pp. 123-27): Double figure illustrating thoracic viscera comprising two figures from Vesalius (Book VI, fig. 1 and fig. 2).

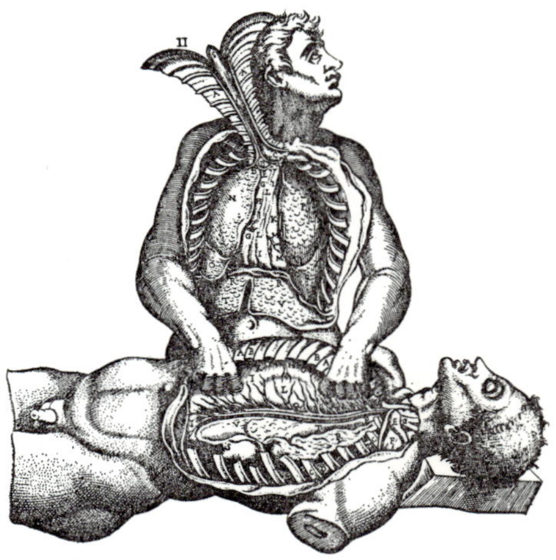

[19] The illustrations of the individual muscles, which were apparently added after 1539, are typical examples.

[20] The repetition of the initials "E" and "F" on p. 329 in Book IV (1543 edition) should also be considered in this context.

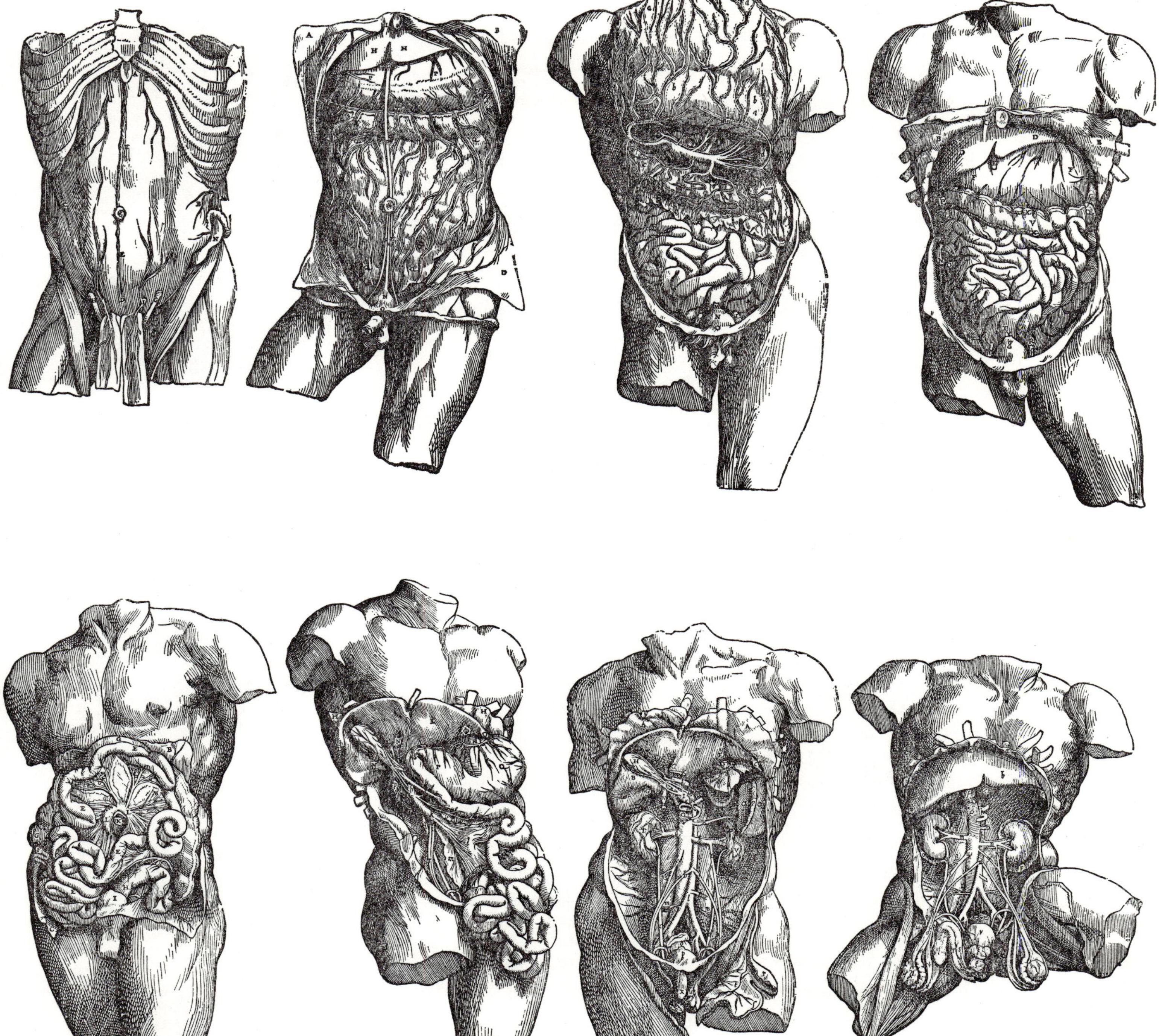

Figures 203 to 210 Vesalius's Fabrica, *1543, Book V: Eight figures illustrating the abdominal viscera. Compare the similar figures in Estienne,* De dissectione *(p. 94).*

details – apart from LEONARDO, we need only think of GERSSDORFF, DRYANDFR, and CANANO – but the success of the *Fabrica* sealed the fate of the full figure as the framework for detail illustration, particularly with regard to the viscera. VESALIUS'S torso was a concession to popular taste, and perhaps a sign of his respect for a tradition which – through his use of this device – was actually prolonged. It was, after all, only an interim solution.

The illustration of individual parts of the body – bones and soft parts, including the tongue and brain – as material objects which cast shadows, indicates that the model must have lain on a table in front of the artist.[21] VESALIUS himself says (on page 562 of the 1543 edition) that omission of the topographical relations, after they have been pictured once, assists the understanding of the observer. The different treatments of shadows in different illustrations may be a clue to distinguishing

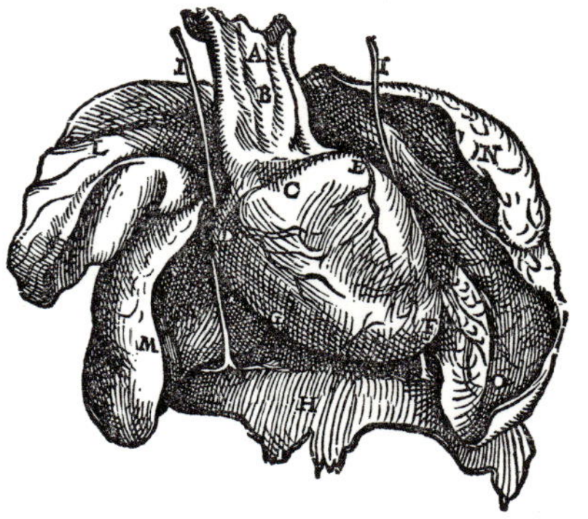

Fig. 212 Andreas Vesalius, 1543: Heart in intact pericardium, surrounded by the lungs and part of the diaphragm. Isolated detail of the thoracic situs.

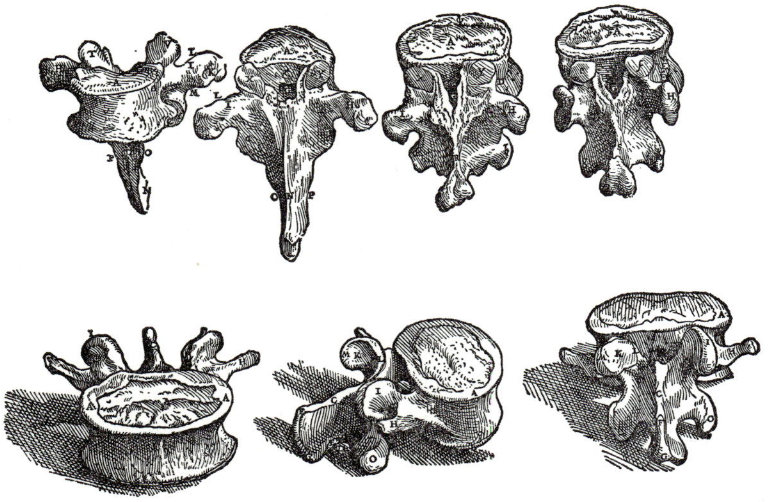

Fig. 211 Illustration of vertebrae from Vesalius's Fabrica. *Top row: without shadowing (Book I, Chap. XVI, figs. 1-4). Bottom row: with shadow-hatching (Book I, Chap. XVII, figs. 1-3).*

the different artists who worked on the *Fabrica.* At least one artist has differentiated between complete shadow (shown by cross-hatching) and half-shadow (shown by simple line-shading). Since this is the technique used on the title page and in the full-figure illustrations of osteology and myology, and since it is also present in a very prominent form in the *Tabulae sex,* these illustrations can be attributed to JAN STEVENSZOON VAN CALCAR.[22]

VESALIUS laid special stress on the shadowing in the illustrations for his work. Not all of his contemporaries, however, were pleased by the appearance of naturalistic shadowing in illustrations of anatomical details. SYLVIUS, who had been VESALIUS'S teacher in Paris, singled out this technique for special reproof. SYLVIUS also criticized the identifying inscriptions used in many of the figures. As we have shown, the Parisian authors of the *De dissectione* had used indication lines to identify

Fig. 213 Andreas Vesalius, 1543: Pericardium opened, otherwise as fig. 212. Both illustrations are abstracted to such an extent that they appear without deep shadows.

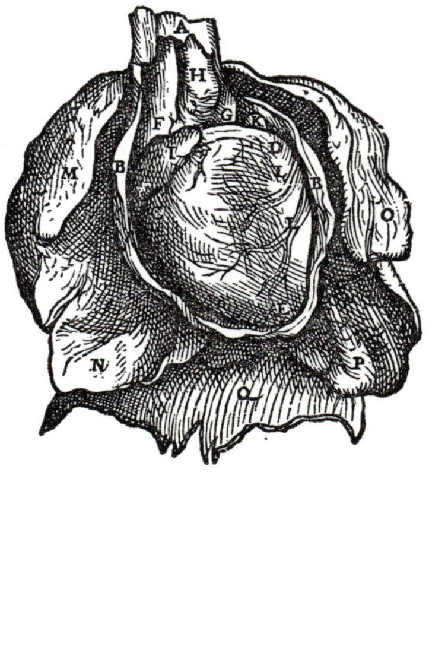

21 The same applies to the plates in the *Epitome* where, for example, the eyes and larynx lie on the ground at the feet of the full figure, which physically stands on the ground.

22 There are several illustrations of lower quality which have primitive shading – in contrast to the large group without shading, for example, the brain, IV, fig. 1; kidney, V, fig. 21.

features in an illustration. This was also the method used in the KETHAM illustrations. In contrast, DRYANDER (1536), or at least one of DRYANDER'S artists, had used letters inscribed on the figure, with an explanatory key provided in the text. This device, which was undoubtedly employed for aesthetic reasons, seems to have first been used in Italy. It was employed by LEONARDO, and is frequently encountered in Italian book illustration of the early 16th century. It is found in the two VITRUVIUS editions published in Venice in 1511 and in Florence in 1513, but it occurs even more extensively, and in a manner quite consistent with its use in the Vesalian anatomies, in the splendid edition published by[23] CESARE CESARIANO[24] in Como in 1519/21. This method was firmly established in medical illustration by VESALIUS, even if he was not the first to use it. The occasional poor legibility (occurring when

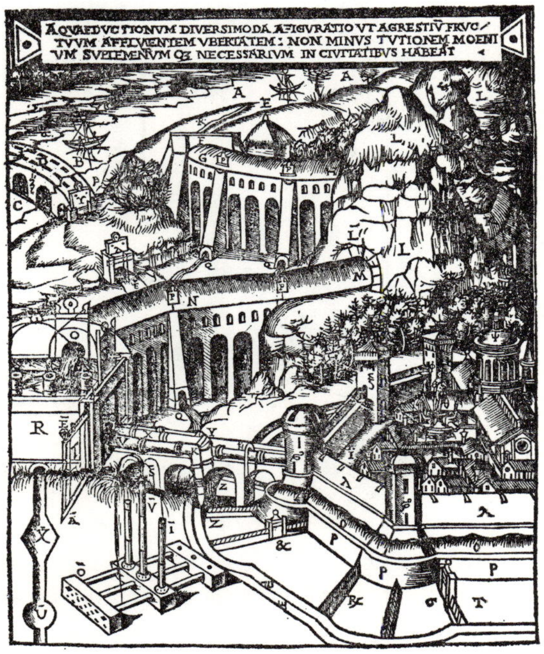

Fig. 214 Cesare Cesariano, illustration using inscribed letters to identify various items, from an edition of Vitruvius, 1519/21. The same technique was used later in Vesalius's Fabrica.

a letter was inscribed on a part of a figure that was already shadowed) was lessened in the second edition of the *Fabrica* by improving the woodblocks. A Basel wood engraver exposed the most indistinct letters with a fine knife.

WILLY WIEGAND – who is the most respected authority on these famous woodcuts, as far as their technical aspects are concerned – printed the *Icones anatomicae* from the old woodblocks at his Bremer Presse in 1935. He wrote that the condition of the woodblocks was "as though they had been cut today."[25] Even the most delicate lines were still absolutely clear except for negligible small abrasions. This is puzzling when we consider that the early editions are held to have run to some three thousand or four thousand copies. WIEGAND assures us, however, that woodblocks do not wear

[23] Or by his followers.
[24] See THIEME-BECKER *VI*, 1912, pp. 312-13.
[25] WIEGAND, *op. cit.*

Fig. 215

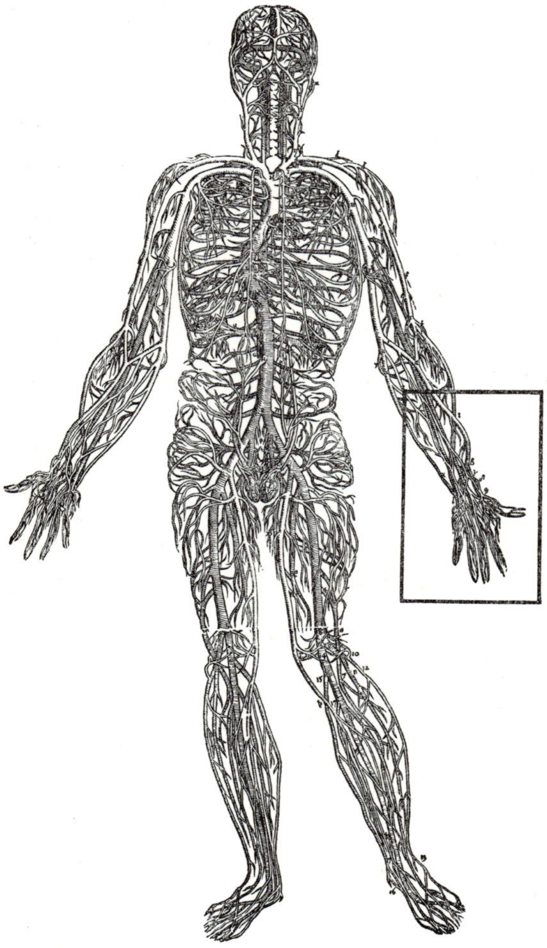

Fig. 216

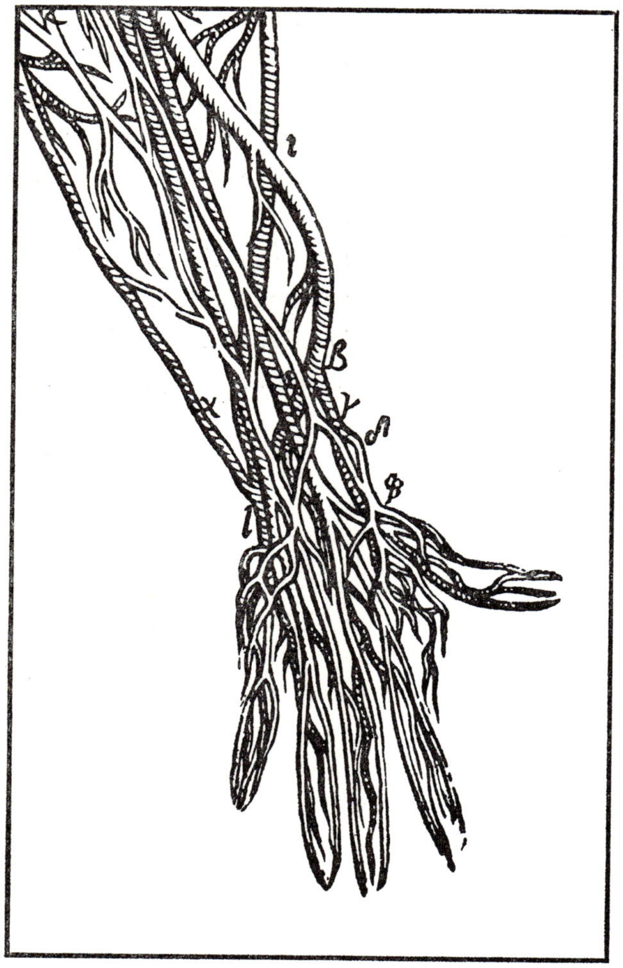

Figures 215 and 216 Vein figure from the third book of the Fabrica. *The detail marked in fig. 215 has been enlarged in fig. 216 to show the inscriptions in small Latin and Greek letters.*

if they are impressed on moist paper, and apparently they wear even less when they are made of birchwood which has been treated with hot linseed oil before engraving. But the care shown by the original printers was only partly responsible for the good preservation of the woodblocks: the excellent craftmanship of the engravers must also be taken into account. The Venetian artists who represented shadow by means of parallel and hatched lines chose to cut obliquely rather than at right angles to the surface, with the result that the reglet gives somewhat during printing and produces incredibly delicate lines.

None of these features of the *Fabrica* which we have examined in this chapter – the type and layout, the use of details rather than full-figure illustrations, the achievement of a three-dimensional effect with shadow and half-shadow, the use of inscribed letters and explanatory keys instead of indication lines – were discovered by VESALIUS or his artists. All of them, however, were used to their full potential in the *Fabrica*, and together they help to make the *Fabrica* the greatest

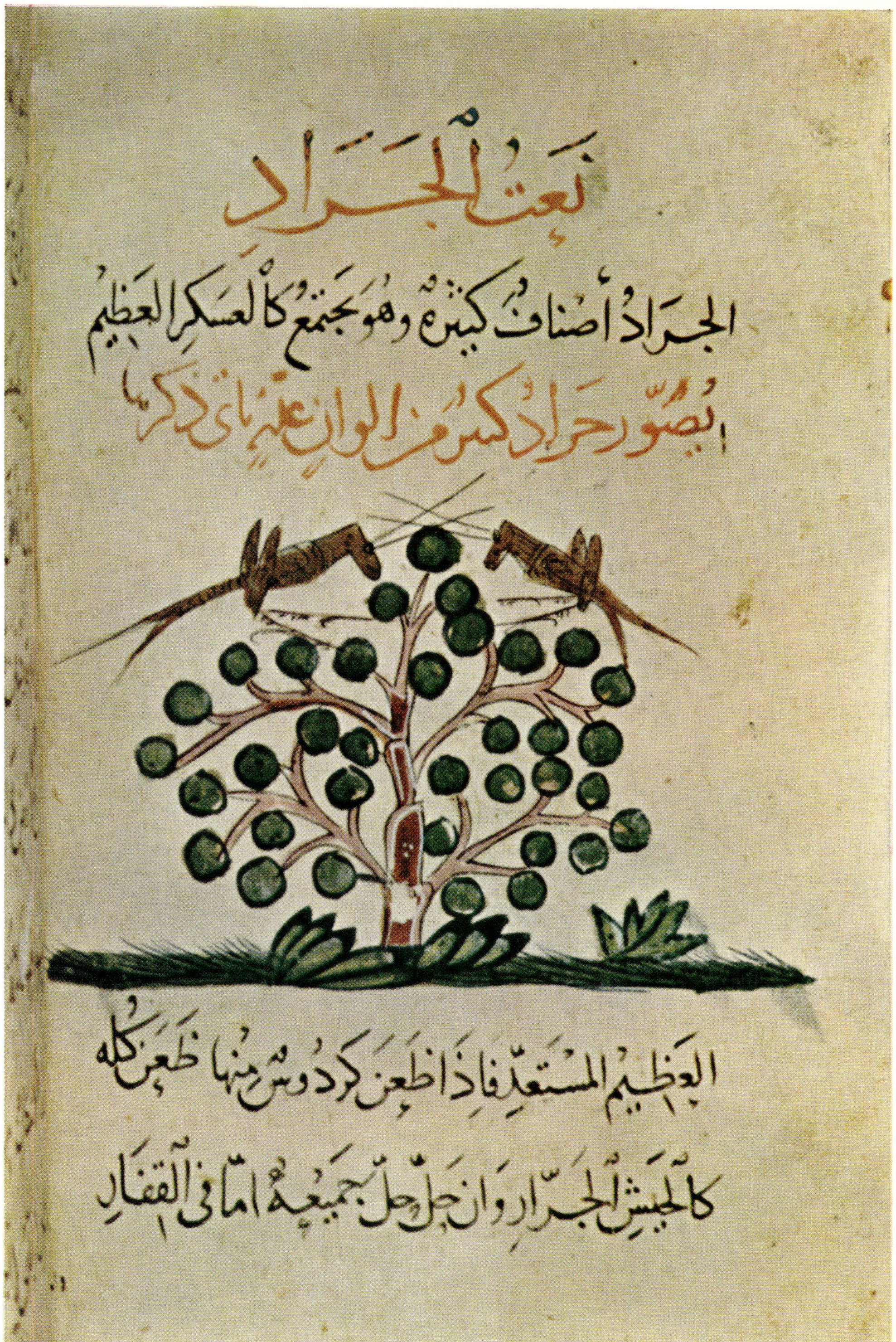

Plate XIX From an Arabic bestiary (Animal Medicaments), *a 13th-century compilation from Aristotle and 'Ubayd Allah B. Jabra'īl B. Bakhtīshū.' MS. Or. 2784, fol. 60 b, British Museum, London.*

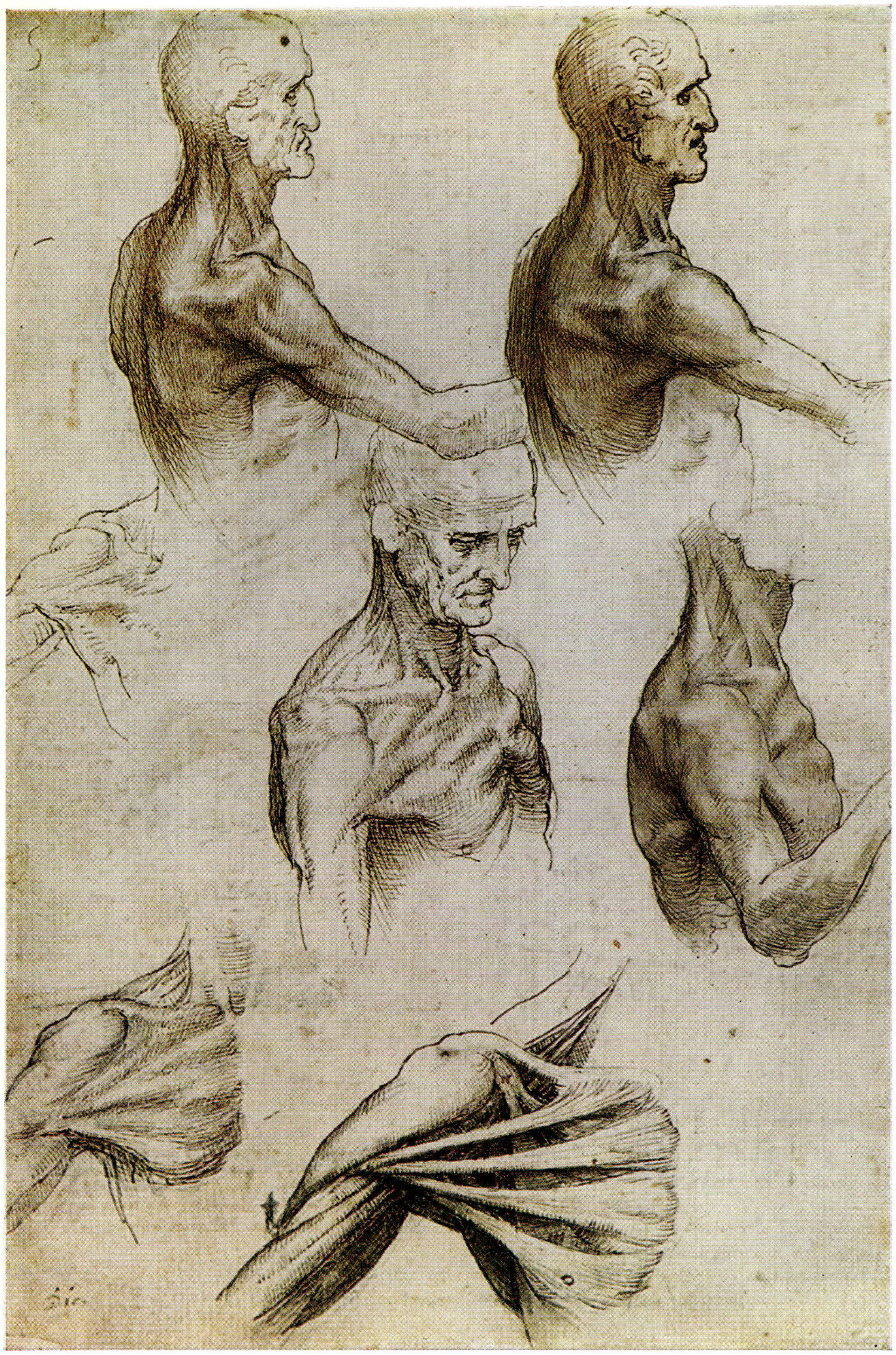

Plate XX Leonardo da Vinci: Study sheet for the anatomy of the shoulder and arm musculature. Fogli A 2^v, Windsor 19001. Pen and ink drawing, circa 1510, The Royal Library, Windsor Castle. By gracious permission of H.M. the Queen, also granted for the Leonardo illustrations reproduced in Plate XXI and on pages 68-74 and page 79.

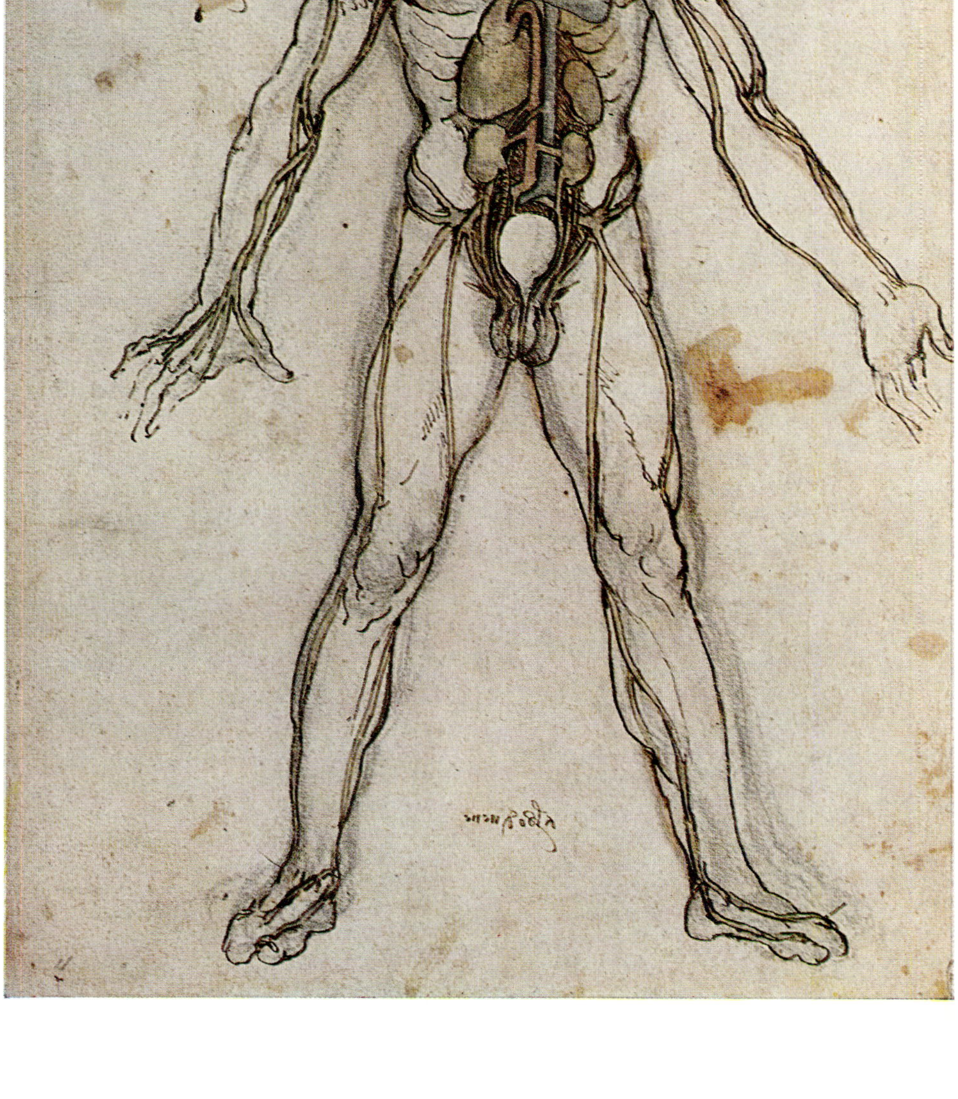

Plate XXI 'Large Vein Figure.' Quaderni V^r, Windsor 12597, before 1500. The deep vessels are 'reconstructed' from Mondino, the superficial vessels reproduced from observation.

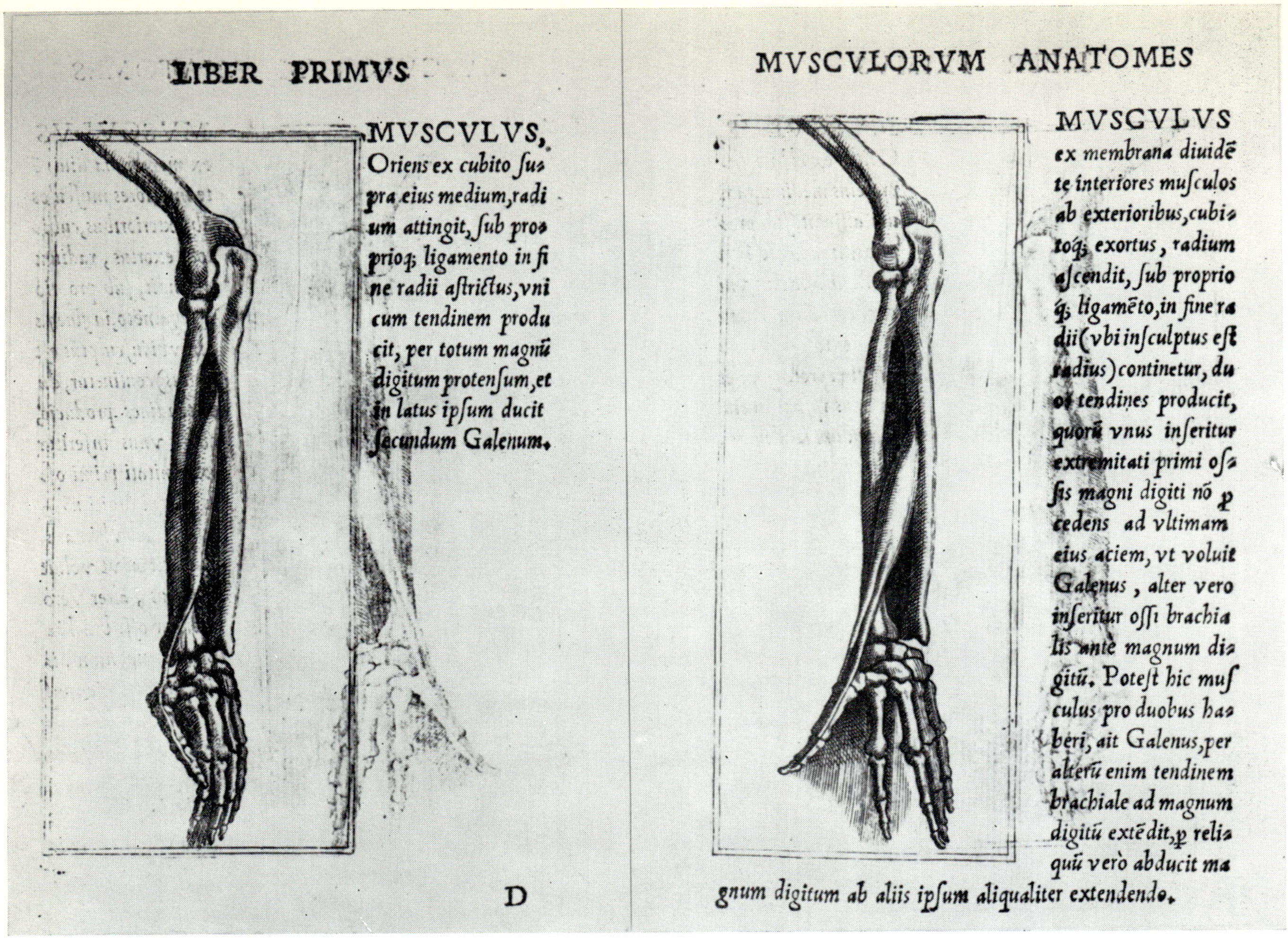
LIBER PRIMVS

MVSCVLVS, Oriens ex cubito supra eius medium, radium attingit, sub proprioq; ligamento in fine radii astrictus, vnicum tendinem producit, per totum magnũ digitum protensum, et in latus ipsum ducit secundum Galenum.

D

MVSCVLORVM ANATOMES

MVSCVLVS ex membrana diuidẽte interiores musculos ab exterioribus, cubitoq; exortus, radium ascendit, sub proprioq; ligamẽto, in fine radii (vbi insculptus est radius) continetur, duos tendines producit, quorũ vnus inseritur extremitati primi ossis magni digiti nõ procedens ad vltimam eius aciem, vt voluit Galenus, alter vero inseritur ossi brachialis ante magnum digitũ. Potest hic musculus pro duobus haberi, ait Galenus, per alterũ enim tendinem brachiale ad magnum digitũ extẽdit, per reliquũ vero abducit magnum digitum ab aliis ipsum aliqualiter extendendo.

Plate XXIIa A sheet from Canano's fragme[nt on] myology (front [and] reverse side).

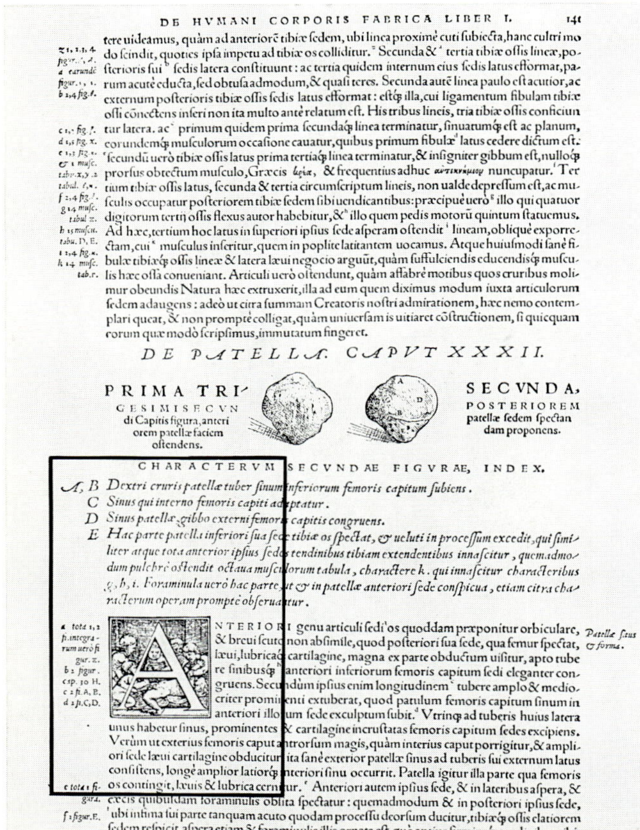
DE HVMANI CORPORIS FABRICA LIBER I. 141

tere uideamus, quàm ad anteriorẽ tibiæ sedem, ubi linea proximè cuti subiecta, hanc cultri modo scindit, quoties ipsa impetu ad tibiæ os colliditur. Secunda & tertia tibiæ ossis lineæ, posterioris sui sedis latera constituunt: ac tertia quidem internum eius sedis latus efformat, parum acutè educta, sed obtusa admodum, & quasi teres. Secunda autẽ linea paulo est acutior, ac externum posterioris tibiæ ossis sedis latus efformat: estq; illa, cui ligamentum fibulam tibiæ ossi cõnectens inseri non ita multo antè relatum est. His tribus lineis, tria tibiæ ossis conficiuntur latera. ac primum quidem prima secundaq; linea terminatur, sinuatumq; est ac planum, corundemq; musculorum occasione cauatur, quibus primum fibulæ latus cedere dictum est. secundũ uerò tibiæ ossis latus prima tertiaq; linea terminatur, & insigniter gibbum est, nulloq; prorsus obtectum musculo, Græcis ἀκρα, & frequentius adhuc ἀντικνήμιον nuncupatur. Tertium tibiæ ossis latus, secunda & tertia circumscriptum lineis, non ualde depressum est, ac musculis occupatur posteriorem tibiæ sedem sibi uendicantibus: præcipuè uerò illo qui quatuor digitorum tertij ossis flexus autor habebitur, & illo quem pedis motorũ quintum statuemus. Ad hæc, tertium hoc latus in superiori ipsius sede asperam ostendit lineam, obliquè exporrectam, cui musculus inseritur, quem in poplite latitantem uocamus. Atque huiusmodi sanè fibulæ tibiæq; ossis lineæ & latera læui negocio arguũt, quàm suffulciendis educendisq; musculis hæc ossa conueniant. Articuli uerò ostendunt, quàm affabrè motibus quos cruribus molimur obeundis Natura hæc extruxerit, illa ad eum quem diximus modum iuxta articulorum sedem adaugens: adeò ut citra summam Creatoris nostri admirationem, hæc nemo contemplari queat, & non promptè colligat, quàm uniuersam is uitiaret cõstructionem, si quicquam eorum quæ modò scripsimus, immutatum fingeret.

DE PATELLA. CAPVT XXXII.

PRIMA TRIGESIMISECVNDI Capitis figura, anteriorem patellæ faciem ostendens.

SECVNDA, POSTERIOREM patellæ sedem spectandam proponens.

CHARACTERVM SECVNDAE FIGVRAE, INDEX.

A, B Dextri cruris patellæ tuber sinum inferiorum femoris capitum subiens.
C Sinus qui interno femoris capiti adaptatur.
D Sinus patellæ, gibbo externi femoris capitis congruens.
E Hac parte patella inferiori sua sede tibiæ os spectat, & ueluti in processum excedit, qui similiter atque tota anterior ipsius sedes tendinibus tibiam extendentibus innascitur, quemadmodum pulchrè ostendit octaua musculorum tabula, charactere k. qui innascitur characteribus g, h, i. Foraminula uerò hac parte, ut & in patellæ anteriori sede conspicua, etiam citra characterum operam promptè obseruatur.

ANTERIORI genu articuli sedi os quoddam præponitur orbiculare, & breui scuto non absimile, quod posteriori sua sede, qua femur spectat, læui, lubricaq; cartilagine, magna ex parte obductum uisitur, apto tubere sinibusq; anteriori inferiorum femoris capitum sedi eleganter congruens. Secundùm ipsius enim longitudinem tubere amplo & mediocriter prominenti extuberat, quod patulum femoris capitum sinum in anteriori illorum sede exculptum subit. Vtrinq; ad tuberis huius latera unus habetur sinus, prominentes & cartilagine incrustatas femoris capitum sedes excipiens. Verùm ut exterius femoris caput antrorsum magis, quàm interius caput porrigitur, & ampliori sede læui cartilagine obducitur, ita sanè exterior patellæ sinus ad tuberis sui externum latus consistens, longè amplior latiorq; interiori sinu occurrit. Patella igitur illa parte qua femoris os contingit, læuis & lubrica cernitur. Anteriori autem ipsius sede, & in lateribus aspera, & cæcis quibusdam foraminulis oblita spectatur: quemadmodum & in posteriori ipsius sede, ubi infima sui parte tanquam acuto quodam processu deorsum ducitur, tibiæq; ossis elatiorem sedem respicit, aspera etiam & foraminulis illis ornata est, quò aptius firmiusq; tendinibus tibiam extendentibus innascatur. Vniuersa enim patella, tota ipsius amplitudine sedeq;, ubi lubrica cartilagine nõ obducitur, tendinibus illis innascitur, nec femori, neq; tibiæ aliter quàm tendinum

Patellæ situs & forma.

Qui patella femoris ossi connectatur.

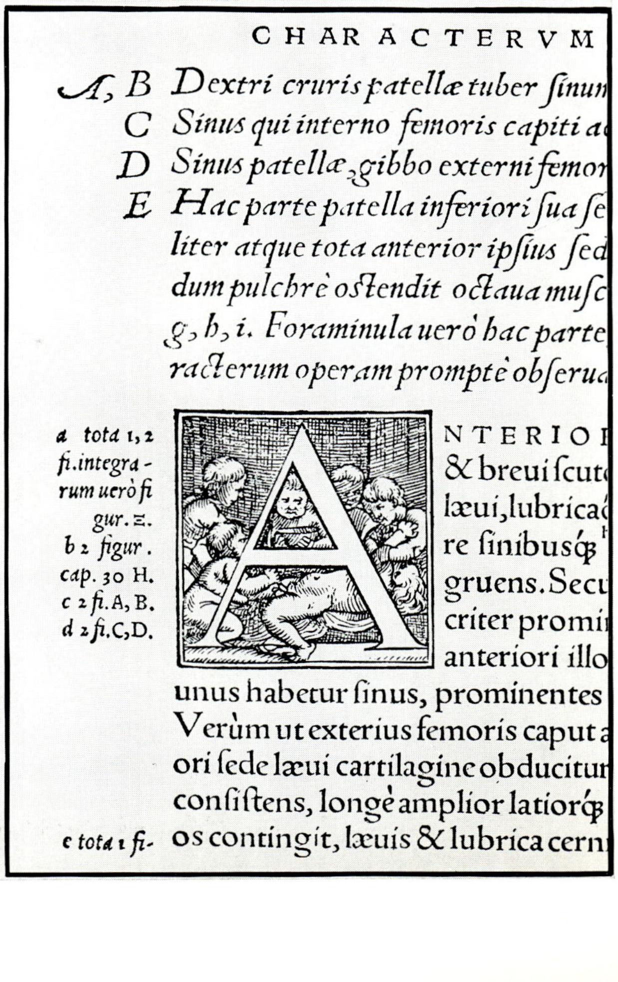
CHARACTERVM

A, B Dextri cruris patellæ tuber sinum
C Sinus qui interno femoris capiti a
D Sinus patellæ, gibbo externi femor
E Hac parte patella inferiori sua se
liter atque tota anterior ipsius sed
dum pulchrè ostendit octaua musc
g, h, i. Foraminula uerò hac parte
racterum operam promptè obserua

a tota 1, 2 fi. integrarum uerò figur. z.
b 2 figur. cap. 30 H.
c 2 fi. A, B.
d 2 fi. C, D.

ANTERIOR
& breui scut
læui, lubrica
re sinibusq;
gruens. Secu
criter promi
anteriori illo
unus habetur sinus, prominentes
Verùm ut exterius femoris caput a
ori sede læui cartilagine obducitur
consistens, longè amplior latiorq;
e tota 1 fi- os contingit, læuis & lubrica cern

Plate XXIIb A page of text from t[he] first book of the Fa[brica] 1543: The top half [and] the detail (right) sh[ow] the key to the lette[rs A] to E inscribed on [...] (ch. 32), illustrating [the] posterior view of the patella. Next to the initial 'A' and the l[...] line there are cross references to other illustrations. Referen[ces] to the textual conte[nt] are given in the ri[ght] hand margin.

Fig. 217

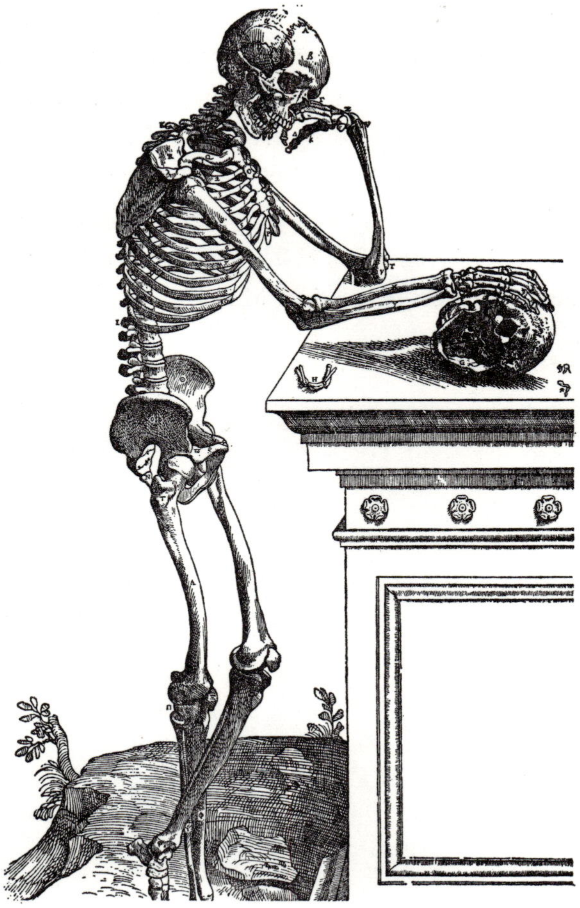

Fig. 218

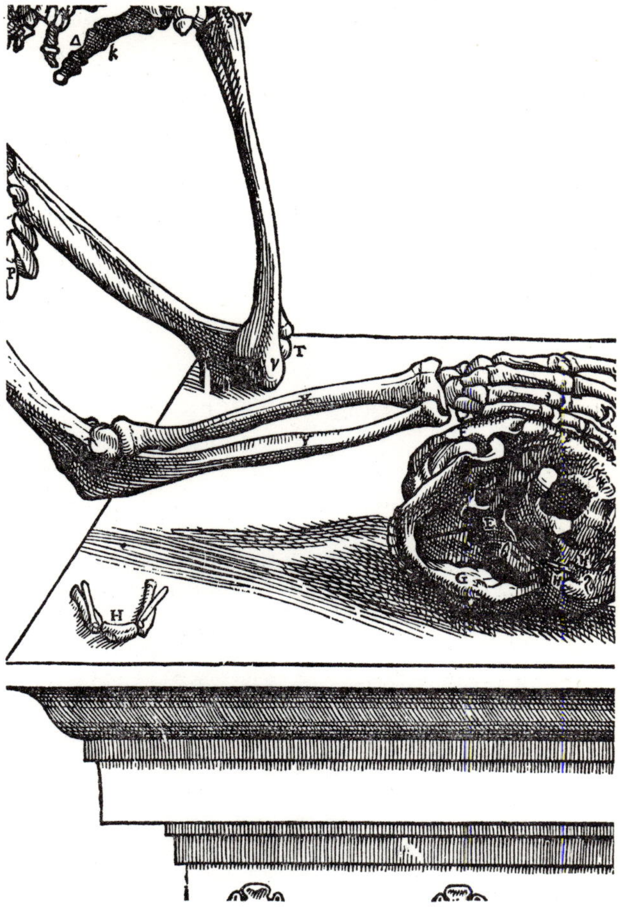

Figures 217 and 218 Second skeleton figure from the first book of the Fabrica *(left). The illustration on the right shows a detail from this figure at a point where the subtle technique of the engraving is impressively revealed.*

of all books in the history of medicine, the first – and perhaps still the best – example of a modern medical textbook.

Such extravagant praise does, of course, require justification. From a modern medical textbook we demand an excellent layout, high-quality paper, easily readable type, and large number of illustrations that are clearly and correctly drawn and well reproduced. Moreover, we expect these illustrations to be integrated into the text by explanatory captions and detailed keys or legends. We may be pleased when printed marginal notes are used – a practice which, unfortunately, is now out of fashion. Finally, we expect a careful index, preferably compiled by the author himself.

VESALIUS provides all this for the readers of his *Fabrica.*[26] But he also provides something that few medical authors since his time have been able to offer: illustrations that are not merely scientifically accurate but artistically superb. Bibliophiles

[26] We are not discussing the text here. It is of equivalent rank, despite its indebtedness to older literature.

count the *Fabrica* among the most beautiful books ever printed. The surprising thing is that the art of book printing was scarcely a hundred years old when this high point was reached. The combination of favorable circumstances that made the *Fabrica* the great work that it is may never be repeated again. Perhaps the fortunate coming together of a gifted and painstaking author, an expert printer, and a group of well-trained artists who found anatomical illustration a challenge and an inspiration, was an instance of the kind of the *felicitas* which VESALIUS said had characterized the Golden Age. With modern hindsight, we may call VESALIUS'S own time the "golden age" of Humanism.[27] The *Fabrica* is a hymn of praise to the harmony in God's supreme object of creation: Man.

[27] See EDELSTEIN, LUDWIG: Andreas Vesalius, the Humanist, in: Bull. Med. *XIV*, 1943, pp. 547-61.

"Plagiarists" of Vesalius

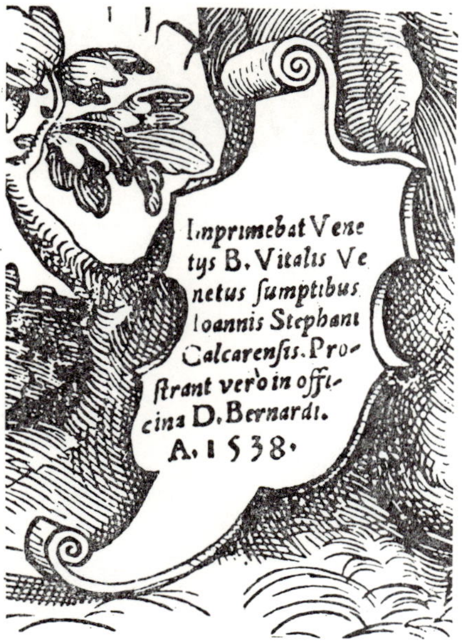

Figures 219 and 220 Impression on the sixth plate (dorsal aspect of skeleton) from Vesalius's loose-leaf anatomy of 1538, and below, Jobst de Necker's copy of 1539. The comparison demonstrates the care with which the Venetian woodcuts were copied in Augsburg.

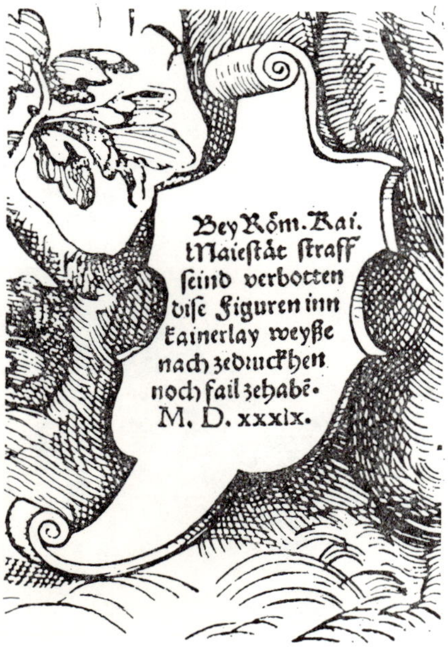

A letter by VESALIUS that was printed at the beginning of the 1543 edition of the *Fabrica* marks the first appearance in the history of medical illustration of the problem of plagiarism. In this letter, VESALIUS accuses authors and publishers in Augsburg, Cologne, Strasbourg, Marburg, Frankfurt, and Paris of having stolen illustrations from his *Tabulae anatomicae* and of having abused his imperial privileges. He actually uses Cicero's word *"plagiarius."* The modern historian is prone to adopt the role of both prosecutor and judge when he observes how certain medical illustrations, and above all anatomical figures, have been repeatedly copied and imitated. As chief witness he calls forward VESALIUS with his celebrated complaint. HARVEY CUSHING[1] undertook the task of identifying all the persons whom, without actually naming them, VESALIUS had accused. This proved to be quite simple in some cases, but impossible in others. And CUSHING was probably quite right to conclude that "it would have been better for VESALIUS's subsequent reputation had this part of his famous letter to OPORINUS been omitted."[2]

The best of these plagiarists was the Augsburg artist JOBST DE NECKER,[3] for whom CUSHING has some sympathy for he admires NECKER'S excellent craftsmanship and his frank way of specifying sources, while at the same time he appreciates the frustration of the injured party. (Of course plagiarism can also be considered as a kind of compliment to the original author.[4]) But the plagiarist can no longer strictly be called so when he transcends the original model with his own ideas, as did the Strasbourg surgeon WALTER RYFF, or when he fully specifies and pays tribute to his source, as did NECKER. Had VESALIUS had the good sense to realize that is was the imitators of his illustrations – and they are to be found in every succeeding century, including the present – who would contribute decisively to the fame of his work, he would never have expressed his anger on paper. Actually, the tendency to imitate a good performance is quite common, especially within medical illustration. There are certain modes of graphic representation which can be considered the best way of rendering specific anatomical details. And why should they not be repeated, merely out of respect for their originator?

One of the "plagiarisms" from VESALIUS that was to have important consequences for medical illustration was the *Compendiosa totius anatomie delineatio aere exarata* by THOMAS GEMINUS,[5] published in London in 1545. *Aere exarata* means "engraved in copper": the illustrations are among the oldest English metal engravings, and the title page is "the first complete title page to be engraved on

[1] CUSHING, HARVEY: A Bio-Bibliography of Andreas Vesalius, New York, 1943, pp. 16-43.
[2] CUSHING, *loc. cit.*, p. 17.
[3] NECKER worked together with HANS BURGKMAIR on the *Triumphzug Kaiser Maximilians* and on the woodcuts for PFINTZING'S edition of *Theuerdanck*. He made an essential contribution to the invention of the colored woodcut, and his craftsmanship was so excellent that he could risk a folio copy of HOLBEIN'S *Totentanz*. See THIEME-BECKER *XXV*, 1931, pp. 377-78.
[4] "The better the work the quicker it was stolen." OLLERENSHAW, ROBERT in: J. Roy. Coll. Surg. Ireland *1*, 1965, p. 173.
[5] Facsimile edition of the English translation of 1553 with an introduction by C. D. O'MALLEY, London, Dawson, 1959.

copper and included in a book."[6] The book is interesting in many respects. It is closely connected with the endeavors of HENRY VIII to raise the standard of English surgery, for which he enlisted the support of JOHN CAIUS, who had lived for several months in the same house as VESALIUS during his studies in Padua.[7]

GEMINUS was soon to be plagiarized himself. Only a few years after the first edition[8] of the oldest copperplate copies of VESALIUS, there appeared in Nuremberg a copy of the copy (see plate XXIIIc). Is was published in 1551 by J. P. FABRICIUS as the *Anatomia Deudsch,* with a forword by JACOB BAUMAN, an elected official of the representative body of Nuremberg surgeons. In common with London and other cities at that time, the larger German towns were striving to improve the professional standards of their surgeons. Accordingly, it was decreed that dissection courses should be held to teach the younger generation and to provide practising surgeons with an opportunity to extend their studies. The participants – and often the instructor as well – required a printed instruction manual, and VESALIUS became the first to meet this urgent need, with his *Epitome.* What VESALIUS said of the *Fabrica* applies also to the *Epitome*: it is highly useful for explaining anatomy even in the absence of a cadaver. The substitute – the illustration – is better than no visiual demonstration at all; and in practice it was quite impossible to find enough cadavers to meet the demand for anatomical dissection. This is the reason why textbooks were suddenly in such great demand in the second half of the 16th century.

It is quite natural that the first illustration of a "modern" anatomical demonstration[9] to be produced in northern Europe was published in Paris and the second in Nuremberg; dissection classes were held frequently in both cities during the middle years of the century, and there were also qualified artists in the service of able publishers in both cities. JOST AMMAN illustrated numerous medical works of the Frankfurt publisher SIEGMUND FEYERABENO, among them the *Opus chyrurgicum* by PARACELSUS. On the title page of the 1565 edition of the *Opus chyrurgicum* there is a picture of a dissection class (fig. 222) which AMMAN must have personally attended in Nuremberg, where he lived and worked.[10] It is the German counterpart

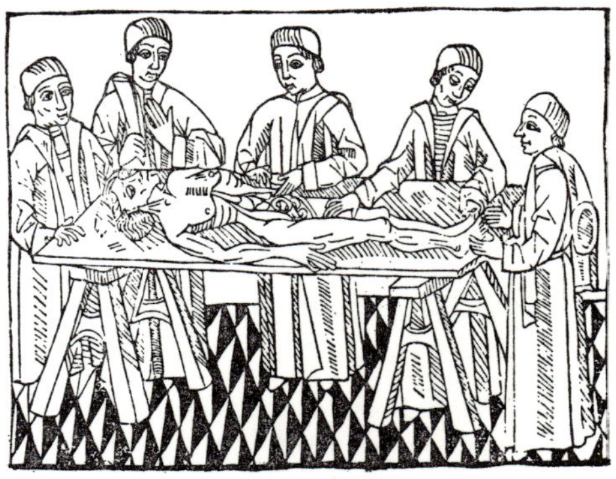

Fig. 221 French anatomy, Lyon, 1482, the oldest known incunabulum of this type. From Bartholomaeus Anglicus, Le propriétaire *des* choses.

Fig. 222 Nuremberg anatomy, circa 1565. Woodcut by Jost Amman in Paracelsus, Opus chyrurgicum, *Frankfurt am Main, 1565.*

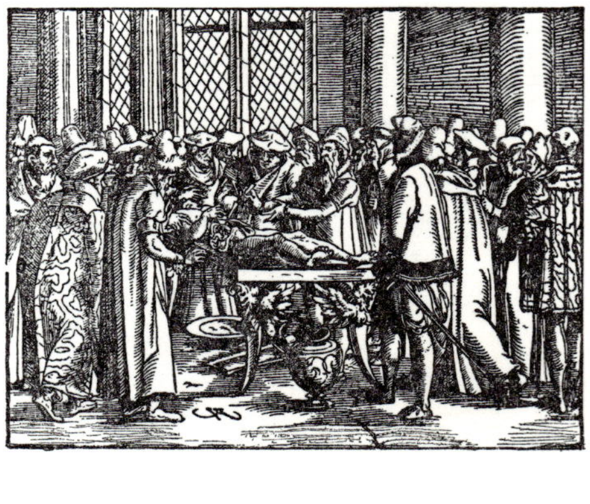

6 See RATH, ERICH: Zur Entwicklung des Kupferstichtitels, in: Buch und Schrift *3*, 1929, p. 53.

7 For an introduction to recent literature treating English anatomy around 1500, see POYNTER, F. N. L.: Anatomie in England im 16. und 17. Jahrhundert, in: Frühe Anatomie, edited by R. HERRLINGER and F. KUDLIEN, Stuttgart, 1967.

8 The plates were printed many times in London between 1552 and 1559, and VESALIUS's name ultimately disappeared from the title page; see CUSHING, pp. 119-30. Around 1560 they were sold in Paris, where further printings were made by the publisher ANDREAS WECHEL. The first two editions, in Latin, do not disclose that the copperplate engravings are of English origin; the third edition of 1569, in French, finally mentions the name of HENRY VIII, but not that of GEMINUS.

9 A picture of an anatomical dissection in the French and English incunabula of the *Bartholomaeus Anglicus,* Lyon, 1482, 1485, etc., and London, 1495, shows a physician next to the cadaver, but no prosector and no lecturer. This illustration undoubtedly belongs within an older tradition. See WOLFF-HEIDEGGER, G. and A. M. CETTO: Die anatomische Sektion in bildlicher Darstellung, Basel/ New York, 1967, Catalogue No. 49, 50, 52, 53, 54 ff.

10 A detailed interpretation is contained in my essay "Die Anatomie des Jost Amman und die Illustration zu Feyerabends Paracelcus-Ausgabe von 1565" in: Sudhoff's Archiv, *37*, 1953, pp.23-38.

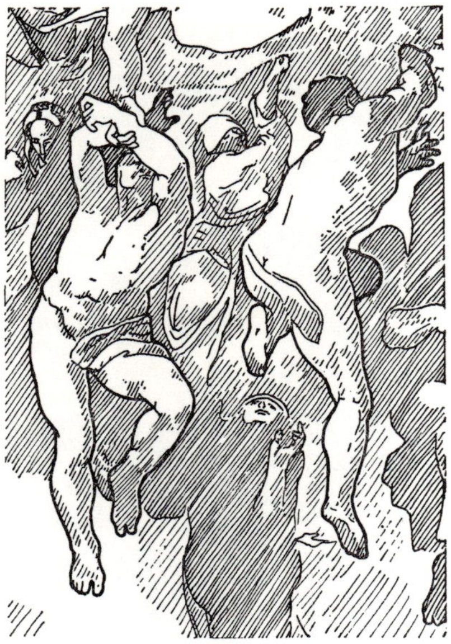

Fig. 223

Figures 223 and 224 Above: outline sketch of a detail from Michelangelo's 'Last Judgment' in the Sistine chapel, Rome, 1508-12. Below: title-page copperplate by G. Becerra for Valverde, Historia de la composicion del cuerpo humano, *Rome, 1556.*

Fig. 224

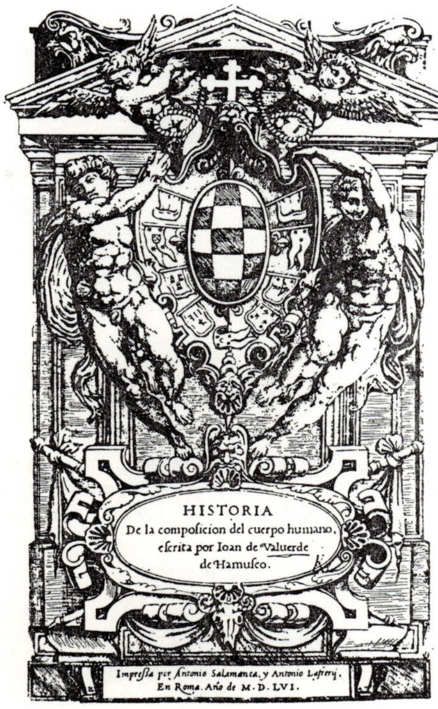

to the title-page woodcut of the *Fabrica* (fig. 184), although it was produced more than twenty years later. The demonstration no longer takes place in a theater, but in a church;[11] nor is the audience dominated by students, but by practising physicians and other academicians; and the anatomist is a surgeon (recognizable by his short robe[12]) rather than a doctor of medicine. However, the spirit of the anatomical demonstration is that of VESALIUS: the anatomist stands by the cadaver demonstrating what he observes, while the surrounding figures discuss what they are being shown.

In his bibliography of the "direct successors" of VESALIUS, CUSHING included the anatomical textbook of JUAN DE VALVERDE DE HAMUSCO, which was the most successful of all the close imitations; it was published between 1556 and 1682 in Italy, Flanders, and Holland. The first edition appeared in Rome in 1556. It was there that the Spaniard VALVERDE met his fellow countryman GASPAR BECERRA, who had worked with MICHELANGELO in the Sistine chapel of the Vatican. He was persuaded by VALVERDE to undertake several drawings for the Spanish textbook. Actually, this work was not really so much a plagiarism[13] of VESALIUS as an improvement on VESALIUS. New features contained in the VALVERDE[14] anatomy were the now famous "flayed figures" (figs. 226-229) and several plates illustrating angiology, cardiology, reproduction, and a pregnancy. It has been traditionally held that BECERRA drew all these illustrations, but not all are worthy of an artist who was so highly reputed at that time. Particularly interesting are the copperplate titles. In the roundelay of the Baroque frontispiece they play a prominent role, despite the different artists and different publishers (figs. 224, 230, 231).

The first of these engraved title pages, undoubtedly by BECERRA (fig. 224), is most closely related to the two "flayed figures" mentioned above – notice the two suspended heraldic figures, which appear to have been directly taken out of MICHELANGELO'S sketchbook (fig. 223). CUSHING is probably right in saying that the figure of St. Bartholomew in the "Last Judgment" of the Sistine chapel is the model for these figures. The combined influences of TITIAN (through VESALIUS) and of MICHELANGELO (through VALVERDE) resulted in a showpiece which caught the imagination of many later graphic artists engaged in medical illustration. However,

[11] We know that some of the anatomical demonstrations in Nuremberg took place in the chapel of the St. Roch cemetery and some in the refectory of the secularized Dominican abbey (COITERS'S dissections, for example).

[12] The short robe of the barber-surgeons.

[13] ALBERTI LOPEZ has listed those alterations in the text which VALVERDE consciously made as corrections of VESALIUS. ALBERTI LOPEZ, LUIS: La anatomia y los anatomistas españoles del Renacimiento, Madrid, 1948. Recent discussion can be found in GUERRA, footnote 10 on p. 105.

[14] Historia de la composicion del cuerpo humano, Rome, 1556; Anatomia del corpo humano, Rome, 1560; Vivae imagines partium corporis humani aereis formis expressae, Antwerp (Plantin), 1566, 1568, 1572; Anatomie, oft levende beelden van de deelen des menschelicken lichaems, Antwerp (Plantijn), 1568; La anatomia del corpo umano novamente ristampata, Venice (Giunti), 1586; Anatome corporis humani nunc primum à MICHAELE COLUMBO latine reddita, Venice (Junta), 1589, 1606.

practically all the remaining figures in the VALVERDE editions that are imitated from VESALIUS – whether they are direct copies or, in a few cases, original designs[15] – testify to a deterioration in quality that set in after VESALIUS. The "flayed figures," or écorchés, are of course exceptions. VALVERDE himself asserts that these figures are not related to VESALIUS and emphasizes that the artist has drawn the shadows with strokes that follow the course of the muscle fibers (see figures 227 and 229). This explanation is quite convincing, even though it can be easily shown that the same trick was used in the *Fabrica.*

The extraordinary influence of the Manneristic taste of the period must be considered separately from the quality of craftmanship. Modern critics have been particularly irritated by the illustration of the abdominal situs encased in a coat of mail (fig. 225).[16] It is my belief that the Roman taste of about 1555 could no longer bear the classical torsos of Venetian derivation, and that that is all there is to it. The occasional practice of providing living heads for dissected corpses (fig. 202) also merely reflected the artistic taste of the time.

What, then, was the reason for the success of the VALVERDE anatomy? It was handier in every respect than VESALIUS'S enormous volume, and also less demanding on the reader, and easier to print – and undoubtedly much cheaper. Even today, this can be the secret behind the success of a medical textbook.

The various editions of this work enable us to consider the effect that the new technique of copperplate engraving had on the field of medical illustration during the last half of the 16th century. Copperplates were not as sturdy as woodblocks, and did not stand up as well under wear. The first two editions of the VALVERDE anatomy had been printed in Rome;[17] the second edition of 1560 was given a new engraved title page (fig. 230), but all the other illustrations remained unchanged. Sometime between 1560 and 1586, the plates – including the 1560 frontispiece – were sold to the JUNTA publishing house in Venice: "nella Stamperia de Giunti" was now inscribed on a new copperplate for the title page of the third edition of 1586, and the title-page copperplate for the 1560 edition was placed in storage. The copperplates for the illustrations were worn, however, and had to be sent to the engraver for restoration. It was necessary to re-engrave all the lines which were no longer deep enough. This proved to be impossible without occasionally lengthening an old line or adding a new one. A careful comparison, especially of enlarged details (figs. 227, 229), shows the contrast between the delicate line of the original 1556 edition and the hard, occasionally doubled line of the restored plate of 1586.

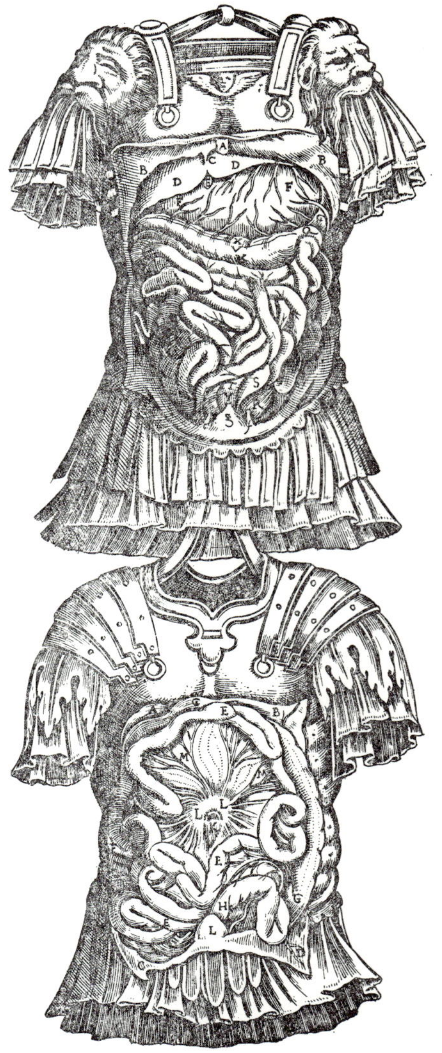

Fig. 225 Valverde: Abdominal viscera in coats of mail. Plate II, Book III of the Antwerp edition of 1568.

Figures 226 and 227 (facing page, top) Valverde de Hamusco, Historia de la composicion del cuerpo humano, *Rome, 1556, Plate I, Book II.*

Figures 228 and 229 (facing page, bottom) Valverde de Hamusco, La anatomia del corpo humano, *Venice, 1586, Plate I, Book II. The plate from 1556 has been reworked.*

15 A list is given by MEYER, A. W. and SHELDON K. WIRT: The Amuscan Illustrations, in: Bull. Hist. Med., Baltimore, *14,* 1943, pp. 667-87. – Criticism in GUERRA, *loc. cit.* He has clearly recognized the method of VALVERDE, who made his corrections by entering them on the illustrations copied from VESALIUS. A copy modified in such a manner is naturally no longer a "copy" in the strict sense of the word.

16 MEYER and WIRT, for example, state that it is "one of the things that amuses and puzzles for it certainly added nothing to anatomical knowledge and did not evidence allegiance to the Master," *loc. cit.,* p. 677.

17 Cf. footnote 14, p. 123.

TAB. PRIMERA DEL LIB. SEGVNDO

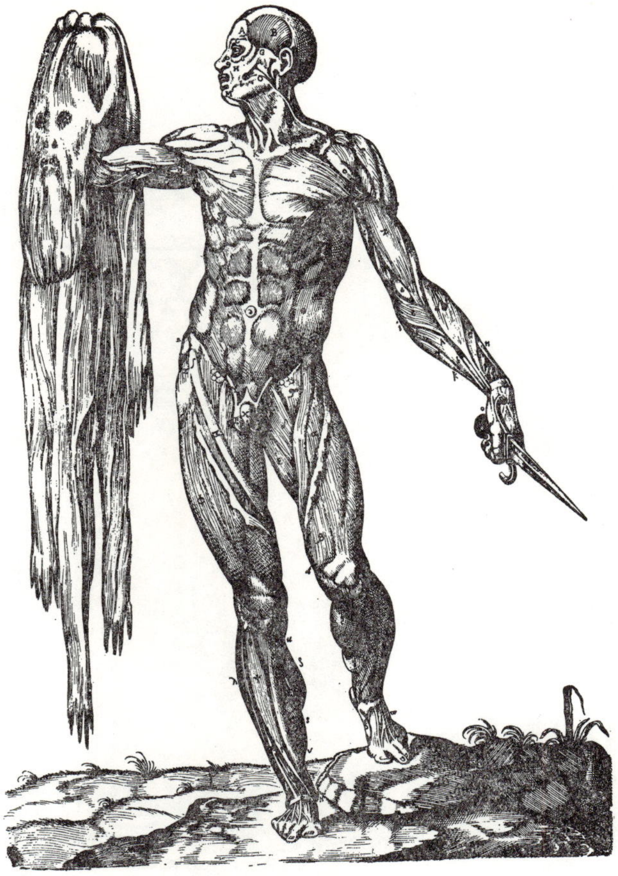

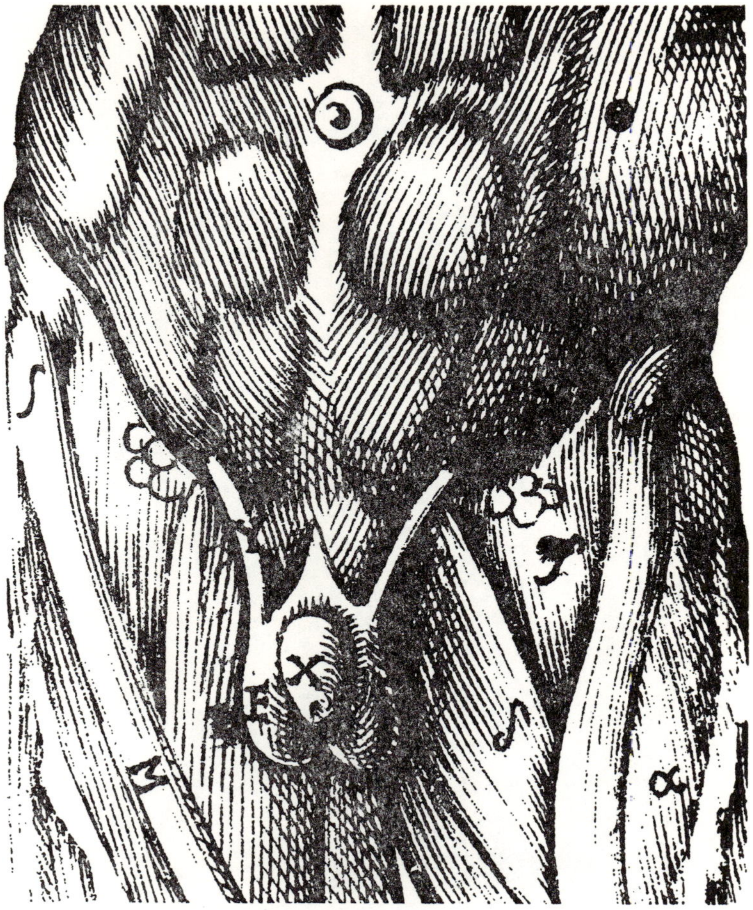

Tauola I. del Lib. II. 64

TABVLA · I · LIBRI · II ·

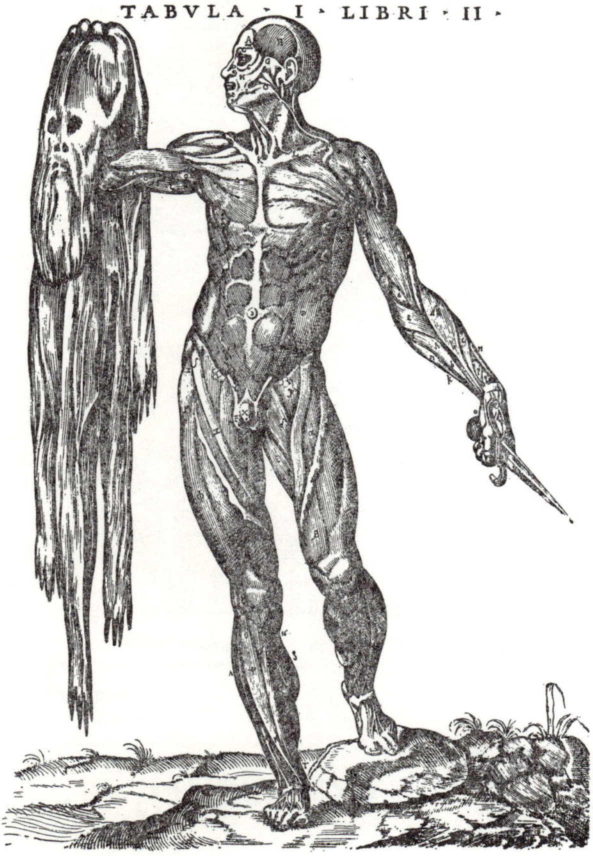

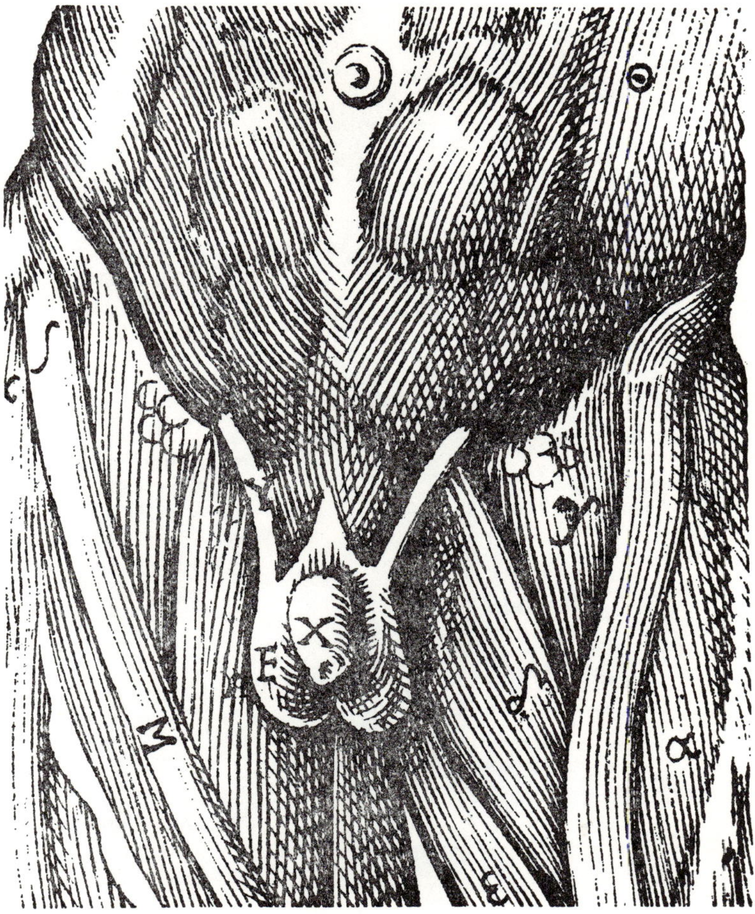

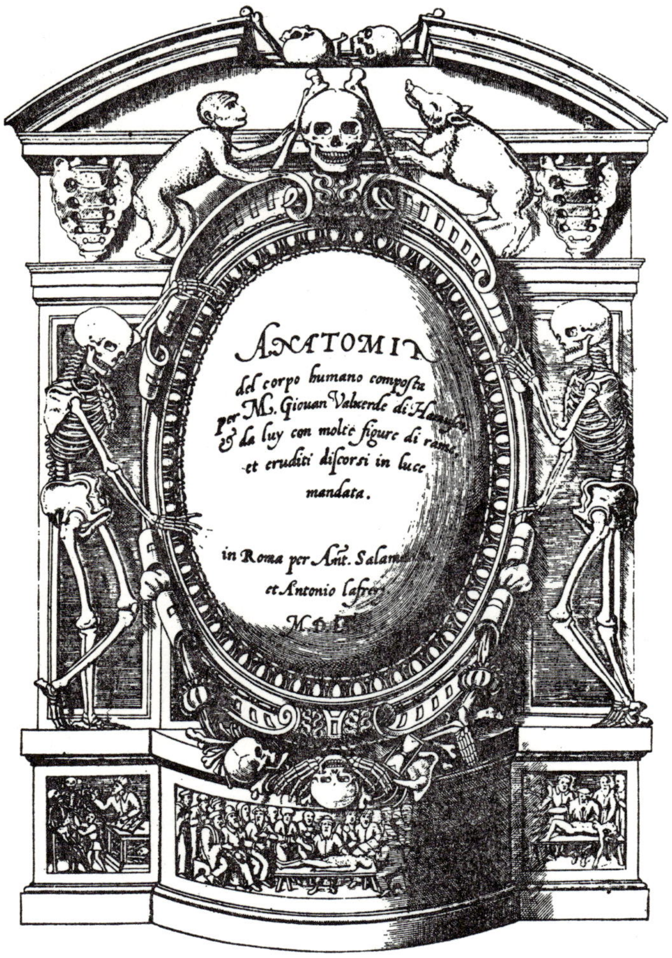

Fig. 230

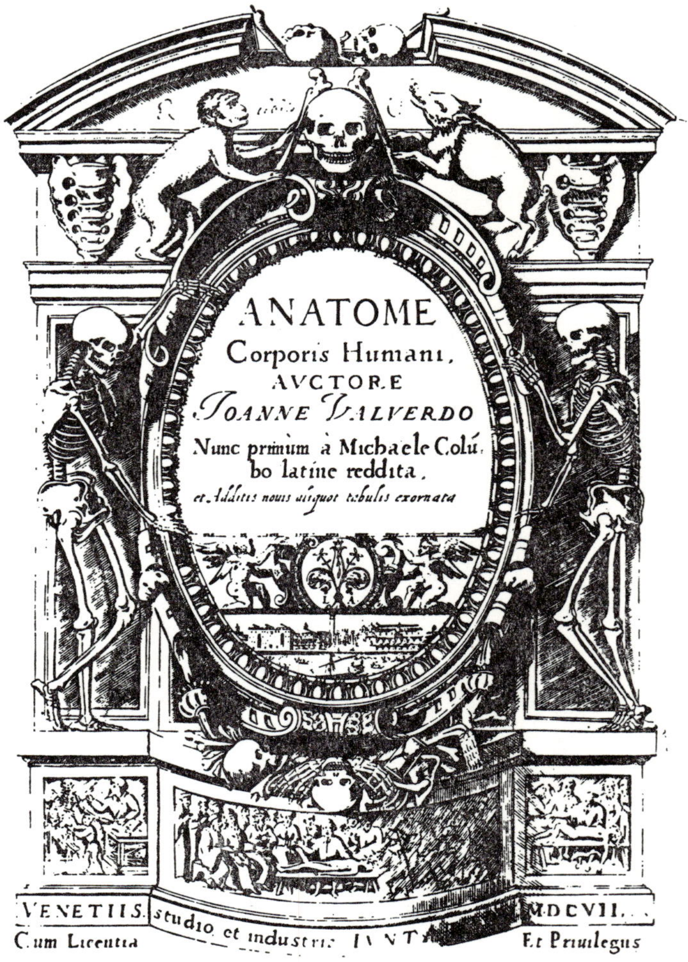

Fig. 232

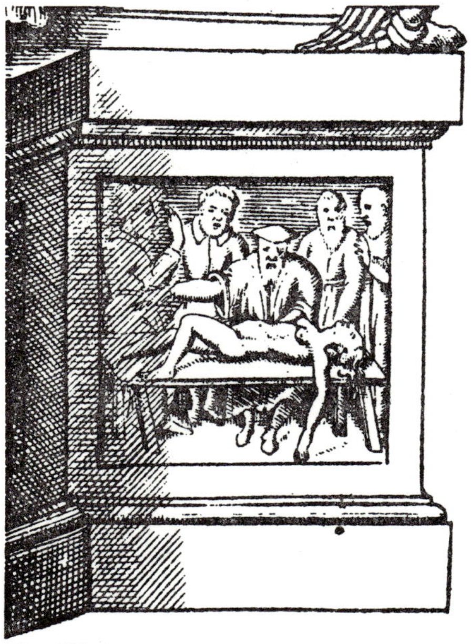

Fig. 231

Figures 230 and 231 Valverde de Hamusco, Anatomia del corpo humano, *Rome (Salamanca-Lafreri), 1560.*

Figures 232 and 233 Valverde, Anatome corporis humani, *Venice (Junta), 1607. The plate from 1560 was reworked. The detail on the lower right shows its condition in 1589. For the 1607 edition only the inserted date of 1589 was altered.*

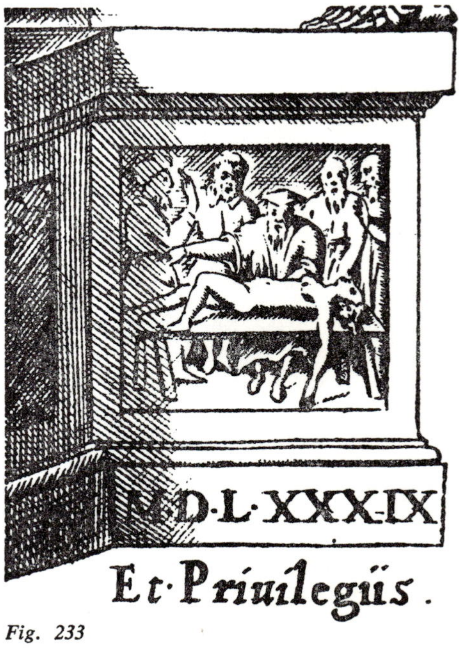

Fig. 233

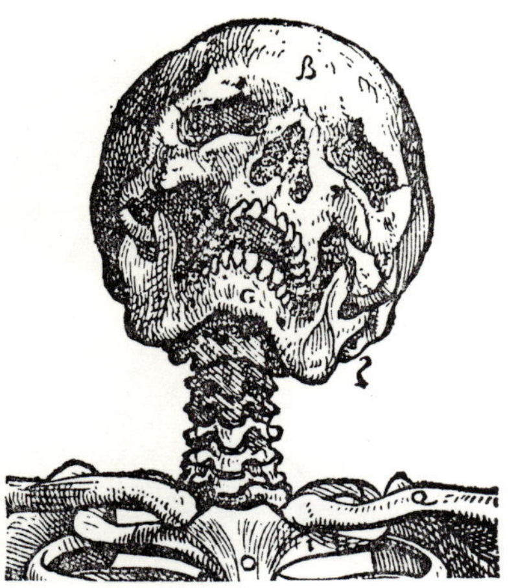

Fig. 234

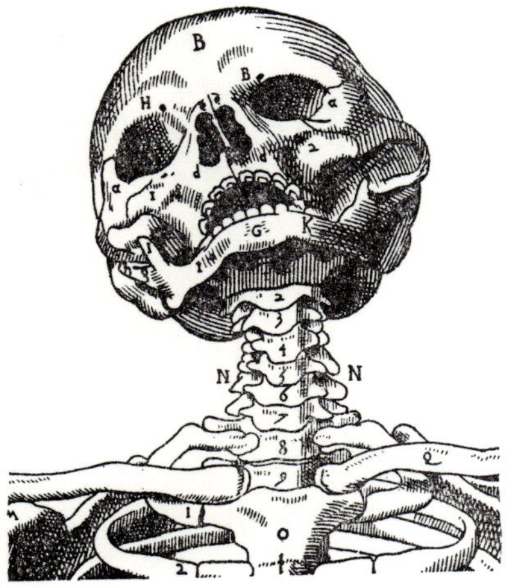

Fig. 235

Figures 234 to 236 Details from the skeletons of Vesalius, 1543, top; Coiter, 1572, center; Platter, 1581, bottom.

Fig. 236

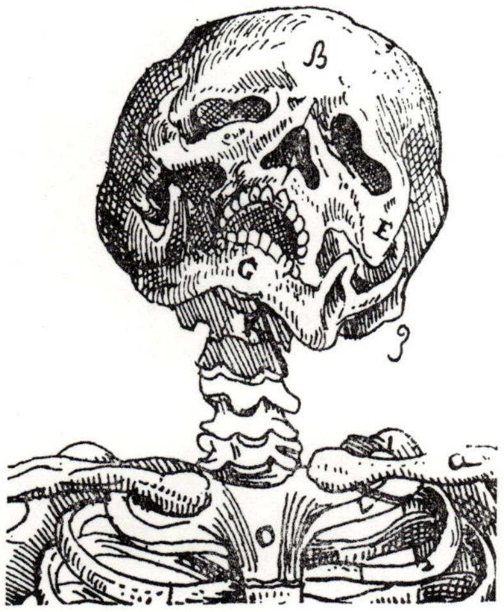

Our contrasted pair of figures also reveals where faults have been improved; for example, next to the letter "E." The restorer has taken the liberty too of using superimposed oblique shading to intensify the parallel shading lines of the original plate.

For the next Junta edition, in 1589, the frontispiece plate from the 1560 edition was taken out of storage. Despite the fact that it was worn, it could still be used after restoration. The inscription of the cartouche, containing the old title, was eradicated. Fortunately, the Roman publishers, Salamanca and Lafreri, had inserted no signature into the ornamental frame, so Junta were able to insert their signature into the cartouche without having to alter anything in the pictorial decoration. Nevertheless, it is still evident that the new title page of 1589 is not entirely homogeneous (fig. 232), for the plate had to be thoroughly reworked. A comparison of one detail – we have reproduced the scene from the lower right corner of the plate (figs. 231, 233) – shows the completely altered shading. The restoration is so different from the original that it looks almost more like a copy than an extensively reworked plate.[18] The fact that the restorer was an inferior typographer is clear from a comparison of the two inscriptions; the Rome engraver had more style.

Valverde had said in his foreword that several of his friends had advised him to use new illustrations rather than copying those of Vesalius, but that he had decided against it. In this way, he said, he avoided confusing readers, who would otherwise have been unable to tell exactly where his opinion and Vesalius's differed. Vesalius's illustrations were so good that it would have seemed a case of envy or jealousy had he not made use of them. Moreover, it was just as easy to improve them (in detail), as it was difficult either to ignore them or to produce better ones. This attitude, which seems so strange to us today, apparently was not thought unusual then. As additional evidence of this fact, we can turn to the works of two German physicians of the last half of the 16th century who deliberately attempted to illustrate their books "according to Vesalius": Volcher Coiter (1534-1576) and Felix Platter (1536-1614).

Coiter is one of the first students of medicine to have drawn the illustrations for his own publications. His *Externarum et internarum principalium humani corporis partium tabulae,*[19] Nuremberg 1572, contains a number of copperplate engravings, some of them imitated from Vesalius and some of them original. The first category includes two skeletons which, as drawings, cannot compete with the models in the *Fabrica,* but which do contain a number of improvements with regard to anatomical detail. Coiter goes as far as to modify the typical pose of the posterior view in order to show the sole of the foot; the result is a "lamenting skeleton" shown in a half-kneeling position.

[18] I should like to thank the custodian of the collection of graphic art at the Kunsthalle of Kiel University, Dr. Johann Schlick, for his expert assistance on this question.

[19] In this context *tabulae* are not illustrated plates, but tables that are part of the text. See Herrlinger, Robert: Volcher Coiter 1534-1576, Nuremberg, Edelmann, 1952.

Fig. 237

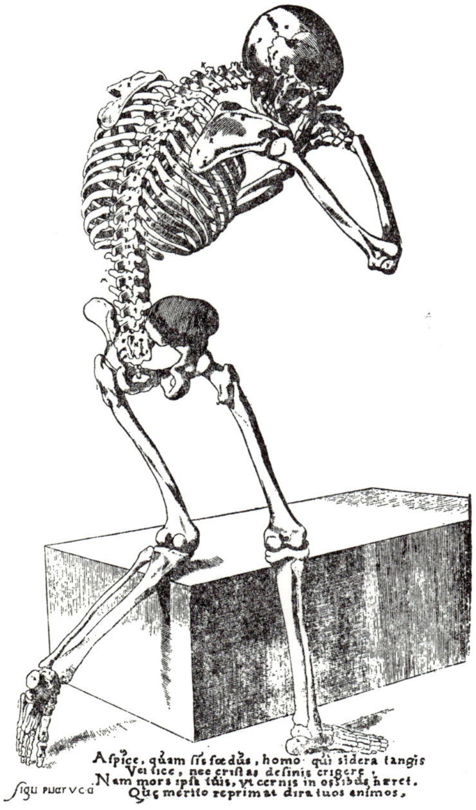

Fig. 238

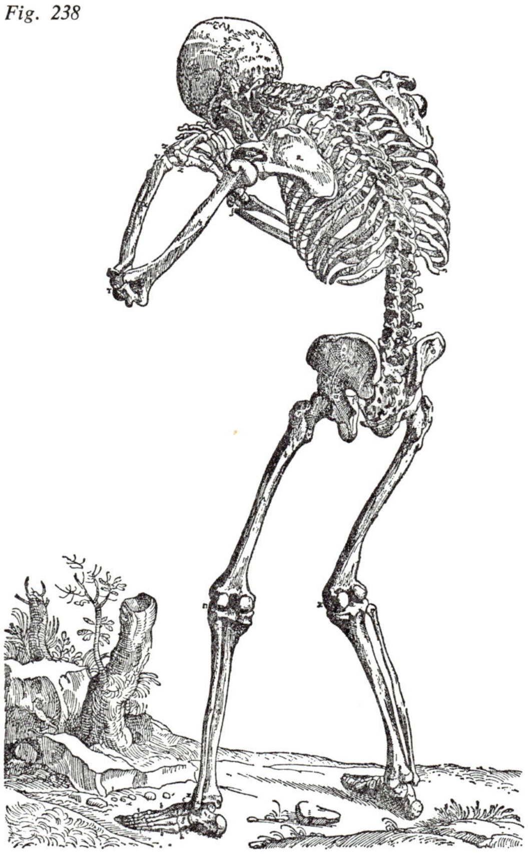

Fig. 239

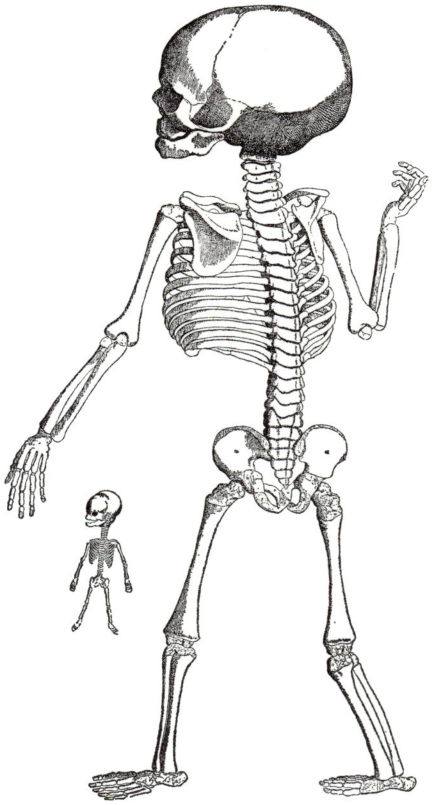

Figures 237 and 238 Skeleton from Coiter, 1572, and Vesalius, 1543. Coiter's skeleton is posed to demonstrate some things – such as the bones of the foot – which are not shown in Vesalius's figure.
Fig. 239 Coiter, 1572: Skeleton of a six-month-old child. Drawn by Coiter himself.
Figures 240 and 241 Interior base of the skull from Vesalius, 1543, and from Coiter, 1572, juxtaposed for comparison.
Fig. 242 Coiter, 1572: Interior base of the skull of a six-month-old child. Drawn by Coiter.

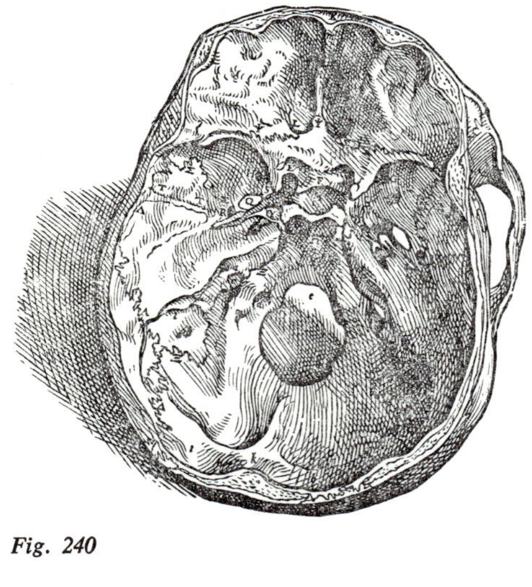

Fig. 240

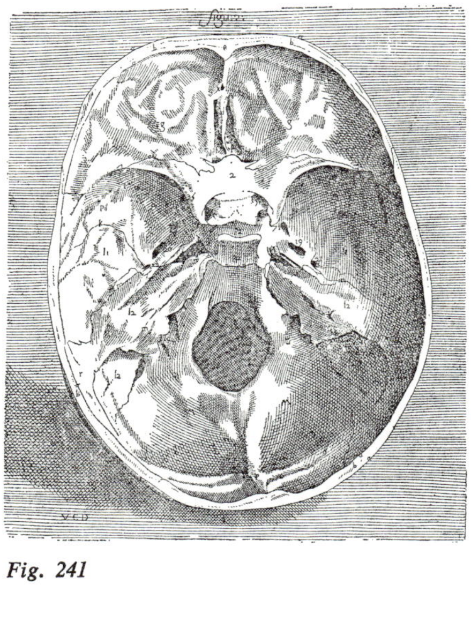

Fig. 241

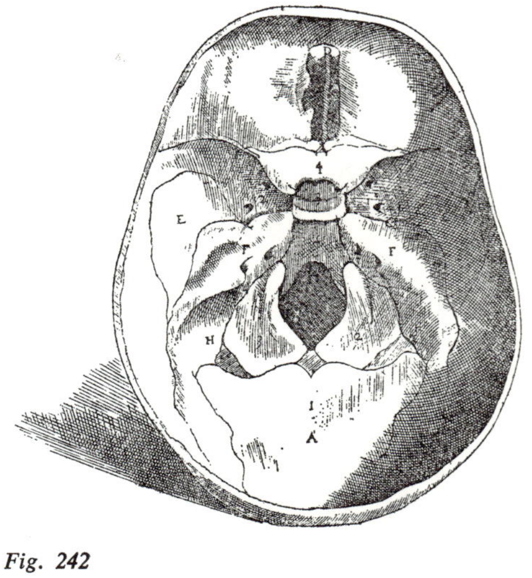

Fig. 242

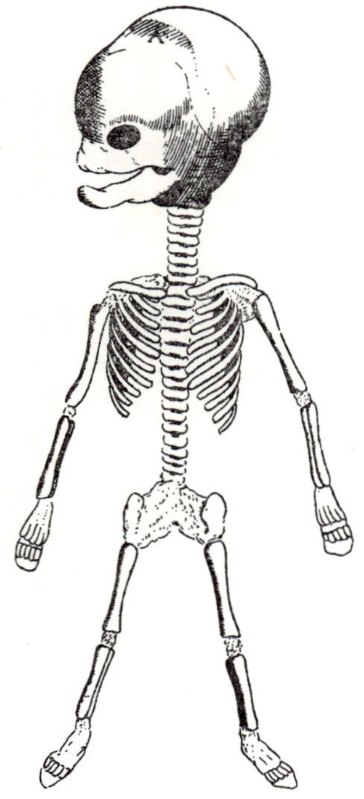

Fig. 243 Coiter, 1572: Skeleton of a three-month miscarriage. Drawn by Coiter.

Fig. 244 Skeleton of a malformed hen. Drawing by Georg Palma in Lectiones Gabrielis Fallopii, *Nuremberg (Gerlach), 1575.*

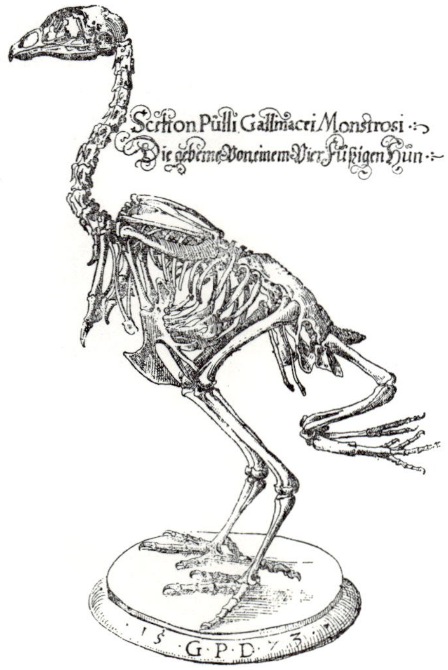

The illustrations of the base of the skull are of excellent quality, superior to the woodcuts of the *Fabrica* in every respect (compare figures 240 and 241). They bear the signature "V.C.D." indicating that they were drawn by COITER himself. Not only does the copperplate engraving achieve more than the woodcut, but the eye of the physician also sees more than the eye of the artist. In order to heighten the three-dimensional effect, COITER uses LEONARDO'S device of setting the object against a shaded background. He also uses the technique of double shading that was employed in the best woodcuts of the *Fabrica.*[20] A shaded background is not used, however, in the illustration showing the base of an infant's skull (fig. 242); COITER probably considered it unnecessary here. In another simply-drawn but effective figure, the skeleton of a three-month fetus (fig. 243), COITER successfully employs parallel-stroke shading and a kind of dotted shading to make two different types of tissue visible.

To his famous critical edition of the *Lectiones Gabrielis Fallopii,* COITER appended a group of illustrations which are not related to the rest of the book; namely, the *Diversorum animalium sceletorum explicationes iconibus illustratae.* The inspiration for this appendix came from ALDROVANDI; however, COITER'S illustrations, most of which he etched himself, are far superior in quality to the zoological illustrations of ALDROVANDI, and they occupy a prominent position in the history of zoology and comparative anatomy.[21] One or two of the animal skeletons in COITER'S book were drawn by GEORG PALMA[22] (fig. 244). KÖNIG has drawn attention to PALMA'S drawing talent [23] and has reproduced a sample. We have included a further sample (plate XXIIIb), which is also an example of the kind of sketches that 16th-century physicians may often have included in their notes as part of the record of their observations. It is quite probable that this practice was encouraged in Montpellier, Padua, Bologna, Tübingen, and elsewhere.

While COITER was in Montpellier in 1556, studying on a grant from Groningen University, he met FELIX PLATTER. They remained in contact even after they took up posts in Nuremberg and Basel, respectively. Both were fascinated by anatomy – which is hardly surprising, considering that the second edition of the *Fabrica* appeared while they were studying. COITER described VESALIUS as "*omnium in re anatomica princeps,*" and PLATTER wrote in his *Corporis humani partium per icones delineatorum explicatio* of 1581 that "*nemo hactenus rectius Vesalio figuras Anatomicas depingi curaverit*" ("no one has improved on the illustrations of VESALIUS"). PLATTER, who lived in Basel, where the *Fabrica* was published and where the printing blocks were still to be found, had practical reasons for not illustrating

[20] As though this were a Nuremberg tradition, the high value accorded to shadow was still evidenced two hundred years later in CH. J. TREW'S *Tabulae osteologicae* of 1767.
[21] COLE, FRANCIS JOSEPH: A History of Comparative Anatomy, London, 1944.
[22] KÖNIG, KLAUS G.: Der Nürnberger Stadtarzt Dr. Georg Palma (1543-1591), i.e. Medizin in Geschichte und Kultur, edited by R. HERRLINGER and K. E. ROTHSCHUH, Vol. I. Stuttgart, 1961.
[23] KÖNIG, *loc. cit.,* pp. 86 ff.

his book with Vesalius's plates, although the successors of the publishers offered to sell them to him; the format would have been too large, the book too thick, and printing too expensive. Platter, however, wanted to write a textbook and a convenient reference work for physicians; accordingly he had Vesalius copied.

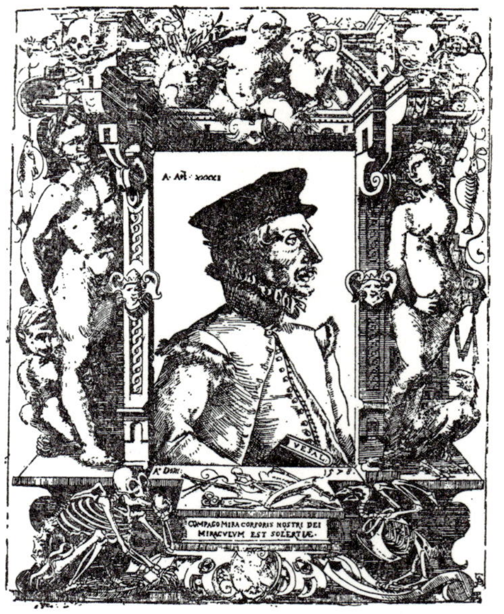

Fig. 245 Abel Stimmer: Portrait of the Basel municipal physician Felix Platter in his 41st year. Etching.

Platter's *Icones* are etchings, the first etchings to be used in medical illustration. Before the invention of lithography, etching was the simplest method available for reproducing line drawings. In an etching, a sketch can be reproduced directly without any need for technical finishing. Parmigianino was a master in this field; and German graphic artists, particularly the so-called "minor masters," were also notably attracted to it. Popular taste, however, for a long time continued to favor woodcuts in book illustration. Platter probably chose etching only because it allowed easier production – a sort of highspeed process – rather than for artistic reasons. The tendency of etching toward sketchlike representation, or graphic abbreviation, may have coincided with the basic objective of Platter's project, but he was eventually dissatisfied with the results of the copying process. This is evident from his "Foreword to the Reader," where, with a show of guilty conscience, he confesses to the extremely casual work of the etching-needle. Apparently the engraver did not follow Platter's detail to the degree required, and in a mood of resignation the author speaks of the *"malevolentia"* of his illustrators. The fact that he speaks in the plural, and adds that he does not wish to mention names, certainly does not help us to answer the question of who was the master responsible. In fact, it would be impossible to identify the etcher at all if the monogram "S.A." did not appear on the portrait of Platter at the front of the *Icones* (fig. 245). This is the monogram of Abel Stimmer of Basel, a brother of the celebrated Tobias. We can see Stimmer's skill at work in the framework around this portrait, where the cumbersome scrollwork and sham architecture of contemporary fashion dissolve into a fanciful organic frame which is far ahead of its time. Such a loose and fanciful approach is, however, obviously unsuitable for exact anatomical illustration. Platter was accordingly obliged to ask the more demanding reader to refer to Vesalius's originals when studying the *Icones*. However, Platter did feel that he had made some valuable contributions with regard to the treatment of the illustrations within the text, regardless of the unsatisfactory quality of the illustrations themselves. In the first place, he assures us that he has put all of the illustrations together at the end of the book, in order to save the reader the trouble of continual page-turning and searching. Moreover, he has been careful to place the explanatory legend for each illustrated plate on the page – and this is indeed a milestone in the history of medical illustration. Platter's illustrations themselves, however, remain totally indebted to Vesalius; and where he appears to have introduced innovations into the *Icones*, closer observation reveals them to be merely amendments, of the kind we noted in Valverde and Coiter.

Figures 246 and 247 Vesalius, 1543, and Platter, 1581: Musculi palpebrarum. Supplemented in Platter by the M. corrugator supercilii which was first described by his friend Coiter in 1572.

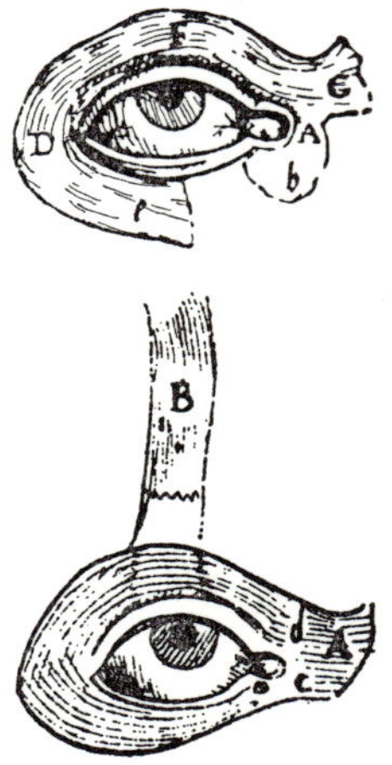

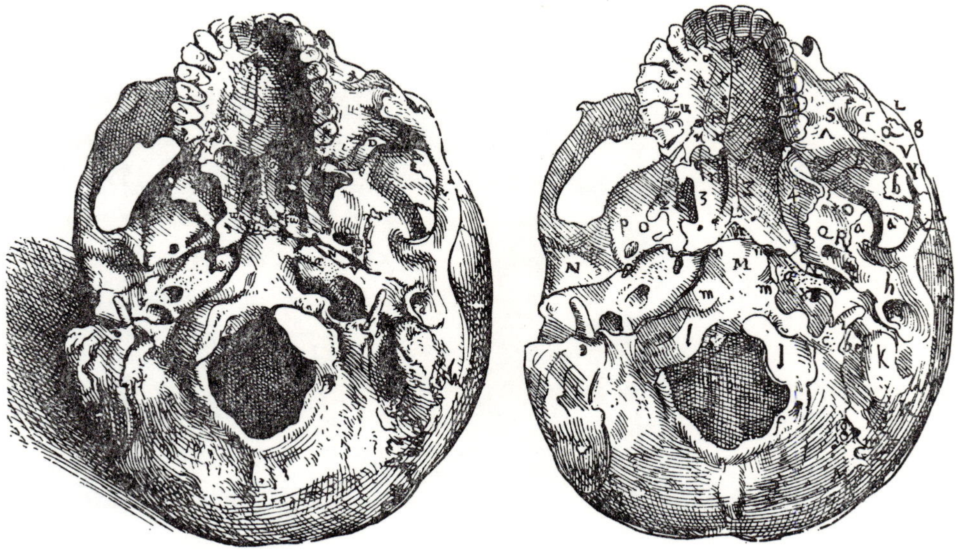

Figures 248 and 249 Left, base of the skull from Vesalius's Fabrica, *1543; right, Platter's etched 'copy', 1581. Several anatomical details suggest that the artist must have had a skull before him. The inscribed letters are almost identical and more legible in Platter's etching, whereas a few supplementary additions were probably suggested by Coiter's far superior illustration, 1572. This was drawn by Coiter from his own dissection quite independently of Vesalius.*

Bartolomeo Eustachio

Even before the second edition of VESALIUS'S *Fabrica* was ready for printing in Basel, a series of copperplate engravings were completed in Rome for BARTOLOMEO EUSTACHIO'S *De dissensionibus ac contraversiis anatomicis.* According to EUSTACHIO, these plates – later known as the *Tabulae anatomicae clarissimi viri* – were completed in the year 1552,[1] and engraved by GIULIO DE MUSI.[2] The book was never published, however, and for a long time it was not clear what had eventually become of the engraved plates. MALPIGHI searched for them, but without success. They were finally rediscovered in 1717 in the possession of the heirs of a certain PIER MATTEO PINI, to whom EUSTACHIO had willed them in 1570, four years before his death. Altogether, only thirty-nine plates were found.[3] Pope Clement XI acquired them and gave them to his personal physician, J. M. LANCISI, who had helped in the search for them. LANCISI then organized the first printing from these copperplates, under the title quoted in brief above.[4] This edition included eight smaller plates which had been used for EUSTACHIO'S *Opuscula anatomica* of 1564. About a dozen further editions were to follow during the 18th century, several from the original plates.[5]

EUSTACHIO'S anatomical illustrations are remarkable in many respects. At least some of them impress the contemporary observer as being amazingly modern. The reason for this is that they are the product of an exceptionally lucid intellect. The series of muscle-figures, for example, are arranged in pairs, in which front and back views (or left-side and right-side views) are shown together. Since the artist was unable to free himself from the traditional poses – which admittedly he handles in a superb manner – thoroughly surrealistic drawings result. All the figures are posed within an unusual frame, three sides of which resemble the geodetic scales sometimes shown on the sides of maps. The numbers on the frame can be taken to provide coordinates for the pictured space, like the coordinates on a sheet of graph paper. This increases the artistic tension between pose and frame, nature and mathematics. EUSTACHIO'S approach is, indeed, the direct antithesis to VESALIUS'S. ALBRECHT VON HALLER clearly stated the essential character of Eustachian illustration: *Eae tabulae ad alios fines factae sunt, quam Vesalianae* ("These plates were made for different purposes than Vesalius's"). The author by no means intended to

1 *Opuscula anatomica,* Venice, 1564. Foreword and Chapter 13 of "De renibus."

2 Neues allg. Künstler-Lexicon, revised by G. K. NAGLER, *11* (2, 1924), p. 152.

3 They are titled "TABULA PRIMA" to "TABULA OCTAVA," whereas the rest are numbered "TAB. IX to "TAB. XXXXVII."

4 The title in full is *Tabulae anatomicae clarissimi viri quas e tenebris tandem vindicatas / et / Sanctissimi Domini* CLEMENTIS XI. *Pont. Max. / Munificentia dono acceptas / praefatione notisque illustravit, ac ipso suae bibliothecae / dedicationis die publici juris fecit /* JO. MARIA LANCISIUS */ intimus cubicularius et archiater pontificius. Romae 1714, ex officina Typographica* FRANCISCI GONZAGAE *in via Lata.* The frontispiece is ornamented with an anatomical scene which shows EUSTACHIO performing a dissection. The copperplate for this title page was done by P. L. GHEZZI, a member of the Accademia di S. Luca, Rome.

5 Bibliographies in CHOULANT, 1852; CHOULANT-FRANK, 1920; and in the facsimile edition of 1944: PAZZINI, ADALBERTO, Introduzione e commento storico alle "Tavole anatomiche di Bartolomeo Eustachio," Rome, Bottega dell' antiquario.

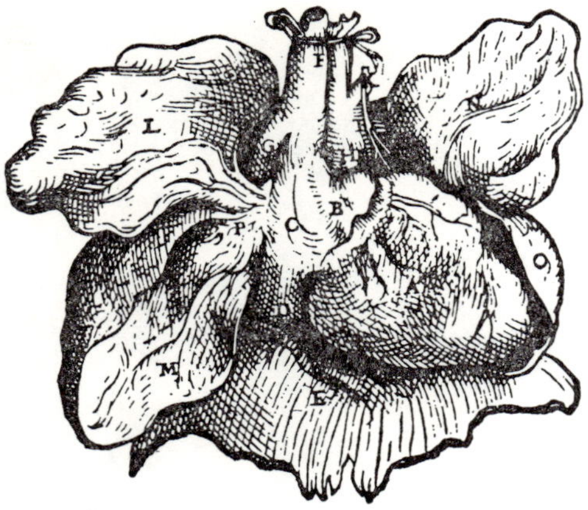

Fig. 250

copy from nature; in fact, it is obvious that everything shown on one of these figures could not be seen at once on the same cadaver, and that it was necessary to combine observations of several dissections within single figures. From numerous autopsies, then, the "standard figure" materializes in the imagination of the anatomist, a generic figure which is no longer a direct copy from nature but a composite of many observations. Although these figures are posed like living beings, their special attraction is lucid geometrical form. This had not been the aim of VESALIUS; he had intended to achieve much more – to provide illustrations so realistic and true to nature that the reader could study anatomical dissection without having recourse to an actual cadaver. EUSTACHIO makes greater demands upon his reader than VESALIUS. SINGER had the feeling that EUSTACHIO'S figures were dead, and those of VESALIUS alive. Comparison demonstrates in more than one case, however,

Figures 250 and 251 Isolated illustration of heart, lungs, and diaphragm in Vesalius (above) and Eustachio (below).
Figures 252 and 253 Two plates from Vesalius's Fabrica, *1543, and Eustachio's* Tabulae anatomicae, *ca. 1550, for comparison.*

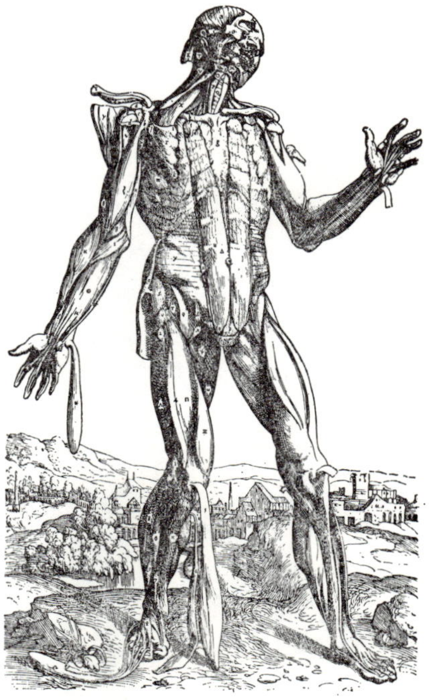

Fig. 252

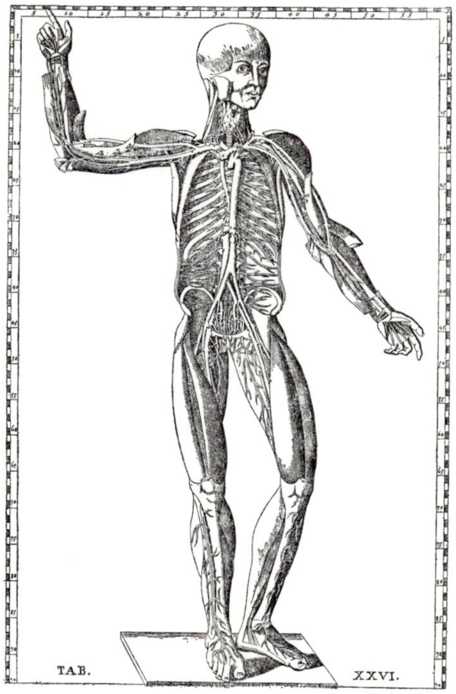

Fig. 253

Fig. 251

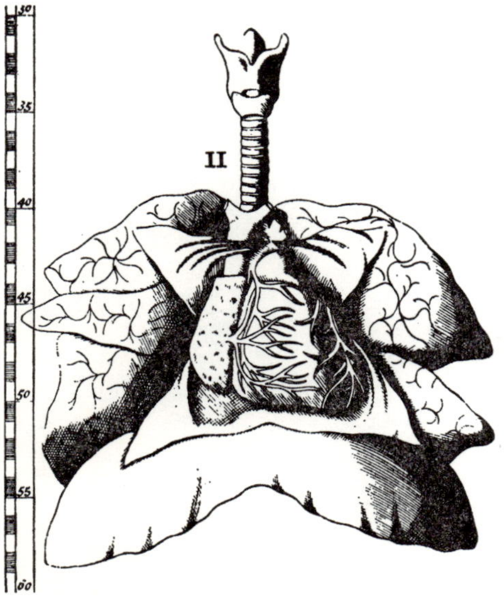

that precisely the opposite is true – VESALIUS'S cadavers are sometimes very convincingly dead indeed.

Copperplate engraving was a technique admirably adapted to EUSTACHIO'S intentions. The achievements possible in what was then the most modern method of reproduction available are shown above all in the greatly admired[6] "Tabula XVIII," (see plate XXVI, p. 138). The plates reached the height of their renown about the middle of the 18th century, after an *Explicatio* had been provided for them by

[6] "The glory of the whole Eustachian collection is a truly magnificent drawing of the Sympathetic System . . . a really great figure." SINGER, Short History, 1957, p. 138.

B. S. ALBINUS, an anatomical colleague of BOERHAAVES in Leyden. The distinguishing feature of this edition, published in 1744 in Leyden, lies in the fact that it contains magnificent copies of all the plates (see figure 255), each furnished with an outline drawing containing inscriptions. This particular method of explaining a drawing was one of the most valuable contributions made to medical illustration by ALBINUS and his excellent graphic artist J. WANDELAAR.

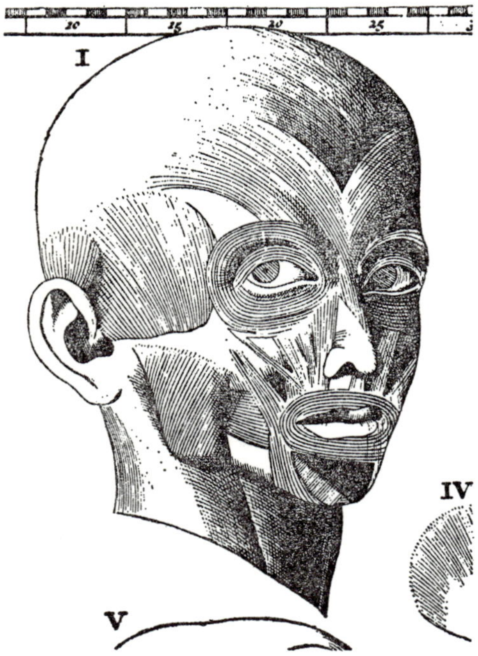

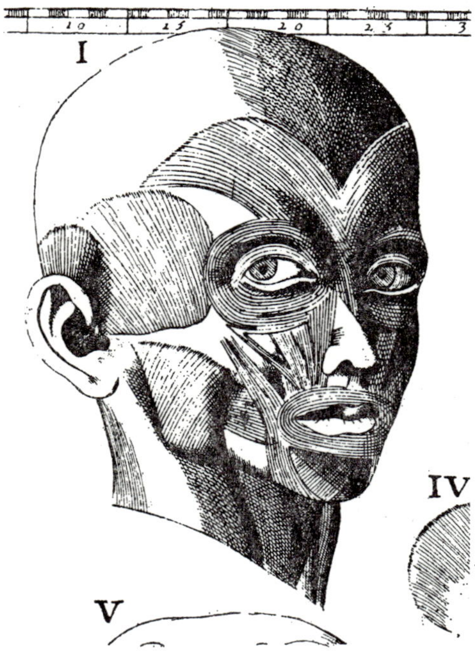

Figures 254 and 255 The same motif engraved by Giulio de Musi (left), circa 1550, a copy of the 1714 edition, and by J. Wandelaar (right) from the 1744 edition.

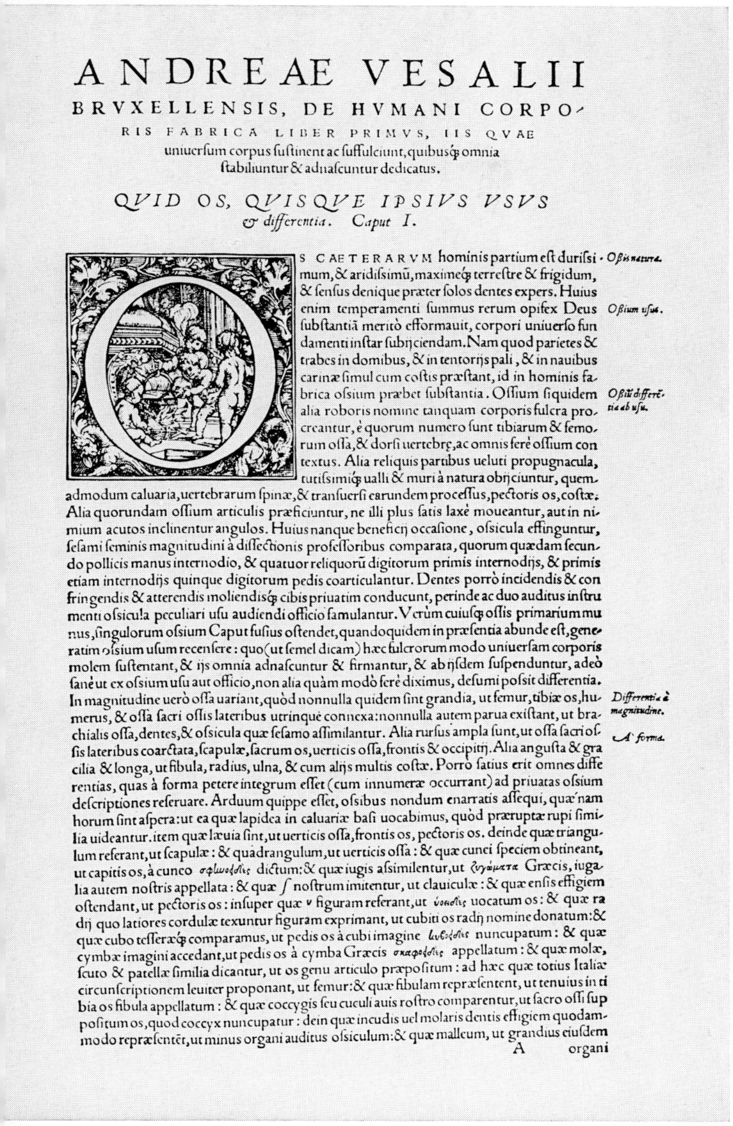

ANDREAE VESALII BRVXELLENSIS, DE HVMANI CORPORIS FABRICA LIBER PRIMVS, IIS QVAE uniuerſum corpus ſuſtinent ac ſuffulciunt, quibusq́ omnia ſtabiliuntur & adnaſcuntur dedicatus.

QVID OS, QVISQVE IPSIVS VSVS & differentia. Caput I.

OS CAETERARVM hominis partium eſt duriſsimum, & aridiſsimũ, maximeq́ terreſtre & frigidum, & ſenſus denique præter ſolos dentes expers. Huius enim temperamenti ſummus rerum opifex Deus ſubſtantiã meritò efformauit, corpori uniuerſo fundamenti inſtar ſubijciendam. Nam quod parietes & trabes in domibus, & in tentorijs pali, & in nauibus carinæ ſimul cum coſtis præſtant, id in hominis fabrica oſsium præbet ſubſtantia. Oſſium ſiquidem alia roboris nomine tanquam corporis fulcra procreantur, è quorum numero ſunt tibiarum & femorum oſſa, & dorſi uertebræ, ac omnis ferè oſſium contextus. Alia reliquis partibus ueluti propugnacula, tutiſsimiq́ ualli & muri à natura obijciuntur, quemadmodum caluaria, uertebrarum ſpinæ, & tranſuerſi earundem proceſſus, pectoris os, coſtæ. Alia quorundam oſſium articulis præficiuntur, ne illi plus ſatis laxè moueantur, aut in nimium acutos inclinentur angulos. Huius nanque beneficij occaſione, oſsicula effinguntur, ſeſami ſeminis magnitudini à diſſectionis profeſſoribus comparata, quorum quædam ſecundo pollicis manus internodio, & quatuor reliquorũ digitorum primis internodijs, & primis etiam internodijs quinque digitorum pedis coarticulantur. Dentes porrò incidendis & confringendis & atterendis moliendisq́ cibis priuatim conducunt, perinde ac duo auditus inſtrumenti oſsicula peculiari uſu audiendi officio famulantur. Verùm cuiuſq́ oſſis primarium munus, ſingulorum oſsium Caput fuſius oſtendet, quandoquidem in præſentia abunde eſt, generatim oſsium uſum recenſere: quo (ut ſemel dicam) hæc fulcrorum modo uniuerſam corporis molem ſuſtentant, & ijs omnia adnaſcuntur & firmantur, & ab ijſdem ſuſpenduntur, adeò ſanè ut ex oſsium uſu aut officio, non alia quàm modò ferè diximus, deſumi poſsit differentia. In magnitudine uerò oſſa uariant, quòd nonnulla quidem ſint grandia, ut femur, tibiæ os, humerus, & oſſa ſacri oſſis lateribus utrinquè connexa: nonnulla autem parua exiſtant, ut brachialis oſſa, dentes, & oſsicula quæ ſeſamo aſſimilantur. Alia rurſus ampla ſunt, ut oſſa ſacri oſſis lateribus coarctata, ſcapulæ, ſacrum os, uerticis oſſa, frontis & occipitij. Alia anguſta & gracilia & longa, ut fibula, radius, ulna, & cum alijs multis coſtæ. Porrò ſatius erit omnes differentias, quas à forma petere integrum eſſet (cum innumeræ occurrant) ad priuatas oſsium deſcriptiones reſeruare. Arduum quippe eſſet, oſsibus nondum enarratis aſſequi, quæ'nam horum ſint aſpera: ut ea quæ lapidea in caluariæ baſi uocabimus, quòd præruptæ rupi ſimilia uideantur. item quæ læuia ſint, ut uerticis oſſa, frontis os, pectoris os. deinde quæ triangulum referant, ut ſcapulæ: & quadrangulum, ut uerticis oſſa: & quæ cunei ſpeciem obtineant, ut capitis os, à cuneo σφηνοειδὴς dictum: & quæ iugis aſsimilentur, ut ζυγώματα Græcis, iugalia autem noſtris appellata: & quæ ſ noſtrum imitentur, ut clauiculæ: & quæ enſis effigiem oſtendant, ut pectoris os: inſuper quæ υ figuram referant, ut ὑοειδὴς uocatum os: & quæ radij quo latiores cordulæ texuntur figuram exprimant, ut cubiti os radij nomine donatum: & quæ cubo teſſeræq́ comparamus, ut pedis os à cubi imagine κυβοειδὴς nuncupatum: & quæ cymbæ imagini accedant, ut pedis os à cymba Græcis σκαφοειδὴς appellatum: & quæ molæ, ſcuto & patellæ ſimilia dicantur, ut os genu articulo prępoſitum: ad hæc quæ totius Italiæ circunſcriptionem leuiter proponant, ut femur: & quæ fibulam repræſentent, ut tenuius in tibia os fibula appellatum: & quæ coccygis ſeu cuculi auis roſtro comparentur, ut ſacro oſſi ſuppoſitum os, quod coccyx nuncupatur: dein quæ incudis uel molaris dentis effigiem quodammodo repræſentẽt, ut minus organi auditus oſsiculum: & quæ malleum, ut grandius eiuſdem

A organi

Oſsis natura.

Oſsium uſus.

Oſsiũ differẽtia ab uſu.

Differentia à magnitudine.

A forma.

Plate XXIIIa The first page of text from Vesalius's Fabrica, *1543.*

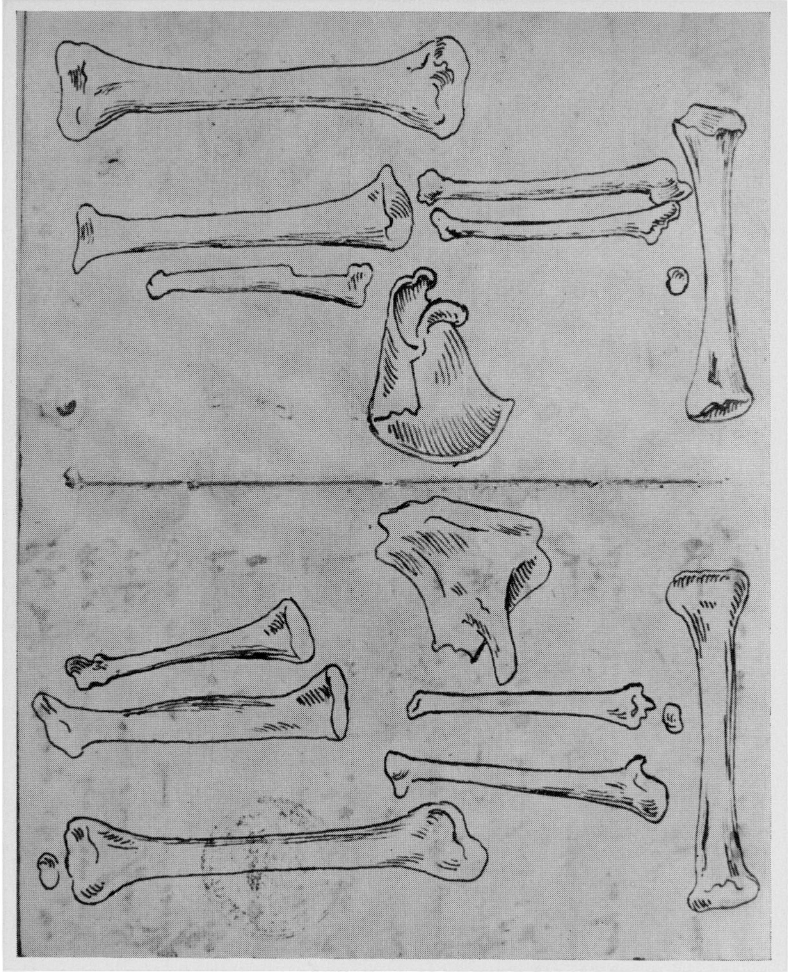

Plate XXIIIb Georg Palma, 1543-1591: Bones of a macerated embryo. Pen and ink drawing for the illustration of a case history, circa 1583, Nuremberg, Stadtbibliothek, St. Med. 11.8°.

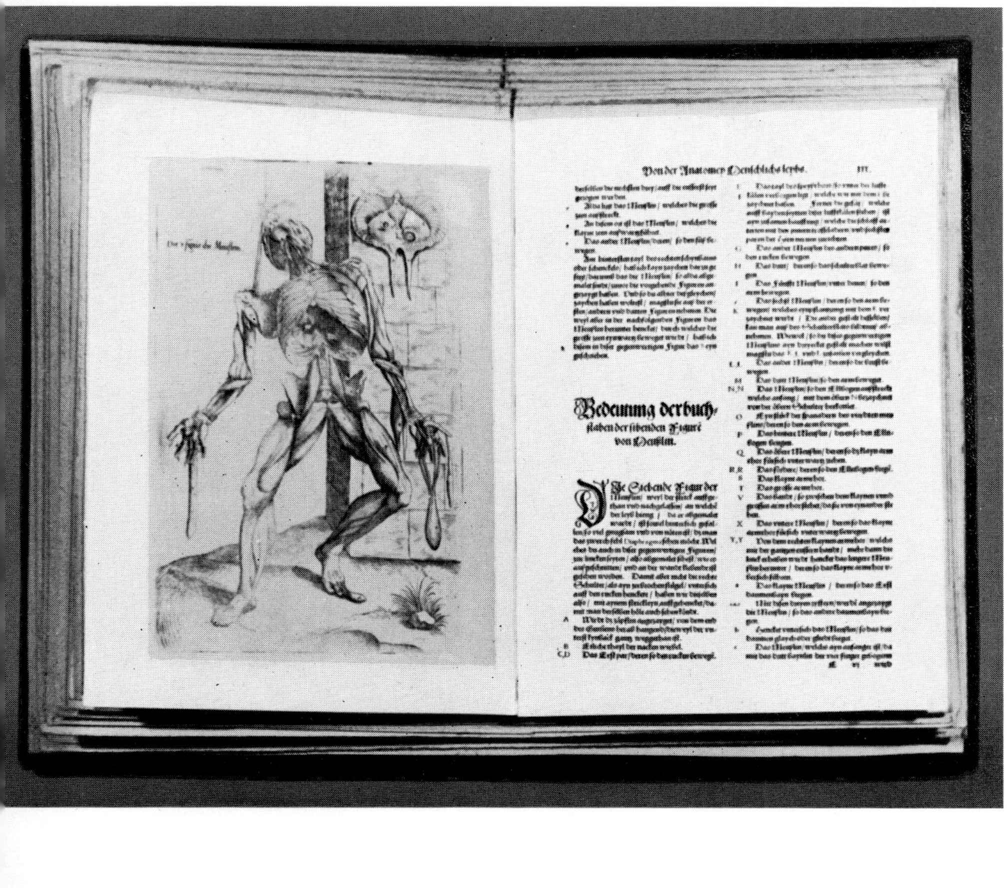

Plate XXIIIc An opened specimen of the extremely rare Anatomia Deudsch, Ein kurtzer Auszug der beschreibung aller glider menschlichs Leybs aus den buchern des Hochgelerten Hern D. Andree Vesalij von Brüssel, *published for surgeons by Jacob Bauman in Nuremberg, 1551.*

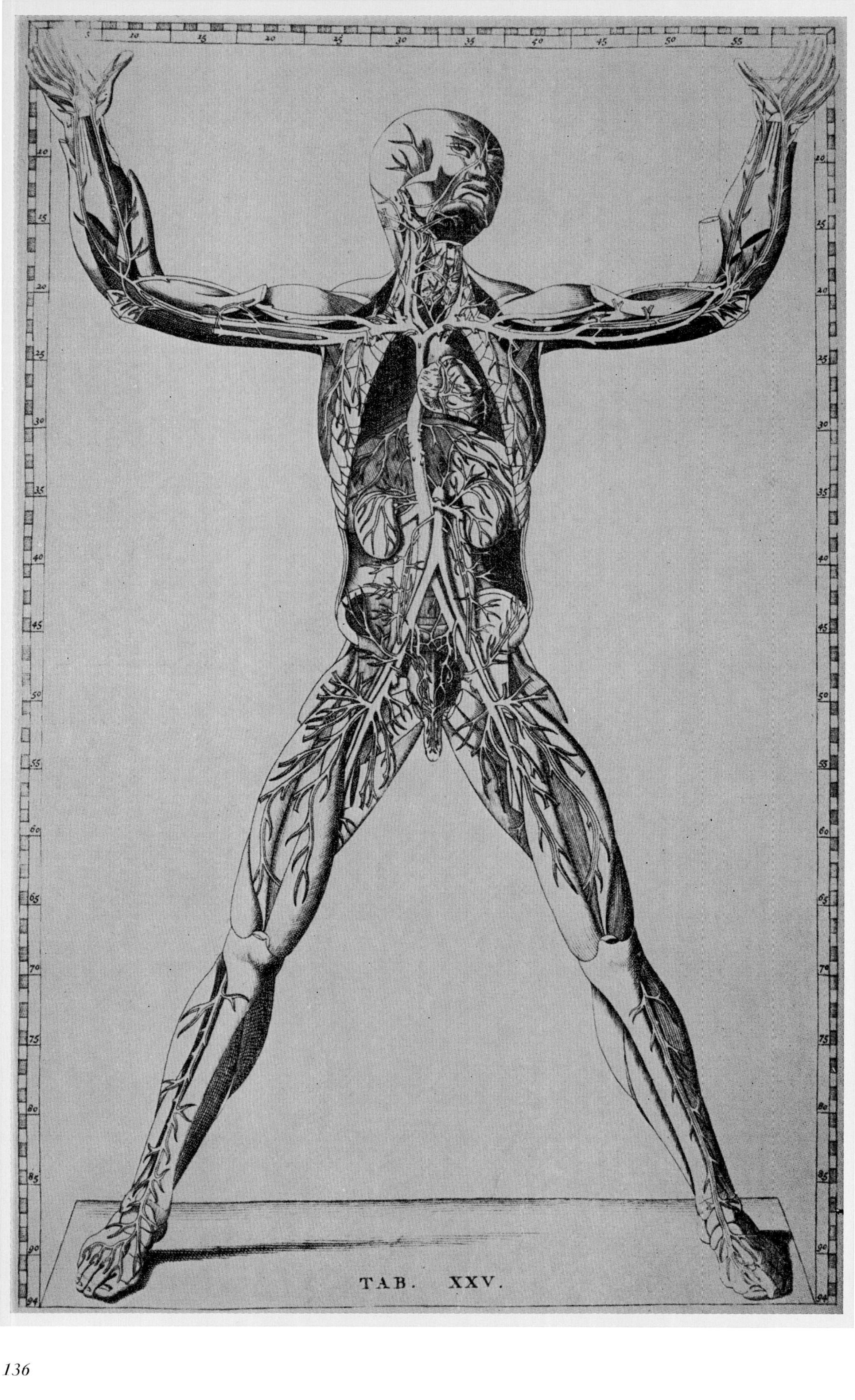

Plate XXIV Bartolomeo Eustachio, Tabulae anatomicae, *tab. XXV. Copperplate engraving by Giulio de Musi, before 1552.*

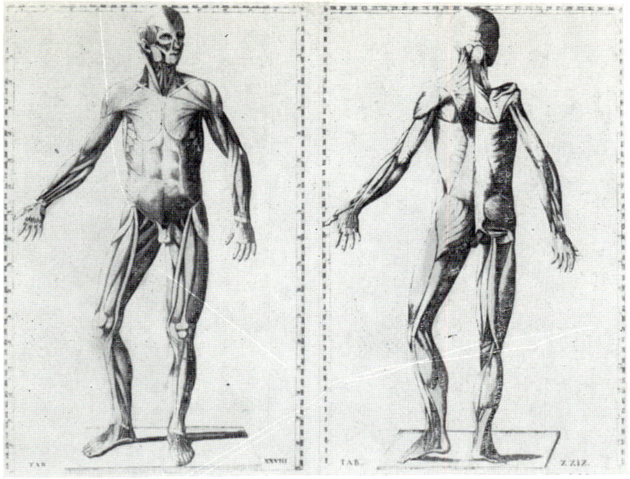
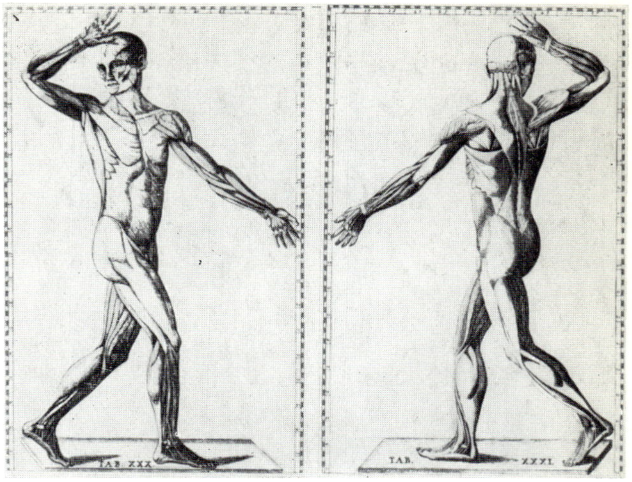
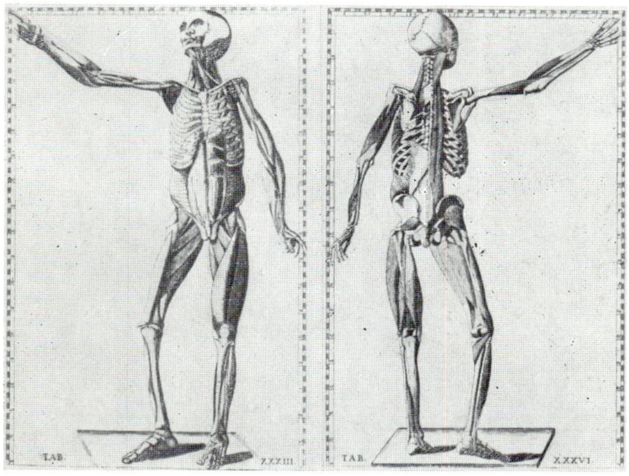
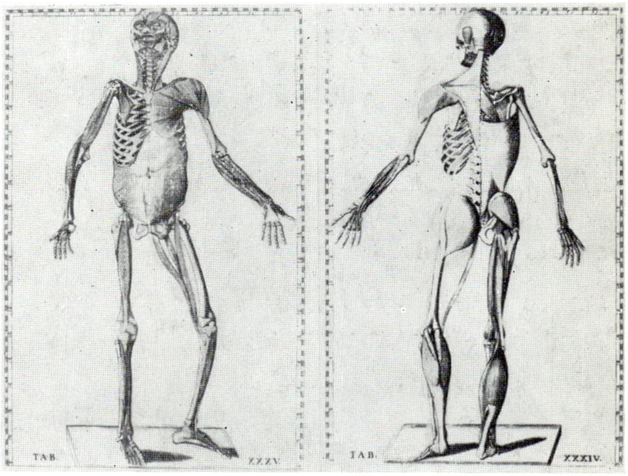
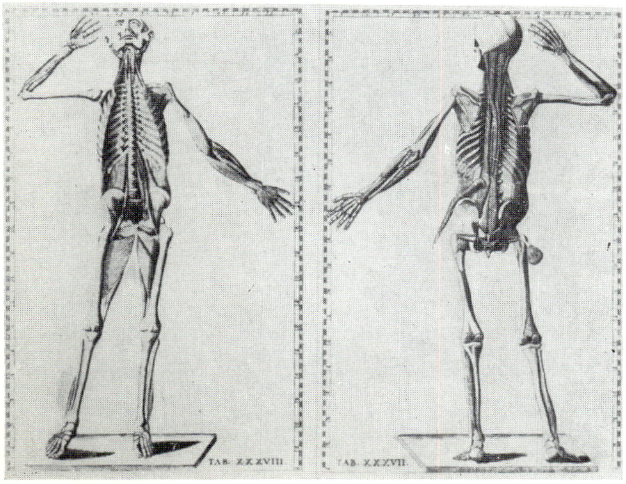
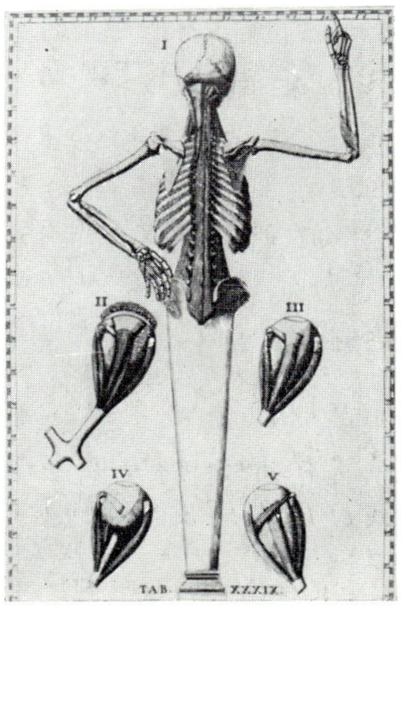

Plate XXV Eleven of the twelve myological tabulae from Bartolomeo Eustachio's Tabulae anatomicae, *ed. by J. M. Lancisi, Rome, 1714. The plates are arranged in pairs: XXVIII + XXIX, XXX + XXXI, XXXIII + XXXVI, XXXV + XXXIV, XXXVIII + XXXVII. Plates XXXII (not reproduced here) and XXXIX have no counterparts.*

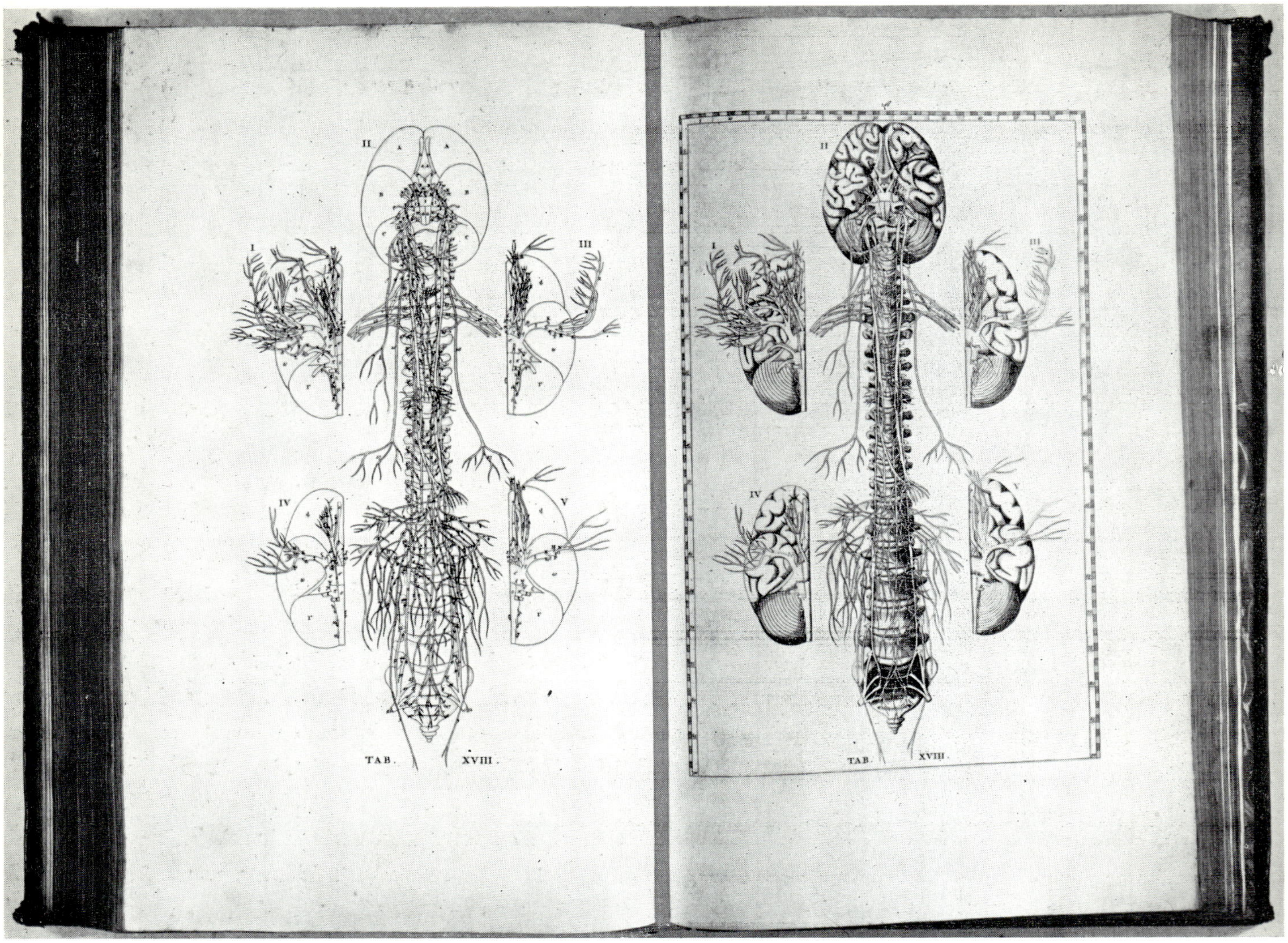

Plate XXVI The Eustachio edition of 1744 with outline sketches and commentaries provided by Bernhard S. Albinus was published in Leyden. The plates are copies of engravings from the Rome edition of 1714.

Other 16th-Century Medical Illustrations

It is easy to get the impression that medical illustration during the 16th century consisted mainly of anatomical illustrations. CHOULANT is to be held partly responsible for this, for he was interested only in anatomical illustration, and his *Geschichte und Bibliographie der anatomischen Abbildung* (1852) has dominated the field of medical iconography for the past century. It is one of the purposes of our present study to break up this monopoly, a monopoly CHOULANT himself certainly did not intend to establish. The special studies of WEINDLER (1908), GOLDSCHMID (1925), and NISSEN (1951) are useful here, but each of these scholars was also interested in a specific and limited subject, just as CHOULANT was. Moreover, there is one branch of medical illustration – the history of surgical illustration – that has not yet been investigated beyond the end of the 15th century.[1]

Surgery

Fig. 256 Instrument cabinet, from Brunschwig, Buch der Cirurgia, *1497.*

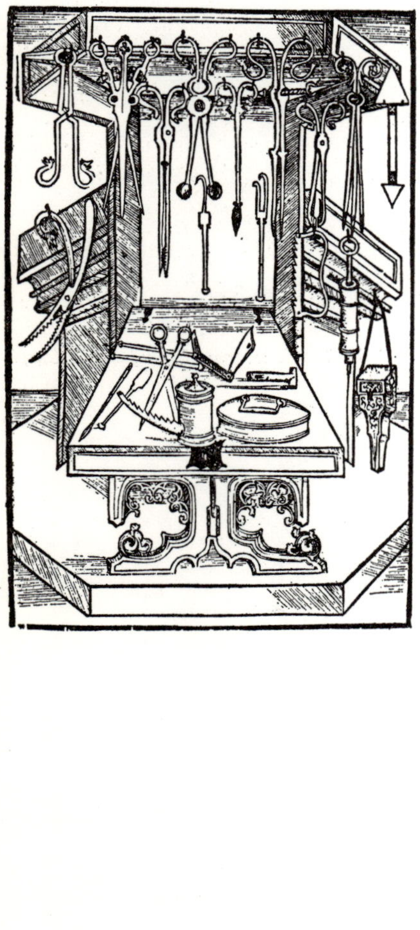

In our treatment of surgical illustration during the Middle Ages, we chose to arrange the material according to the different themes presented in the illustrations. This seemed appropriate to the subject, and it corresponded to SUDHOFF'S treatment. But even this traditional approach could not ignore the fact that together with schematic and semi-schematic illustration, there was also a tradition of naturalistic illustration that had persisted since antiquity, even though naturalism was somewhat at odds with the formal idiom of the medieval period. Essentially, symbolism and naturalism are antagonistic artistic methods. Only at certain supreme moments in the history of art has a synthesis of the two succeeded. With regard to subject matter and aim, the essential nature of practical graphic art in science and medicine is most conducive to such a synthesis.

Surgery is manual work; surgical illustration therefore shows manual operations and implements. In an age which makes it possible for the plastic arts to represent human actions realistically and naturalistically – we are using these terms synonymously here – the illustration of surgical operations will become increasingly important. We can see this happening in 16th-century medical illustration. In addition to purely instructive drawings showing surgical techniques, there are also a number of descriptive scenes that occasionally have narrative elements or elements of an eyewitness report.

Accordingly, 16th-century surgical illustration can be arranged into three general groups: (1) instruments and equipment, (2) techniques of handling the equipment, and (3) surgical operations, often including the procedures followed both in examination and in operation.

1. *Instruments and equipment.* The surgical textbooks of this epoch are full of illustrations of instruments and surgical equipment. Late medieval paintings devot-

[1] HUARD, PIERRE and M. D. GRMEK: Mille Ans de Chirurgie en Occident, Paris, Roger Dacosta, 1966. This superbly illustrated work, which appeared after the completion of my manuscript, can provide the reader with additional relevant illustrations.

ed increasing attention to objects that man holds in his hands. Then, in the Renaissance, the pleasure of discovering new technical aids, which was quite characteristic of that period, resulted in the invention of many new surgical instruments. For these inventions to become known and put to wide use, they had to be illustrated. In the 16th century, this development breaks into medicine with the force of a tidal wave.

Illustrations of surgical instruments had appeared only very rarely in medieval manuscripts, and then usually only in manuscripts influenced by the Arabic tradition[2] (see plate XVIIIa, p. 98). In the 15th century, BRUNSCHWIG (1497) allowed us to look into his instrument cabinet (fig. 256), but his forceps,[3] clamps, and trephines were drawn merely in outline, not in exact detail. Some of BRUNSCHWIG'S illustrations are clearly derived from the Moorish tradition (fig. 257), as are those contained in the surgical textbook of the master JAN YPERMAN, a work in manuscript form which fell into oblivion during the period of the incunabula. The slightly younger Frenchman, GUY DE CHAULIAC, who had studied in Montpellier, Bologna, and Paris, and had practiced in the Rhone Valley – especially at the papal court in Avignon – was just as familiar with the Arab physicians as with all his important contemporaries. However, the splendid pictures of instruments in the GUIDO editions of the 16th century are not by GUY DE CHAULIAC himself, but date from the 14th century rather than the 16th, as SUDHOFF demonstrated[4] by comparing them with those in several manuscripts. Similarly, the illustrations in the Junta edition of 1546 also belong to an earlier tradition, as do those in JOUBERT'S revised edition, Lyon, 1585, which was used by GURLT.[5] The earlier Venetian editions, in common with those of 1519, contain no illustrations. Representative of the earliest illustrations of surgical instruments which, as genuine originals, came directly from the author to the presses, are the trephines in the *Tractatus perutilis et completus de fractura cranei* of BERENGARIO DA CARPI, 1535, who was also a pioneer in the field of anatomical illustration. The artist must have had the instruments displayed on a table in front of him while he was preparing the designs for the engraver. The handle of the trephine bow is shown separate from the six adaptable heads, as in a technical drawing (fig. 258). Any instrument-maker would be capable of working from such drawings.

2. *Techniques for using surgical instruments and equipment.* It is obviously sensible to illustrate the way an instrument is to be used, in addition to showing the instrument itself. There is a series of instruments illustrated for the first time in HANS VON GERSSDORFF'S *Feldtbuch der Wundtartzney*, published in Strasbourg in 1517; the artist here progresses beyond BRUNSCHWIG in drawing the tools in full

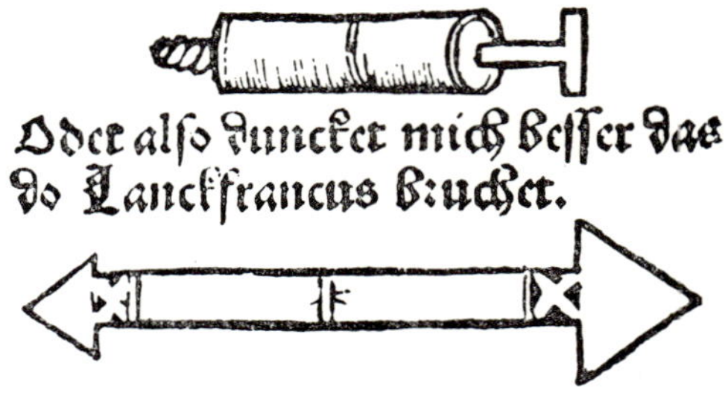

Fig. 257 Arabic instrument (double lancet), taken from Lanfranco by Brunschwig. The instrument also hangs in Brunschwig's instrument cabinet.

Fig. 258 Trephine, from Berengario da Carpi, 1535.

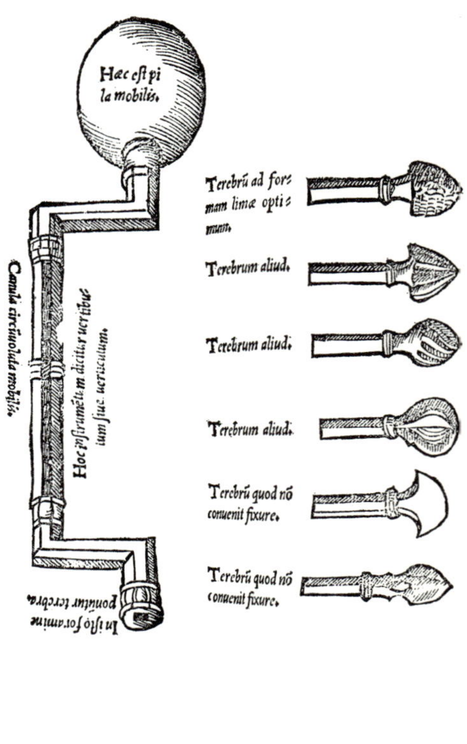

[2] See p. 44.
[3] At the top left of BRUNSCHWIG'S instrument cabinet there hangs an "almisdac," a type of obstetrical cranioclast which appears to have been directly taken from an ABULCASIS incunabula. See SUDHOFF, Studien 11/12, p. 53, fig. 15.
[4] SUDHOFF, Studien 11/12, *loc. cit.*, pp. 87-90.
[5] GURLT, E.: Geschichte der Chirurgie II, 1898, plate VI.

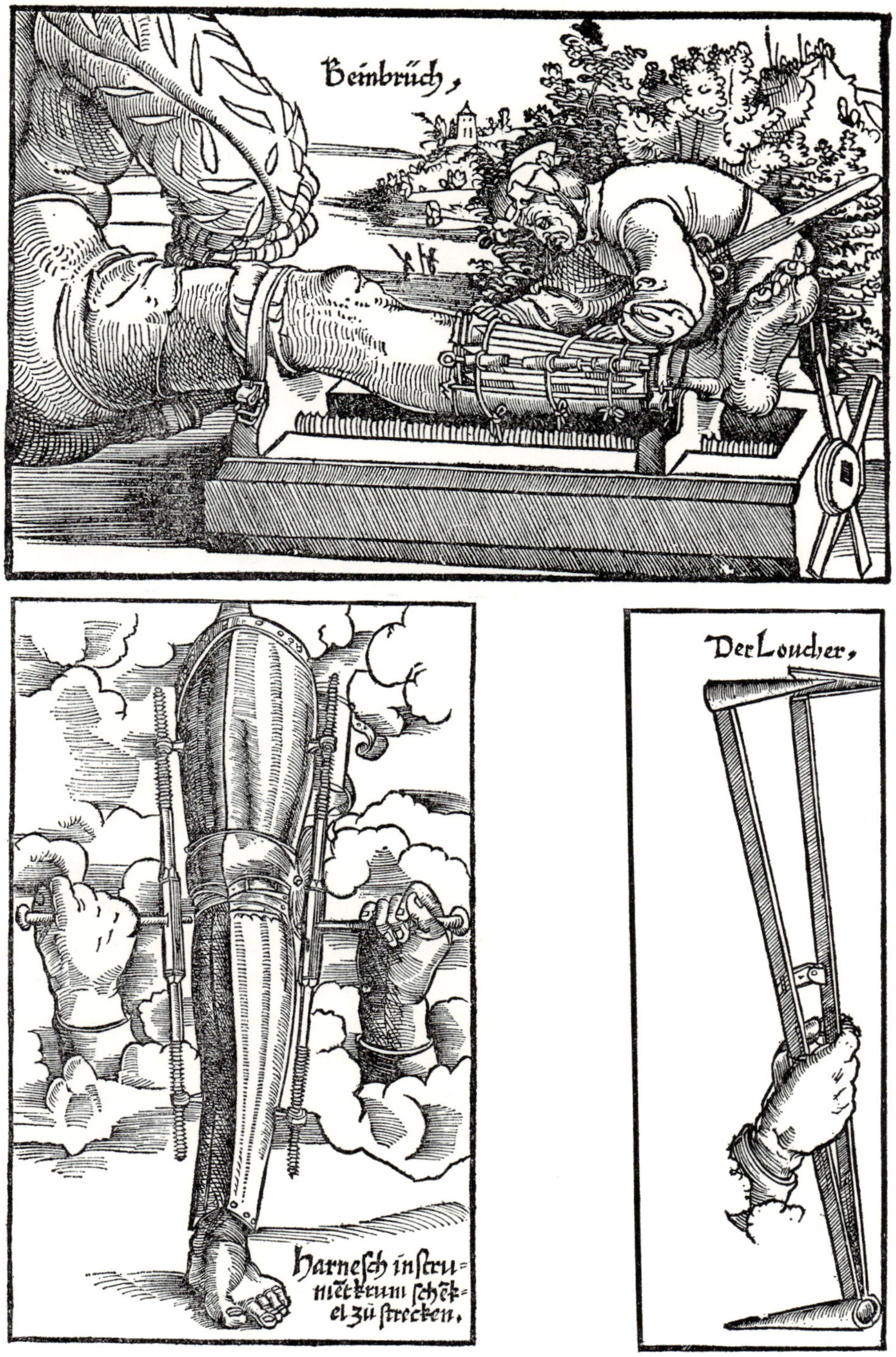

Fig. 259 Hans Wächtlin(?): Surgical instruments and apparatus in use. From Gerssdorff, Feldtbuch der Wundtartzney, *Strasbourg, 1517.*

three-dimensional detail and in demonstrating the use of one instrument, a retractor ("Der Loucher") used for keeping narrow wounds open during surgery (fig. 259). Some of the equipment, for instance that used to stretch a fractured limb, would not have been intelligible at all unless it had been illustrated in use. Both the Hippocratic splint and the *ambe*, a lever with a rounded edge at the end for fitting against the axilla in the resetting of a dislocated shoulder joint (fig. 262), became standard illustrations in German surgical texts after GERSSDORFF'S work appeared. This also applies to the stretching equipment for treating stiffened knee and elbow joints (fig. 259). One of the most impressive illustrations of this type is GERSSDORFF'S picture of his apparatus for treating depressed fractures of the skull (fig. 260). This head is an example of the finest woodcut graphic art of the early 16th century. We have referred only to the early stages of 16th-century illustration here. By the end of the century, a great many other illustrations had appeared that showed instruments and equipment in use – for instance, in the works of RYFF, GUIDI, MAGGI, PARÉ, FABRICIUS AB ACQUAPENDENTE, TAGLIACOZZI, and FABRITIUS HILDANUS.

3. *Surgical operations and procedures*. The surgical literature which we have just mentioned is full of illustrations of surgical procedures.[6] There are single pictures, as well as series of pictures showing the sequence of the individual manual operations and their results. The most extensive series of illustrations, however, are contained not in a book but in a manuscript, the *Practica copiosa* of 1559 by the surgeon CASPAR STROMAYR of Lindau. This work is a textbook on herniology with appendices on gynecology and ophthalmology. Embracing medical examination, surgical operation in all its phases, and post-operative therapy, this book contains the most complete pictorial representation of hernia treatment ever attempted.[7]

The illustrations in GERSSDORFF'S *Feldtbuch* belong to the early phase of 16th-century medical illustration and represent one of its high points. In addition to instruments and indications of their use, it also contains numerous surgical scenes, which however are not actually intended to convey technical information about surgical procedures. In view of their vividness and of the fact that they are only loosely integrated into the text, they may be described as reports. As such, they represent an impressive step forward in the history of illustration, especially when they are compared with the incunabula woodcuts in BRUNSCHWIG'S *Cirurgia* of 1497, which were "naturalistic" only in a very qualified sense.

But it would be wrong to say that naturalistic representation was without precedent at that time. The pictorial report, or scene based upon observation, was by no means

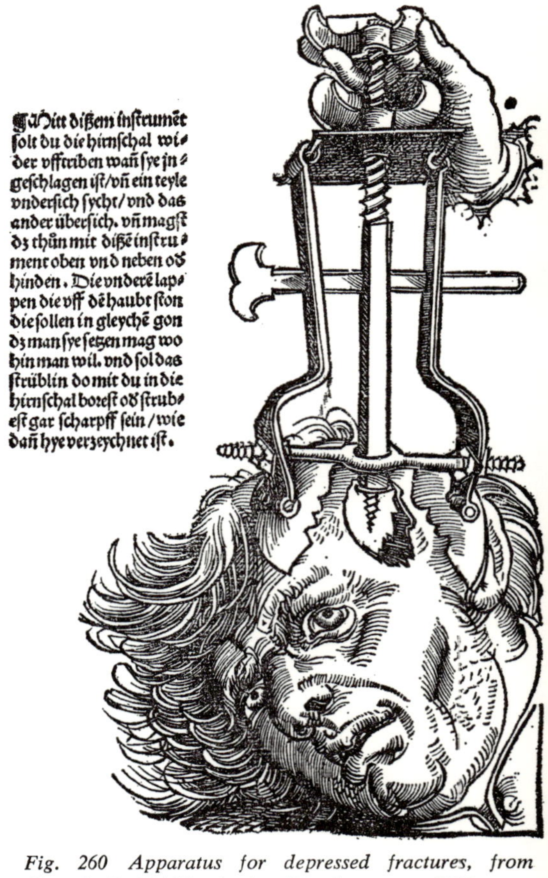

Fig. 260 Apparatus for depressed fractures, from Gerssdorff, Feldtbuch der Wundtartzney, *1517.*

Fig. 261 Application of a seton ('setaceum' to the neck, from Fabritius Hildanus, Observationes *I-C, Frankfurt am Main, 1610. Knife and needle are especially prominent in the original.*

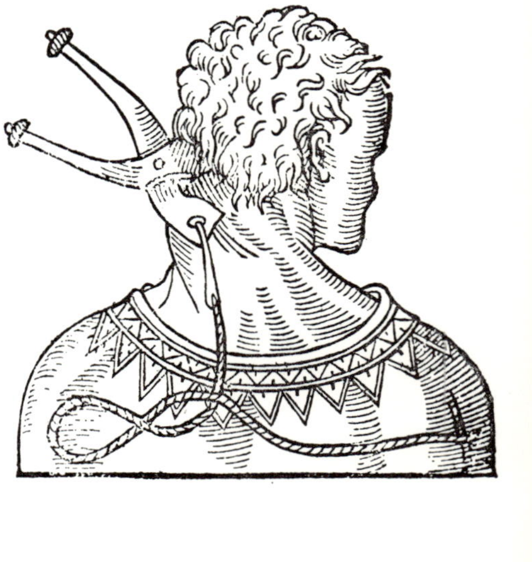

[6] At the Department of Prints and Engravings of the British Museum there is also an illustrated book (Ms. 197 d. 2) which, among a variety of other items, contains pictures of sixteen surgical instruments. This work has previously been misjudged with regard to its origins. It bears the names of the two Tübingen artists FÜLLMAURER and MEYER – erroneously read as KULLMAURER and MEHER – who are known to have been the artists for LEONHART FUCHS'S Historia Stirpium and New Kreüterbuoch, Basel, Isingrin, 1542/43. Catalogue references indicate that the work is a fragment of a surgery textbook which was never printed. Cf. ROTT, HANS: Quellen und Forschungen zur südwest-deutschen und schweizerischen Kunstgeschichte im 15. und 16. Jahrhundert, *2*, 1934, p. LVI, and MACKINNEY (see p. 16, footnote 21), p. 44 and pp. 138-39.

[7] Modern facsimile edition by WALTER V. BRUNN: Die Handschrift des Schnitt- und Augenarztes Caspar Stromayr in Lindau im Bodensee, Berlin, 1925.

[8] THIEME-BECKER *35*, 1942, pp. 233-35. H. ROTTINGER, the editor, has no reservations about attributing all the woodcuts in GERSSDORFF'S Chirurgia to the master responsible for the HOCK situs of 1517.

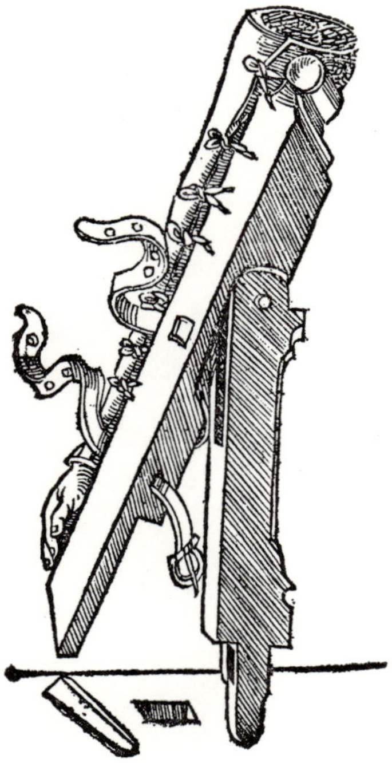

Fig. 262 'Ambe,' from Walter Ryff, Die gross Chirurgei, *Frankfurt, 1545. Reversed and reduced copy from Gerssdorff, 1517.*

Fig. 263 An amputation, from Gerssdorff, Feldtbuch der Wundtartzney, *1517.*

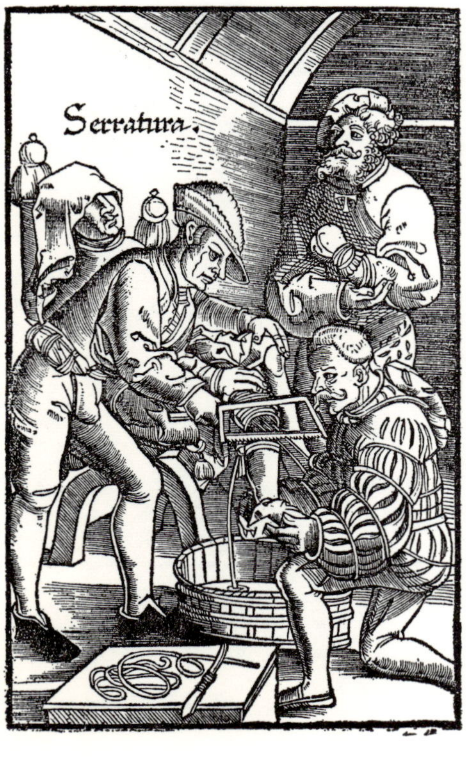

new at the beginning of the 16th century. A 13th-century Viennese codex (Codex lat. 93) contained a large number of physician-and-patient scenes which reflected everyday life (see plate VII). We can also look again at the realistic miniatures of the 14th-century Leyden manuscript (Voss lat. 3), a few of which are reproduced in plate XV.

A direct line leads from the work of the early 16th-century artist who did the illustrations for GERSSDORFF'S book, who is traditionally identified as HANS WÄCHTLIN,[8] to the work of the so-called PETRARCH MASTER,[9] an engraver who worked in Augsburg around 1520. The magnificent series of pictures for the *Von der Artzney bayder Glück, des guten und widerwärtigen,* Augsburg, 1532 – the German translation of PETRARCH'S *De remediis utriusque fortunae* – contains no actual medical illustration, except for a borrowed woodcut. One of the main illustrations, however (which SCHEIDIG dates as being from 1519/20), is worthy of inclusion in a book on medical history: it is the most moving of all depictions of the plague (fig. 264). The recently opened axillary bubo of the dying patient makes this scene into a medical document. Several illustrations from the Augsburg publishing house of STAYNER may be attributed to the same master.[10] Incidentally, the borrowed illustration in the *Artzney bayder Glück* is a zodiac figure that had already been used in a LANFRANCHI edition by GRIMM & WIRSUNG.[11] The traditional zodiac-man, shown here in the position of a crucified figure, is covered with eruptions, presumably caused by a syphilitic infection.

The most beautiful textbook of surgery to be printed in the 16th century was the *Chirurgia è Graeco in Latinum conversa* of VIDUS VIDIUS, Paris, 1544. Its date of publication puts it close in time to VESALIUS'S *Fabrica,* the finest textbook of anatomy produced in the 16th century. ERNST GURLT, however, in his unparalleled *Geschichte der Chirurgie* of 1898, has only this to say about the illustrations in VIDIUS'S extraordinary work: "The illustrations, which in part have been copied from very old manuscripts, are interesting because they show how a mid-16th-century artist conceived the instruments, bandages, machines, and mechanical operations which had been described by older authors." Curiously, GURLT was already acquainted[12] with the fully illustrated edition of the Florentine manuscript of the *Peri arthron* (the NICETAS manuscript, Laurenziana LXXIV, 7), which the Greek scholar HERMANN SCHOENE had published in 1896, but he did not recognize the historical connection between the 10th-century Byzantine miniatures of this manuscript and the 16th-century woodcuts in the *Chirurgia* of VIDIUS, which we

[9] THIEME-BECKER *37*, 1959, p. 270. THEODOR MUSPER, in 1922, opposed the theory that the Petrarch Master is HANS WEIDITZ. Cf. also W. RYTZ in his accompanying text, pp. 36-41, to the facsimile edition of the "Pflanzen-aquarelle des HANS WEIDITZ aus dem Jahre 1529," Bern, Paul Haupt Verlag, 1936; and SCHEIDIG, WALTER: Die Holzschnitte des Petrarcha-Meisters, Berlin, Henschelverlag, 1955.

[10] See KRISTELLER: Kupferstich und Holzschnitt in vier Jahrhunderten, p. 224; SCHEIDIG, p. 318; MUSPER, H. Th.: Der Holzschnitt in fünf Jahrhunderten, Stuttgart, 1964, pp. 183-84.

[11] LANFRANCUS: Kleine Wundartzney. Cf. SCHEIDIG, p. 318.

[12] GURLT (see footnote 5 on p. 140), Vol. I, p. 130.

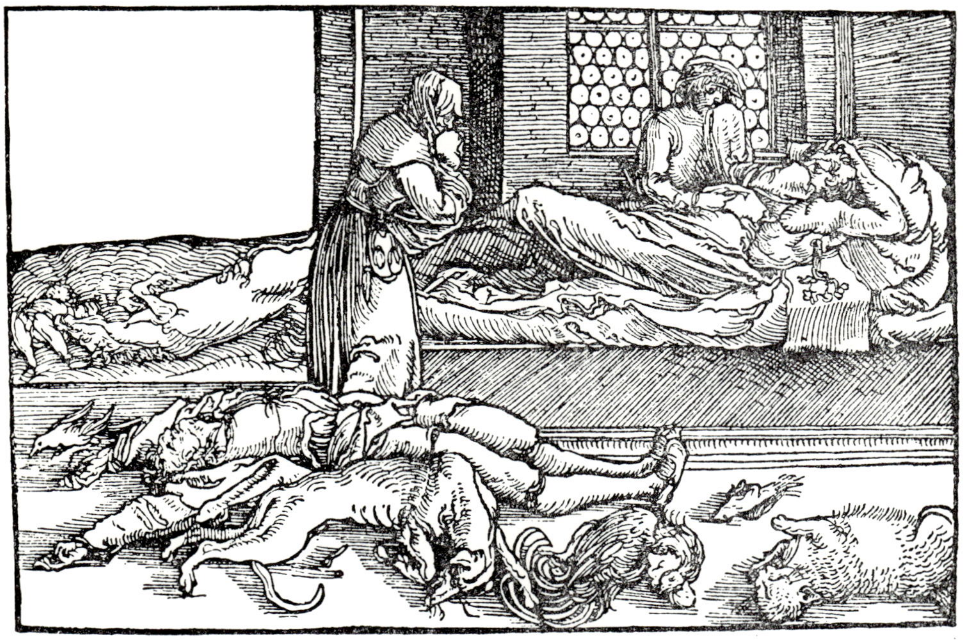

Fig. 264 The plague ('Von dem Sterben oder Pestilenz, die sehr weit tobt und währet'). The white space at the top left originally contained the two saints of the plague-stricken, Sebastian and Roch. The woodcut was finished in 1519/20 but was not printed until 1532, after the Protestant Reformation in Augsburg. From Francesco Petrarca, Von der Artzney bayder Glück, *1532.*

discussed in the chapter on antiquity (see p. 15). Irrespective of the question of whether or not Vidius's illustrations owed their inspiration indirectly to Nicetas,[13] the illustrations do prove that the 16th-century popular interest in all things Greek extended even to illustrated texts that had come down – or supposedly come down – from Greek antiquity. The success of the rediscovered Nicetas illustrations for the *Peri arthron* was so complete that copies of the illustrations were used not only in the Basel edition of the complete works of Galen, which was published by Froben in 1562 at an outlay worthy of such an edition, but also in a spate of Paré editions and Spanish copies published towards the end of the century. Some of the newly drawn illustrations adhered closely to the 10th-century miniatures, but others translated the 10th-century scenes into scenes that conformed more closely to 16th-century artistic taste (compare the two illustrations showing the treatment of a dislocated jaw, plate XXVIII).

Many other surgical scenes shown in 16th-century books were also copied again and again, slightly modified in each successive copy. For example, one of Gerssdorff's woodcuts was copied in Giovanni Andrea della Croce's *Chirurgiae universalis opus,* Venice, 1573; the style becomes Italian, and the figures of the German mercenaries are replaced by Turks.[14] On the other hand, this beautifully illustrated Italian surgical textbook contains original illustrations for

Fig. 265 Zodiac figure; woodcut from Petrarca, Von der Artzney bayder Glück, *1532.*

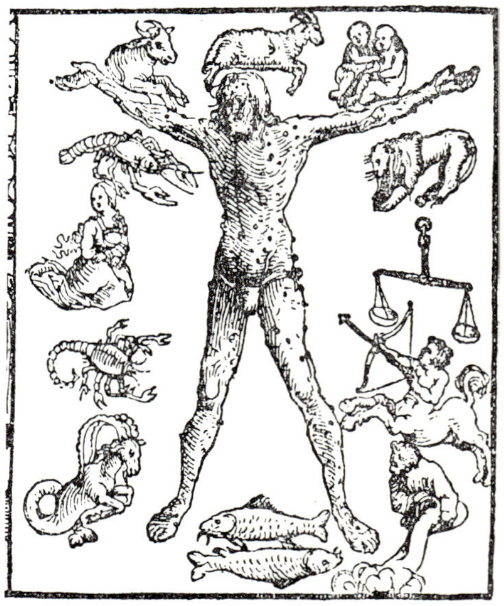

[13] Kellett, C. E.: The Chirurgia of Vidus Vidius, 1544. An occasional lecture May, 1959, in: Mannerism and Medical Illustration. Lectures given at the University of Los Angeles, October 1961, private printing n. d., cf. p. 16.

[14] In the field of medical illustration, the influence of German woodcuts on Venetian artists can scarcely be underestimated.

cranial surgery, which in turn served as models for numerous later illustrations in the same field.

Having completed a brief survey of the treatment of surgical scenes in early 16th-century medical books, we now reach the late phase of classical woodcut illustration, which culminated in VESALIUS'S *Fabrica*. It is worthwhile to digress here for a few paragraphs to consider the fate of woodblock printing in general after the middle of the 16th century. As we have already mentioned (p. 113), the woodblocks used by OPORINUS for the second edition of the *Fabrica* (1555) were extraordinarily good. They were enthusiastically praised by WILLY WIEGAND in 1936 after he had succeeded in making prints at his Bremer Presse which were sometimes even of

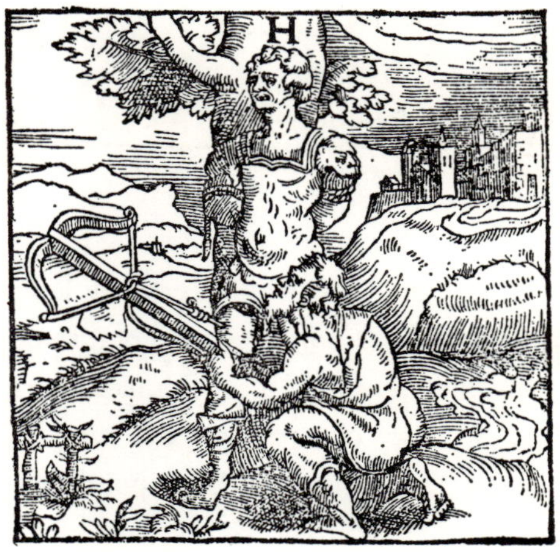

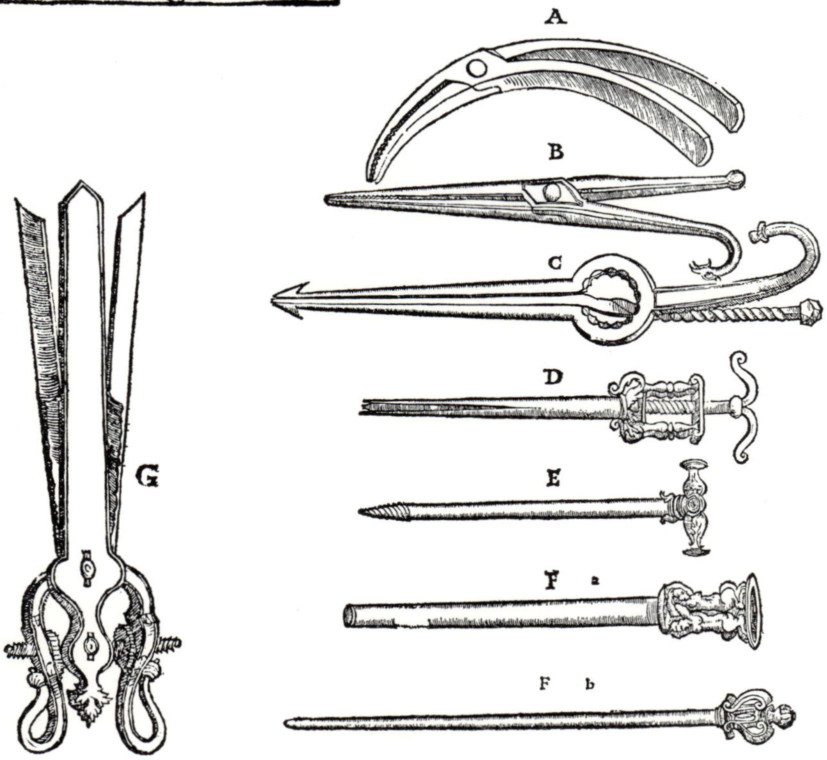

Figures 266 and 267 Surgical instruments (right) and surgical cross-bow (above) for the extraction of arrows. From the Ars Chirurgica *of Guido von Chauliac, Venice, 1546; copied from Gerssdorff, 1519. The drawings of the instruments were probably just as useful to instrument-makers as to surgeons.*

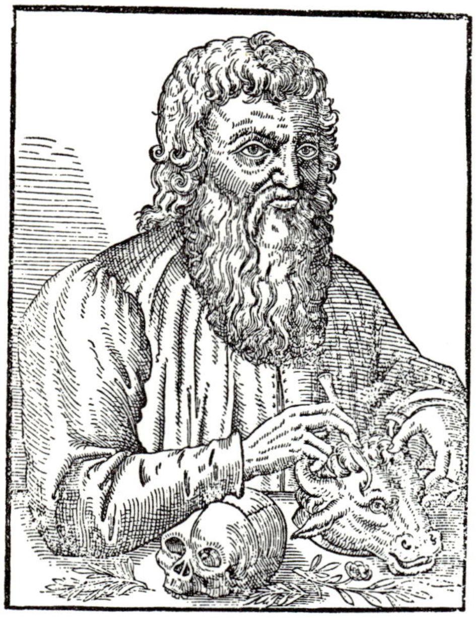

Fig. 268

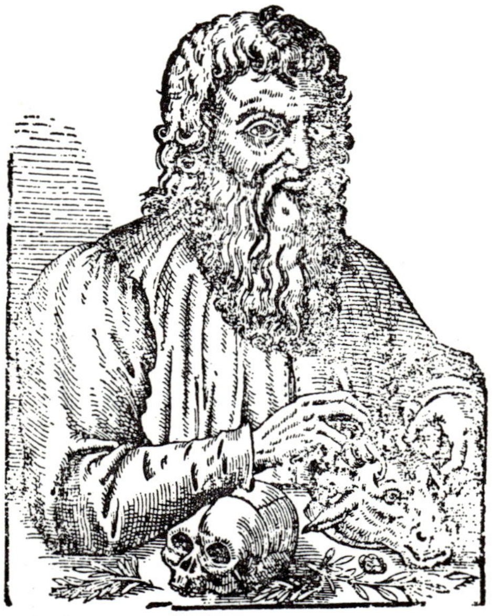

Fig. 269

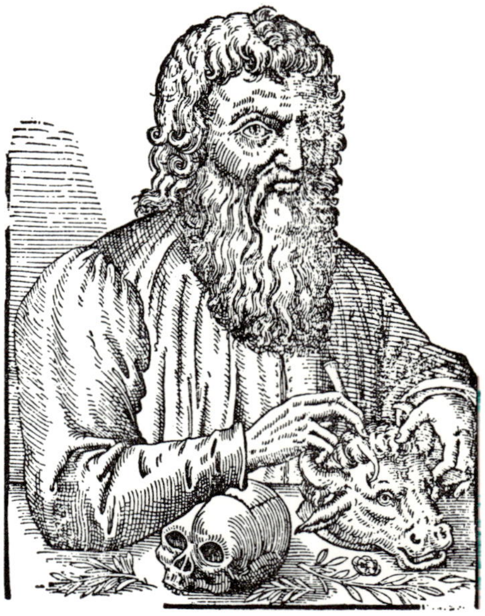

Fig. 270

Figures 268 to 270 Showing the condition of the same printing block in 1594, 1610, and 1635, respectively, from the Frankfurt printing shop of Johannes Feyerabend and his successors. Fig. 269 is a poorly executed print from a woodblock which produced a relatively better print twenty-five years later (fig. 270).

higher quality than those of the 1543 and 1555 editions. This would certainly have been impossible had the material and the technique of the engraver not conformed so well to the demands of this craft. It is quite evident, however, that with increasing mass-production, publishers became content to use cheaper woods, simpler preparation, and a less careful engraving technique. Moreover, the large publishers at the end of the 16th century did not hesitate to go on printing from a woodblock until it literally fell apart. The results of this can be seen when several different editions, or several impressions from the same woodblock appearing in different books, are placed together for comparison.

Let us take one example (figs. 268-270). The Frankfurt printer JOHANNES FEYERABEND had woodcuts made for his complete edition of PARÉ'S *Opera chirurgica* which were copied from many different sources – VESALIUS, for example, was shamelessly plundered – and which unfortunately did not often match the originals in artistic quality. The book appeared in 1594. On page 836 there is an imaginary portrait titled "Hippocratis Coi medicorum principis," a bungling piece of work. In the year 1610 a *Thesaurus chirurgiae,* an anthology of the most important surgical literature of the second half of the 16th century from PARÉ to FABRITIUS HILDANUS, was published at the printing shop of NICOLAUS HOFFMANN, FEYERABEND'S successor. It was compiled by the municipal physician of Frankfurt, PETER UFFENBACH. On page 647 of this bestseller, printed by what at that time was a world-famous publishing house, FEYERABEND'S portrait of Hippocrates reappears. But by this time, as a result of the presumably large number of copies printed for the first Frankfurt edition of PARÉ and for UFFENBACH'S German translation of the same year, the woodblock was so overworked that half the frame is now missing.

Fig. 271 An example of the poor condition of some woodblocks employed for the mass editions of the 16th century, from W. Ryff, Feldt und Stattbuch Bewerter Wundtartzney, *1556. In 1551, the upper border was still intact and the lower virtually undamaged, although the righthand strip was already broken.*

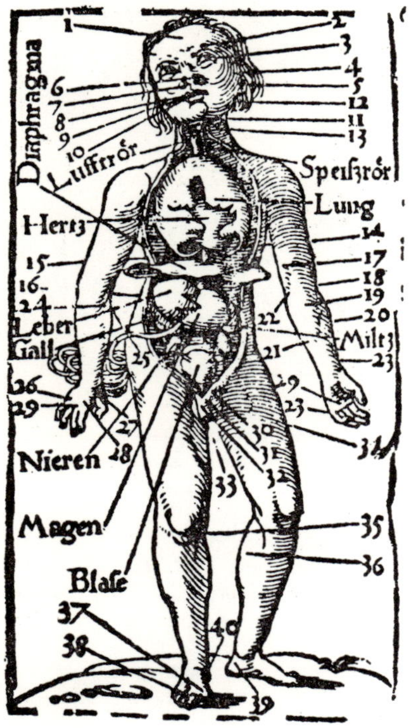

Fig. 272 Fabritius Hildanus, Observationes I-C, *printed in the* Thesaurus Chirurgiae *published by Peter Uffenbach, Frankfurt, 1610. Anus praeternaturalis after an impalement wound, observed in 1602.*

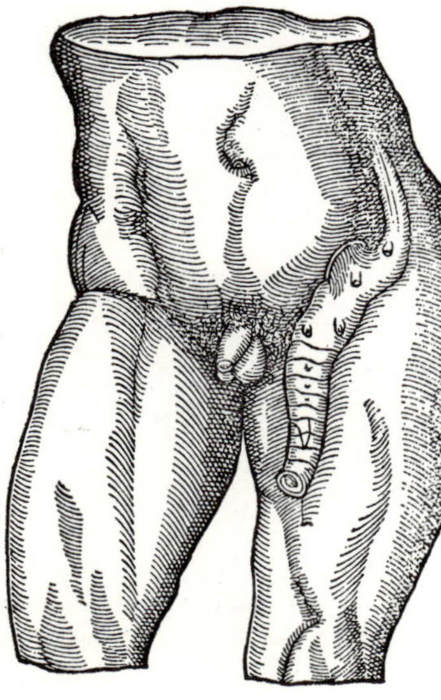

Admittedly, the original designer had used poor technical judgment in engraving the frame as a fragile line. But even the printing surface is in a sorry state and full of scratches. In spite of this, the woodblock survived this edition, although the frame broke again during this printing, and it only just managed to remain level. The eventual condition of the block is demonstrated by the second edition of the German translation, published by CASPAR RÖTTELL in Frankfurt in 1635. The "True and actual portrait of the most excellent and princely of all physicians / Hippocrates from the island of Cos," who is none other than our paltry pseudo-Hippocrates of 1594, has suffered the loss of yet another centimeter of frame. Similar wear can be observed in the successive editions of another book published by FEYERABEND, J. RUEFF'S *Hebammenbuch,* which went through half a dozen printings; and CHARLES SINGER has called attention to the same phenomenon in the successive printings from the woodblocks for KETHAM'S *Fasciculus medicinae,* which were used for many years in the workshop of the GREGORI brothers. Such observations were also made by RÖTTINGER[15] in studying the Frankfurt plagiarisms of BERENGARIO published in the mid-16th century.

Let us now return to the question of surgical illustration during the latter part of the 16th century. In July 1559, the municipal surgeon of Lindau, CASPAR STROMAYR, dedicated to his Zurich colleague PETTER HAFFNER the textbook on herniology which was mentioned briefly on page 142. The amusement felt by the modern reader of this work derives in some part from the fact that both in the diagnostic section (where various types of fractures are illustrated) and in the operative section (which demonstrates a series of surgical operations) the artist has gone to the trouble of preparing full-figure illustrations and complete surgical scenes in order to present information that a modern illustrator would show in a simple detail. The application of bandages and the minutely detailed representation of the postoperative therapy, which for STROMAYR was apparently – and quite rightly – just as important as operational procedure, might justify a few of the elaborately represented scenes, even according to modern standards. However, the artist obviously made sketches of operations on many different patients in order to collect enough material to illustrate all of the stages of one particular kind of operation, and so the reader is somewhat astonished at the rapid changes in personnel in the finished series of illustrations – only the surgeon retains his role throughout; a new patient and a new team of assistants suddenly appear in almost each successive picture.

A number of other texts containing original illustrations also appeared during the second half of the 16th century. A counterpart to STROMAYR'S herniology text is a manuscript on lithotomy compiled in 1575 by the surgeon GEORG BARTISCH of Dresden, who presumably also wrote the text and furnished it with his own

15 RÖTTINGER, HEINRICH: Der Frankfurter Buchholzschnitt 1530-1550, Stud. z. dtsch. Kulturgesch. 293, Strasbourg, 1933.

illustrations.[16] Despite the fact that it was dedicated to August, Elector of Saxony, this work was never published. However, the author's *Augendienst*,[17] a similar illustrated textbook on cataract operations, was printed in 1583. The woodcuts for this book were done after watercolors painted by BARTISCH himself (fig. 273). Similar artistic intentions can be found in the work of WILHELM FABRY, the municipal surgeon of Bern. He can certainly be counted among the "scientific" surgeons of his time and, in a sense, is a German counterpart to PARÉ. His *Observationum et curationum chirurgicarum centuria I*, as well as his later books, contains carefully managed illustrations, among which there are examples of a type of medical illustration that made its first appearance about 1600: the illustration of pathological findings. The illustrator of this book fell back on the old solution of using a torso or half-figure when it was necessary to depict only one part of the human body (see figure 272).

This was the situation, then, until the end of the century, when a work appeared that was simultaneously the conclusion of the early period of surgical illustration and the prelude to the developments that were to take place in the 17th century: GASPARE TAGLIACOZZI'S *De curtorum chirurgia per insitionem*, the first textbook of plastic surgery, published in Bologna in 1597.[18] The twenty-two illustrated plates contained at the end of the book are woodcuts of mediocre technical quality, but they reveal considerable artistic skill. The arrangement is well thought out: the most important instruments, the first three stages of the operation for restoring the nose, two separate plates showing the two most important bandages, two further plates demonstrating their use in the decisive phase of the operation, and finally the removal of the bandage and flap of skin. (Some, but not all, of these illustrations are reproduced in figure 275.) Other plates illustrate the third part of the operation for shaping the nostrils (see figure 274). At the very end, plastic surgery of the lips and ears is explained by means of simple line-drawings. The anonymous artist is unable to dispense with the full-figure illustrations except in the few plates where he portrays heads represented as antique busts!

The scenes are oriented toward didactic representation – they are not drawn from life, and they are not crowded with irrelevant detail. They represent one of the two basic types of illustration which have been considered since LEONARDO and VESALIUS: the general case as opposed to the individual case. The German surgeons STROMAYR and BARTISCH, of course, chose the latter, and showed operations taking place in specific surroundings and involving recognizable individuals.

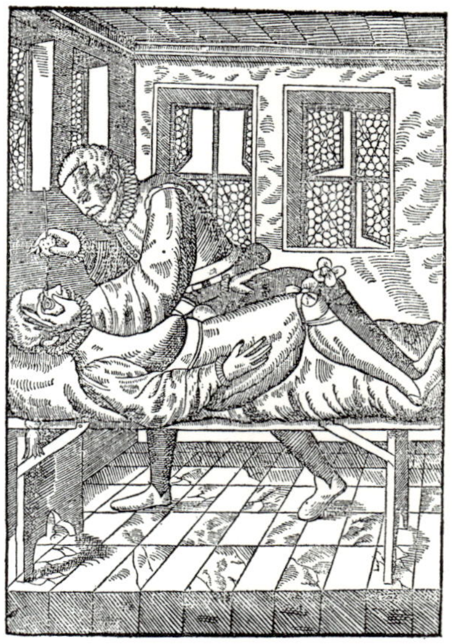

Fig. 273 Woodcut, from Georg Bartisch, Augendienst, *Dresden, 1583. After a watercolor by the author.*

Fig. 274 Detail from plate XX in Tagliacozzi, De curtorum chirurgia, *1597. The hatching on a drape is cleverly exploited as relief background for the demonstration of a post-operative dressing.*

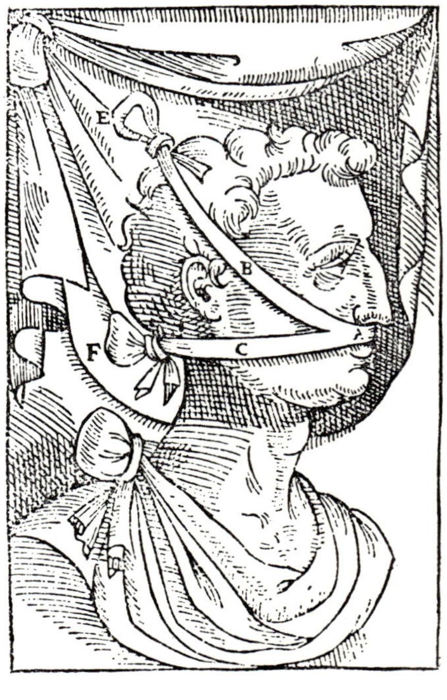

Fig. 275 (opposite page) Twelve of the fifteen figures illustrating the operating technique for plastic surgery of the nose, from Tagliacozzi, De curtorum chirurgia, *1597.*

16 MANKIEWICZ, OTTO: Kunstbuch des Blasenn Steines verfasset durch GEORGIUM BARTISCH vonn Koenigsbrück, Berlin, Oscar Coblentz, 1905.

17 See HAESER, HEINRICH: Lehrbuch der Geschichte der Medizin und der epidemischen Krankheiten, 3rd edition, Vol. 2, Jena, 1881, p. 201.

18 GNUDI, MARTHA TEACH and JEROME PIERCE WEBSTER: The Life and Times of Gaspare Tagliacozzi, Surgeon of Bologna, 1545-1599, New York, Herbert Reichner, n.d. [1950].

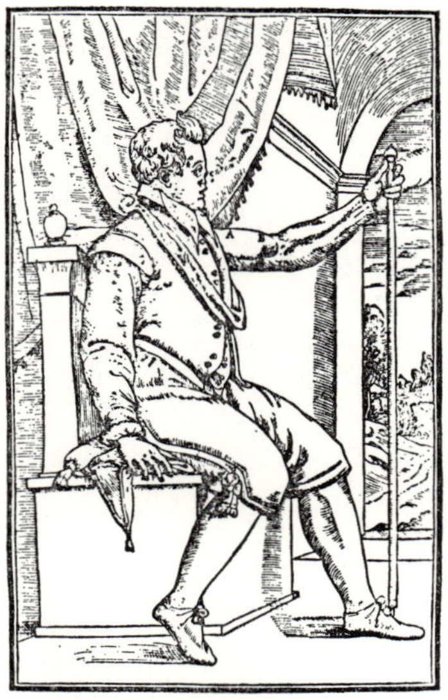
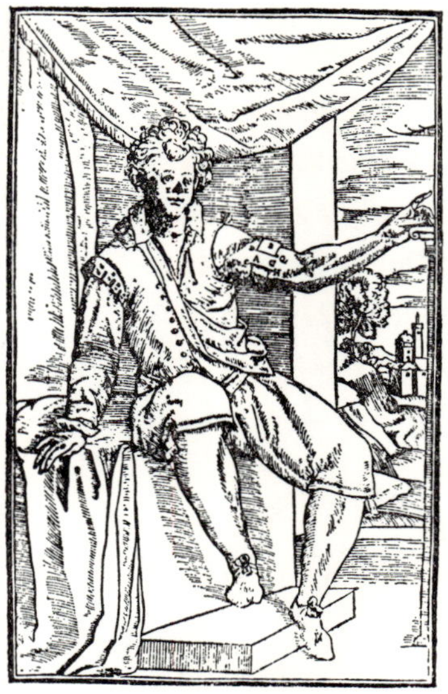
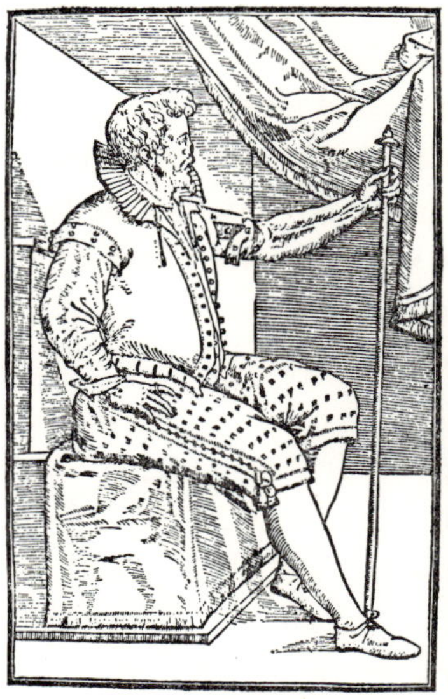
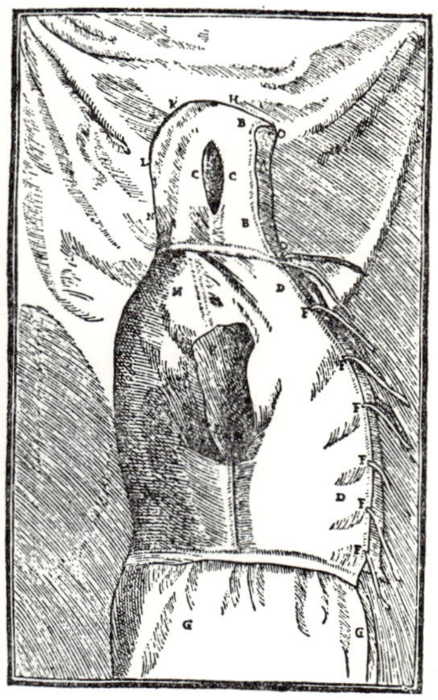
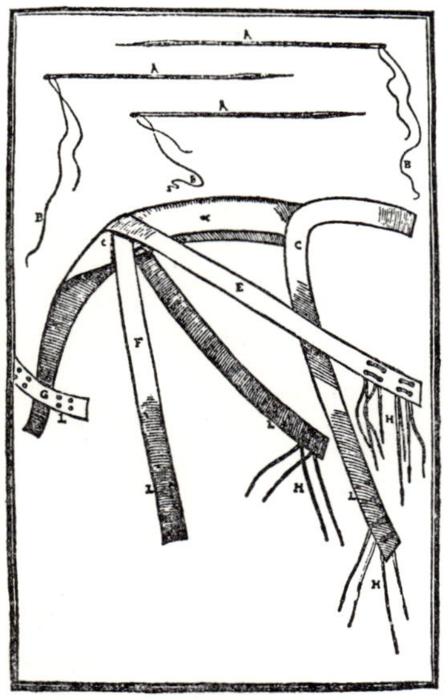
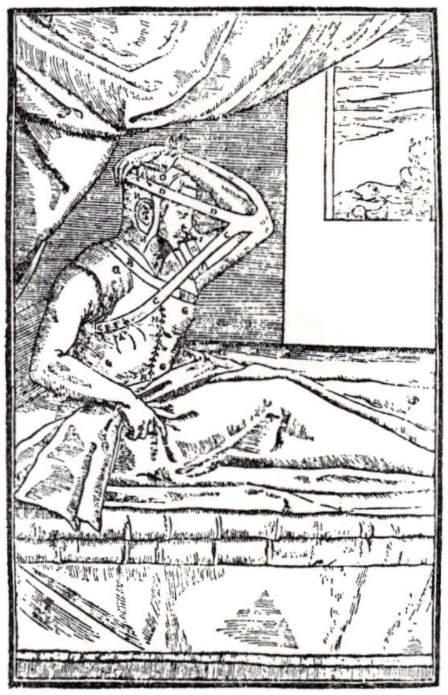
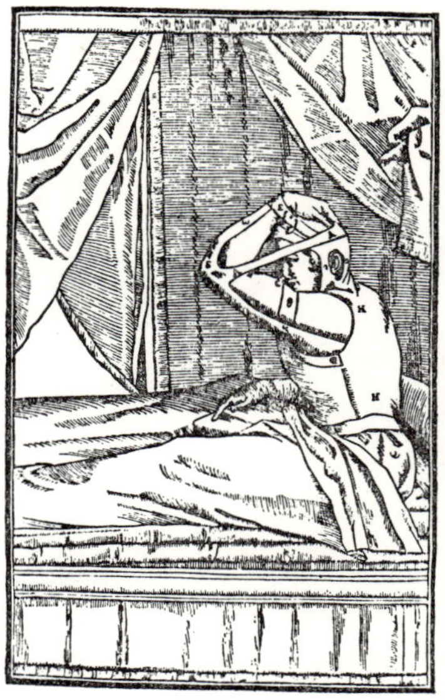
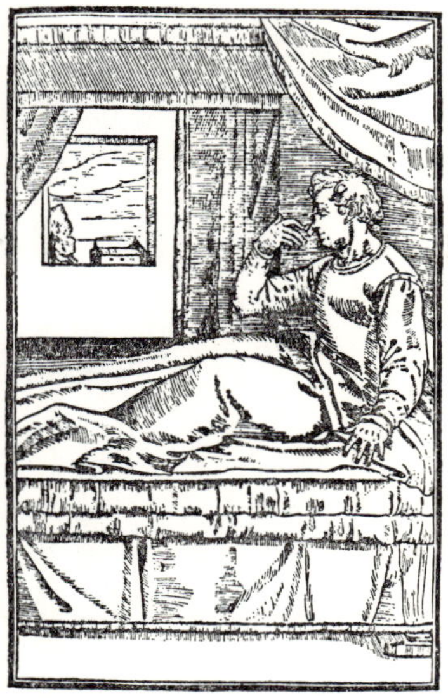
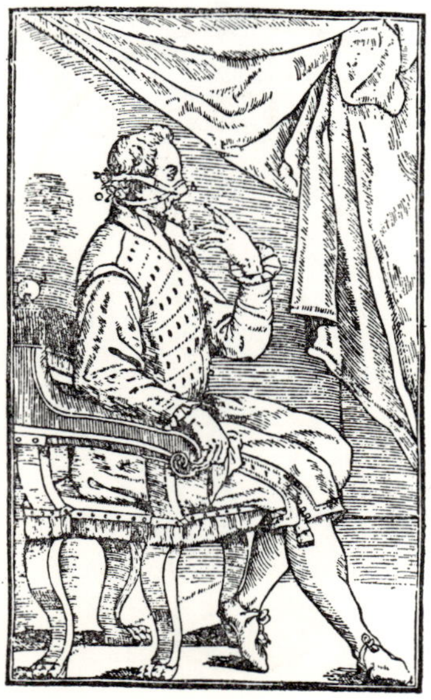
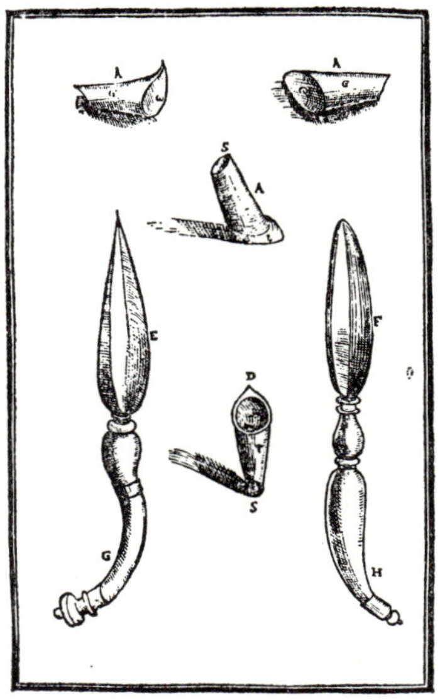
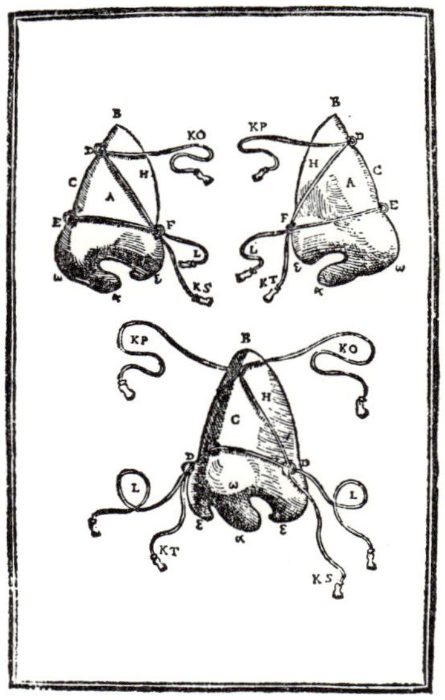
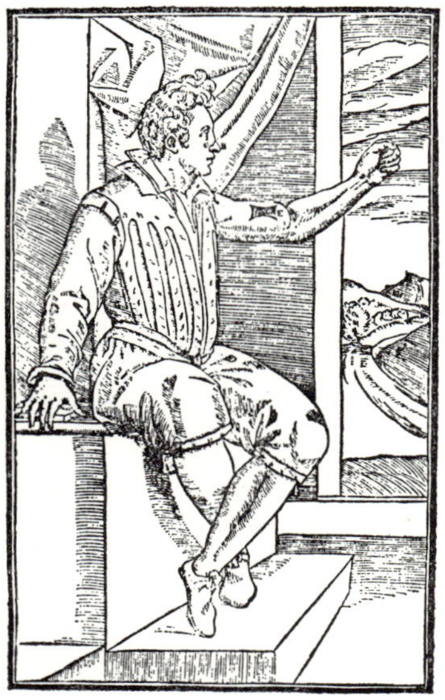

Pathological anatomy; obstetrics

Most other types of 16th-century medical illustration lagged far behind anatomical and surgical illustration. There was very little illustration of pathological anatomy in the modern sense, apart from teratology. GOLDSCHMID,[19] who vainly looked for relevant material, filled his gaps with examples which do not actually belong to medical illustration. However, a cystic mole is to be found in PARÉ (fig. 277) and a horseshoe kidney in BOTALLO (fig. 276).

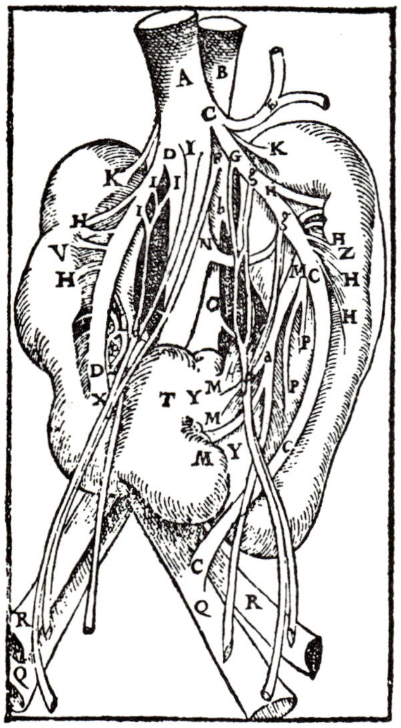

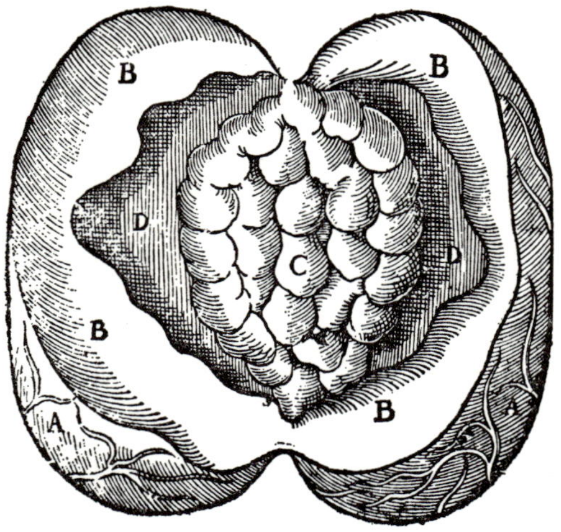

Fig. 277 Cystic mole, from A. Paré, Opera chirurgica, *Franfurt am Main, 1594.*

Fig. 276 Horseshoe kidney, from L. Botallo, Observationes anatomicae *(Observatio I: De monstroso rene).*

Fig. 278 Podalic presentation, from E. Rösslin, De partu hominis, *Frankfurt am Main, 1543; the illustration first appeared in Rösslin's* Rosengarten, *1513.*

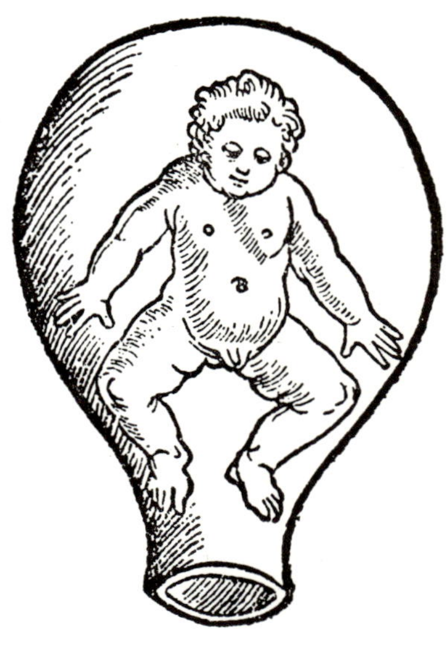

In obstetrics,[20] illustrations showing the positions of the fetus in the uterus – a type of illustration that goes all the way back to SORANOS and MOSCHION (see page 20) – were still the most common kind. During the Middle Ages an Arabic version[21] had been widely used, characterized by the strict geometrical figures and vivid coloring typical of Arabic art. A pregnancy figure belongs to the repertoire of several otherwise purely anatomical textbooks (BERENGARIO and ESTIENNE) or general textbooks (KETHAM). We have come across this type of figure on numerous occasions. There was still only scant literature on obstetrics during the 16th century. The works most frequently published were JACOB RUEFF'S *De conceptu et generatione*

19 GOLDSCHMID, EDGAR: Entwicklung und Bibliographie der pathologisch-anatomischen Abbildung, Leipzig, Hiersemann, 1925.

20 WEINDLER, FRITZ: Geschichte der gynäkologisch-anatomischen Abbildung, Dresden, Zahn und Jaensch, 1908.

21 WEINDLER: figs. 17-20. WEINDLER has not considered the possibility of Arabic origin, nor has GUSTAV KLEIN, the finder of the Munich Cod. lat. 161, or SUDHOFF.

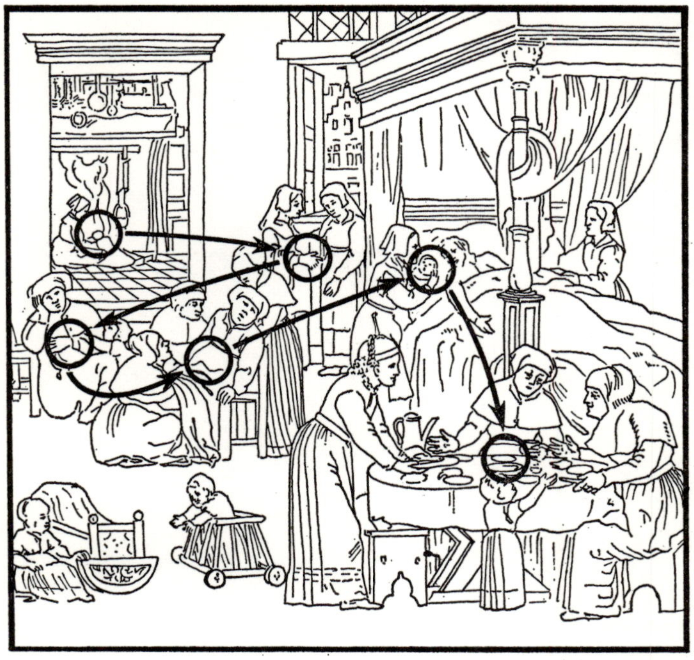 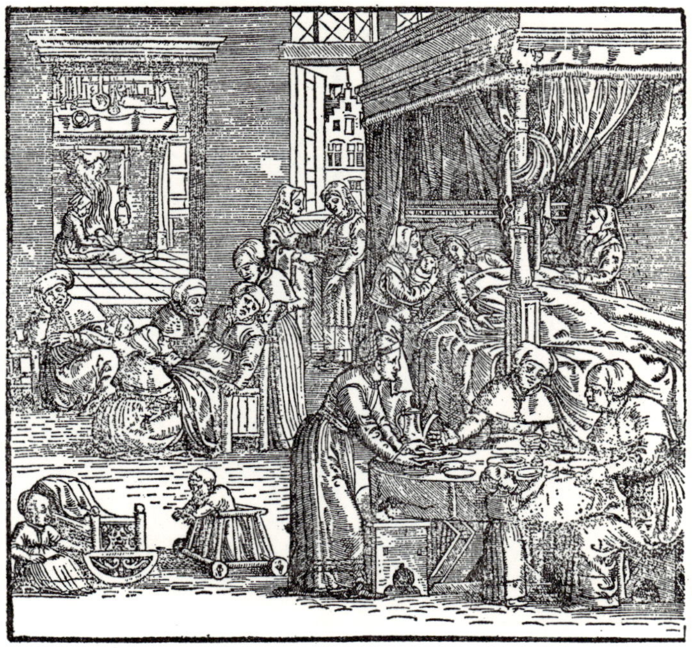

Figures 280 and 281 Consecutive stages of a confinement, from the hearth to the child-bed, and the mother's first meal at the table after childbirth. From Walter Ryff, Frawen Rosengarten, *Frankfurt, 1545.*
The scene in the background can be understood equally well as the last of the series.

Fig. 279 Twins, from Gynaeciorum . . . commentarii, *Basel (Waldkirch), 1586. Originally based on Rueff.*

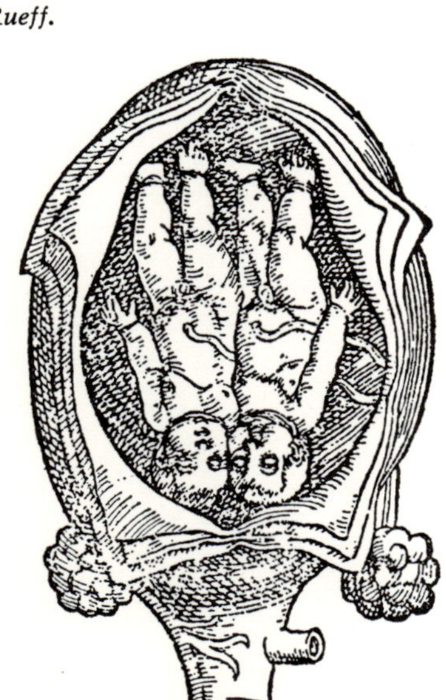

hominis (published in German as *Ein schön lustig Trostbüchle von den empfangknussen und geburten der menschen,* Zurich, 1554) and EUCHARIUS RÖSSLIN'S *Der swangern Frawen und Hebammen Rosengarten,* 1513. RÖSSLIN and RUEFF were the municipal physicians of Worms and Zurich, respectively. The fetal figures in the illustrations of these 16th-century books are drawn as children, not adults (compare figures 278 and 279 with the illustration by MOSCHION, plate V), and all manner of anatomical details now enliven the uterus.[22] Like 16th-century surgical books, these books too are enlivened by complicated scenes; and, again, two different approaches can be distinguished. The first approach is the eyewitness report, i.e. the representation of a specific lying-in room at a specific moment, for example *intra partum.* The second is the late Gothic technique of simultaneous representation of consecutive scenes, with which we are well acquainted from ecclesiastical altar-paintings, and which was still cultivated in the 16th century as a popular kind of explanatory picture. WALTER RYFF'S *Frawen Rosengarten,* Frankfurt, 1545, delights the reader with a title-page woodcut containing a combination of six scenes in one (figs. 280, 281). It shows the stages of pregnancy in six small consecutive scenes in which the pregnant woman can be actually followed through each stage until she is confined to the child-bed. DAGOBERT FREY has made a number of shrewd observations on the principles of this type of demonstration.[23]

[22] SUDHOFF, KARL: Kindslagen in Miniaturen, Schnitten und Stichen vom 12. bis ins 18. Jahrhundert, in: Tradition und Naturbeobachtung, i.e. Stud. Gesch. Med. *1,* 1907.
[23] FREY, DAGOBERT: Kunstwissenschaftliche Grundfragen, Vienna, 1946, pp. 34 ff.

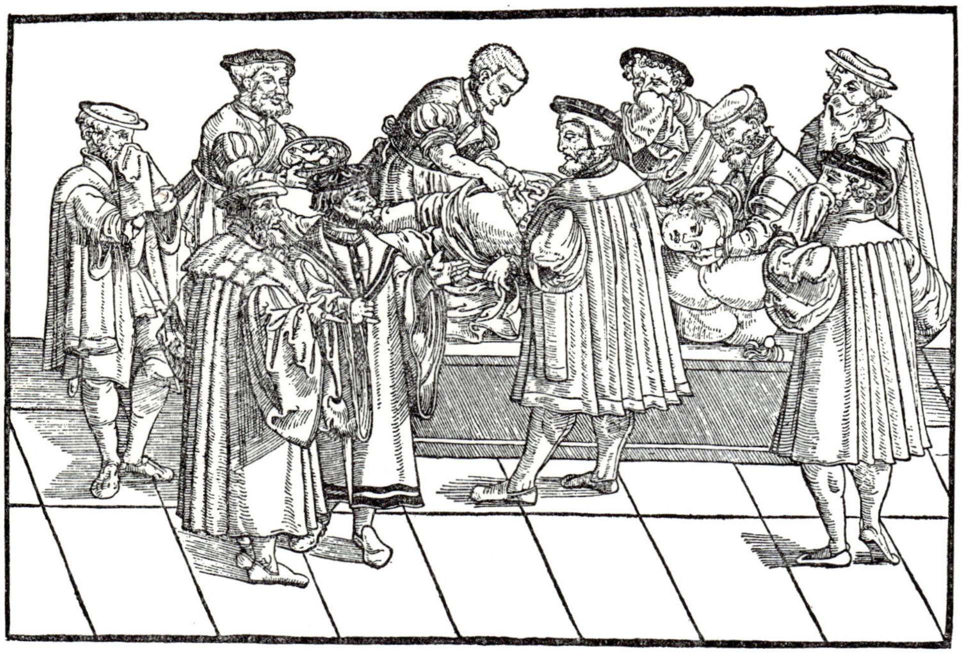

Fig. 282 The memorable Caesarean section on the proprietress of the 'Roten Krebs' in Vienna to facilitate delivery of a child which had been dead for four years. Performed by the Viennese municipal physician Paul Dirlewang in the presence of Professor Cornax and his colleagues. Anonymous pamphlet, Vienna, 1550.

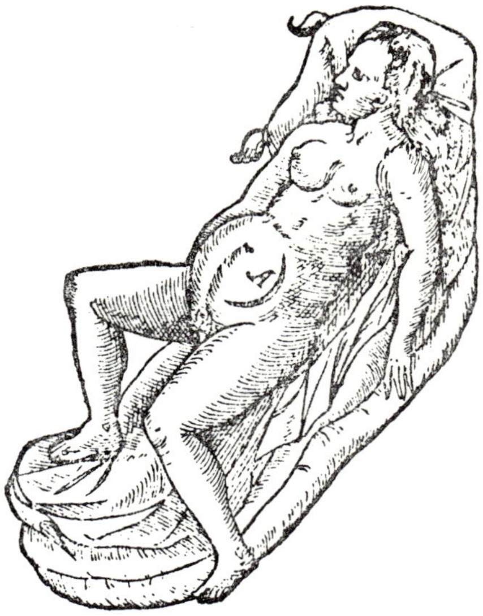

Fig. 283 Position of the pregnant woman and demonstration of the incision for a Caesarean section. From Boudewijn Ronsse, Miscellanea, *Leyden, 1590.*

A comparison between the eyewitness report of a sensational obstetrical operation performed in Vienna in 1549 (fig. 282) and the scientific description of a Caesarean section on a living patient, which dispenses with the scene and shows only the incision line (fig. 283), once again demonstrates two basically different approaches to obstetrical illustration.

Teratology

The first printed illustrations for teratology already appear in the incunabula (p. 48). Among them there is a pair of twins joined at the forehead, which is considered to be the oldest medical illustration still in existence to have been drawn from life. This also points to a development which extends into the present. The intentions of these incunabula were not to present useful medical information. Virtually all pictures of deformed infants, and we know of original watercolors[24] and numerous pamphlets with woodcuts, were not produced for physicians but for the people, largely for merely journalistic purposes and sometimes for political reasons.[25] An exception to this is represented by the publication of a pamphlet recording the birth of Siamese twins in Landshut (fig. 284); the children lived for

[24] Martin, Alfred: Die Jost Ammannsche Federzeichnung einer Doppelmissbildung in der Wickiana der Stadtbibliothek zu Zürich, in: Amman, Aug. F.: Geschichte der Familie Ammann von Zürich, Vol. 2, Zürich, 1911.

[25] Holländer, Eugen: Wunder, Wundergeburt und Wundergestalt, Stuttgart, 1921.

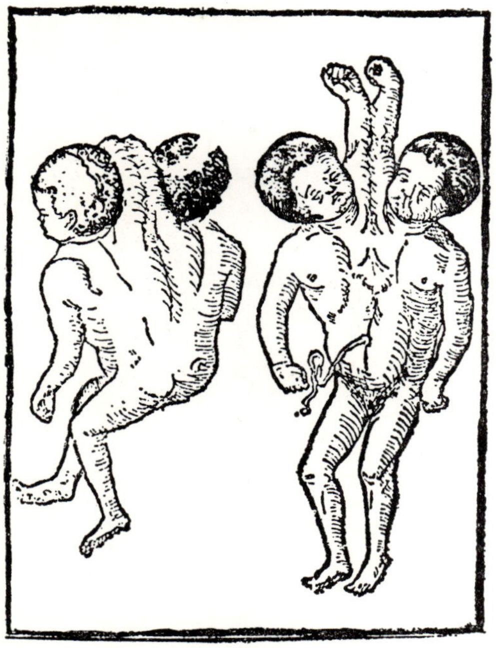

Fig. 284 Siamese twins born in Landshut, 1517.

only half an hour. The author of this report was a physician who arranged for a surgeon to perform the section.[26] In 1512 ALBRECHT DÜRER made a drawing, which was reprinted numerous times, of a quite similar case which occurred in Esslingen; DÜRER had learned of the event by hearsay. On the other hand, HANS BURGKMAIR, the Augsburg painter and graphic artist, seems to have drawn from life two views of a three-legged infant born in Tettnang in 1516. In 1597 a pamphlet appeared in Cologne recording for the first time a "miraculous, frightful birth never before heard of or seen," which was illustrated in an engraving showing the infant after its death;[27] apparently this was an instance of a sympus birth.[28]

[26] HOLLÄNDER: pp. 65-66.
[27] HOLLÄNDER: fig. 200.
[28] GRUBER, GEORG, B.: Historisches und Aktuelles über das Sirenen-Problem in der Medizin, in: Nova Acta Leopoldina N.F. *17*, 1955, No. 117.

Fig. 285 Copperplate engravings in a pamphlet describing and illustrating a sympus; Cologne, 1597.

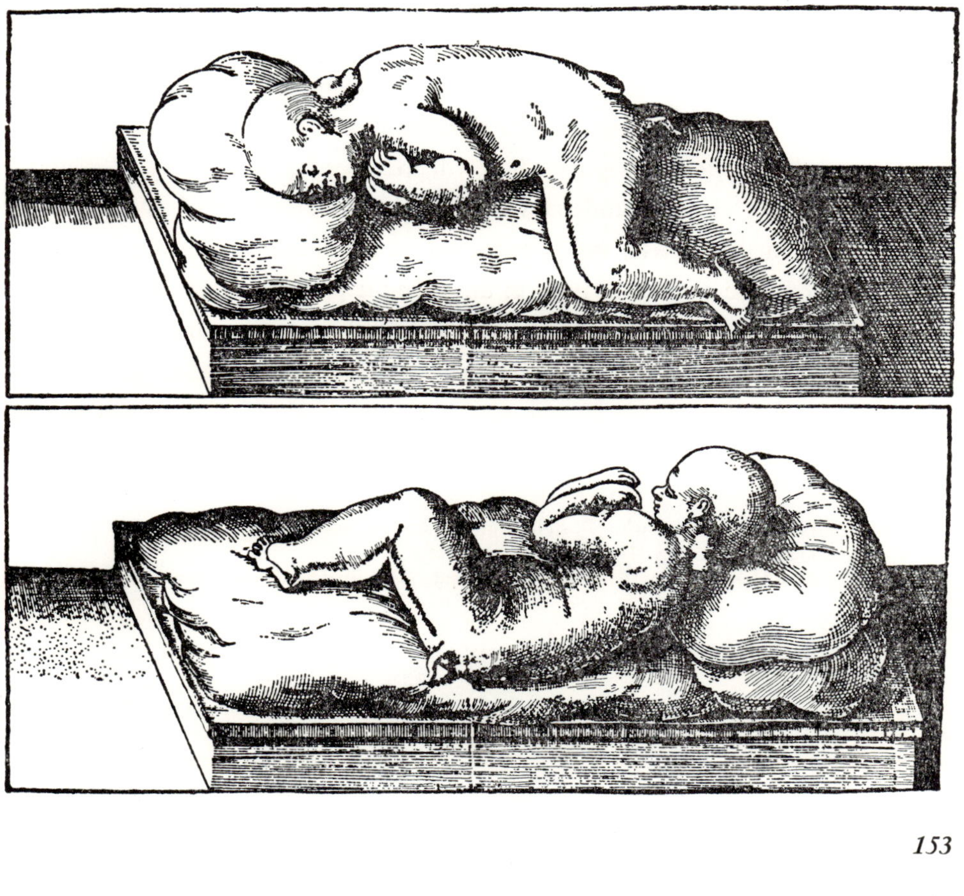

In the 16th century, herbals still fell within the field of medical illustration. Thanks to the pioneering work of Claus Nissen, who has explored this category of literature very thoroughly,[29] I can restrict my remarks here to a summary of the main features of herbal illustration. My summary is, of course, indebted to Nissen. The conflict in medical illustration between the realistic approach, in which a scene or a subject is copied faithfully from life, and the generalizing approach, in which a more or less abstract representation of the subject is given, is evidenced very clearly by a comparison[30] of the two most important 16th-century herbals: those of Weiditz-Brunfels (1530-36) and of Fuchs (1542).

Although a few anatomical illustrations drawn from life were added to the stock of traditional medieval illustrations at the beginning of the 16th century, such as the new anatomical illustrations in the Mondino editions (see p. 40), it was not until the third decade that the real breakthrough occurred with a folio volume containing full-page illustrations taken from life. In this respect botany was several years ahead of anatomy; considering its subject, of course, this is hardly surprising. Around 1528 the Strasbourg publisher Johann Schott (see pp. 54 ff.) engaged Hans Weiditz,[31] a well-known designer and wood engraver, to make a series of illustrations of medicinal plants. Otto Brunfels, a Strasbourg physician, wrote a corresponding text; and in 1530 the *Herbarum vivae Eicones* appeared as a volume in folio with eighty-six woodcuts by Weiditz. A second volume followed in 1531, and a third in 1536.[32] The original drawings of the plants were done as watercolor pen-and-ink sketches. In 1930, sixty-four of the originals were found in the Botanical Institute in Bern, together with other papers left by Felix Platter. It is especially clear from these original sketches that Weiditz drew his plants just as he found them, often damaged or half withered (see fig. 286).

On the contrary, the illustrations for the *Historia stirpium* of the Tübingen physician Leonhart Fuchs, which appeared at the Isingrin workshop in Basel in 1542, are of quite a different type. In this case the preparation of the illustrations was directed by the author, who was an experienced anatomist and physician. His two artists, Albrecht Meyer and Heinrich Füllmaurer, worked in Tübingen under his close supervision.[33] Fuchs, who was a dogmatic Humanist, had worked for years on the arrangement of his material. Rather than having his artists make

[29] Nissen, Claus: Die botanische Buchillustration. Ihre Geschichte und Bibliographie. Vol. I: Geschichte, Stuttgart 1950. Vol. II: Bibliographie, Stuttgart, 1951.

[30] Rytz, W.: Das Herbar Felix Platters, in: Verhandl. Naturforsch. Gesch., Basel *44*, I, 1933, pp. 83 ff.

[31] Thieme-Becker *35*, 1942, pp. 269-71. The article is by H. Röttinger (see footnote 8, p. 142); Röttinger vehemently defends the theory that Weiditz is the so-called Petrarch Master. Nissen (1950), p. 39.

[32] In 1534, an edition of Vol. I and II followed in quarto, for which Schott partly used the woodblocks retrieved from his plagiarist Egenolff in Frankfurt am Main after a successful lawsuit tried at the supreme court.

[33] Rott (footnote 6 on p. 142).

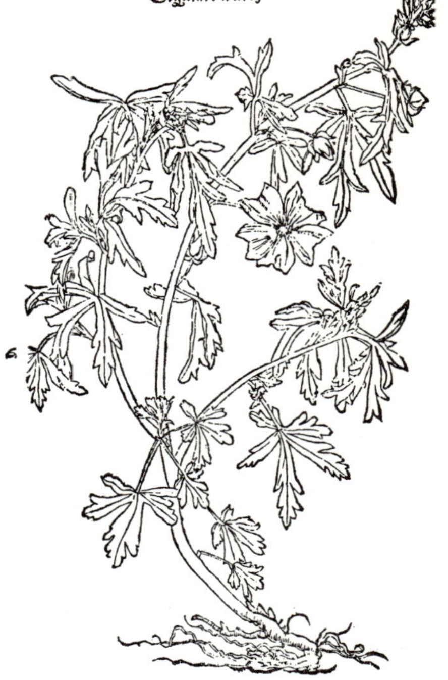

Fig. 286

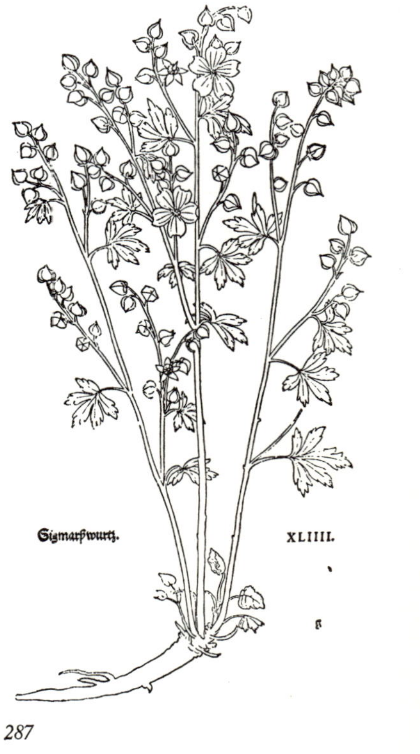

Fig. 287

Figures 286 and 287 Drawings of the mallow, from Brunfels, 1530, and Fuchs, 1542.

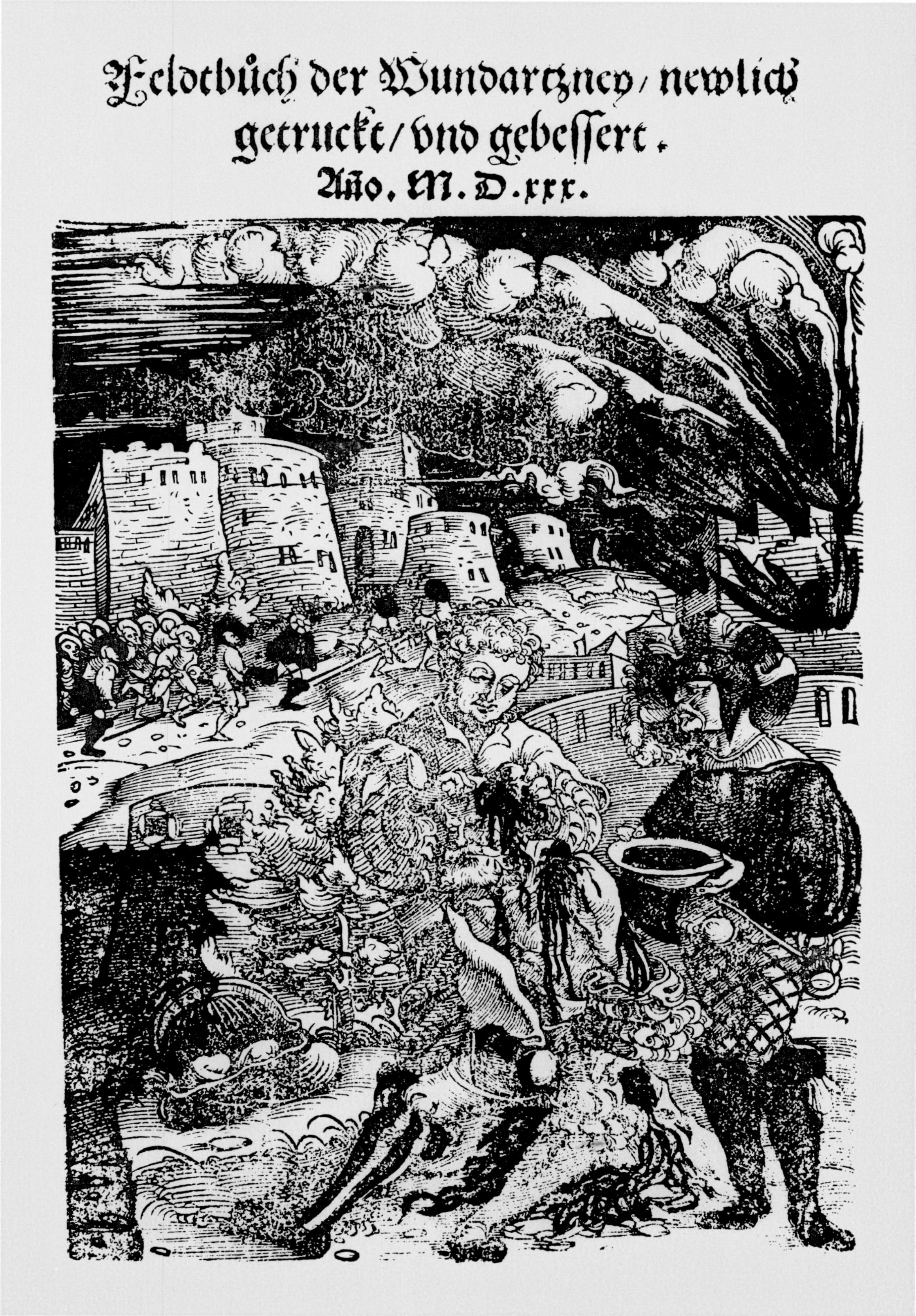

Plate XXVII Two-colored woodcut title page for Gerssdorff's Feldtbuch, *Strasbourg edition, 1530. Fire and blood contrast vividly with the black of the drawing by Hans Wächtlin.*

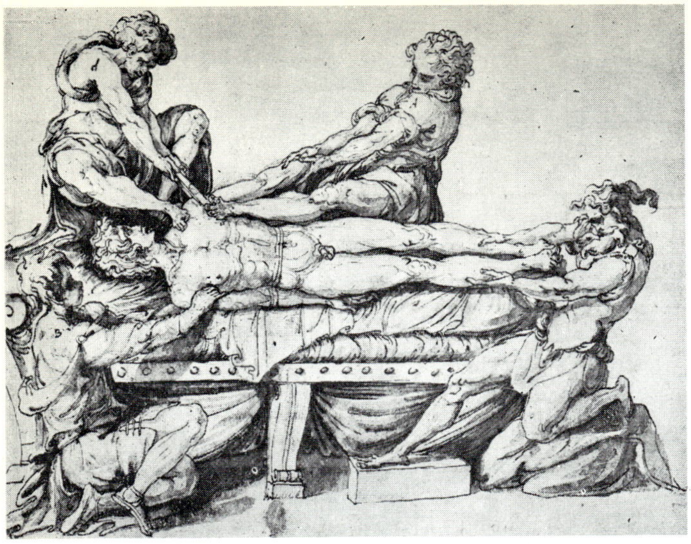

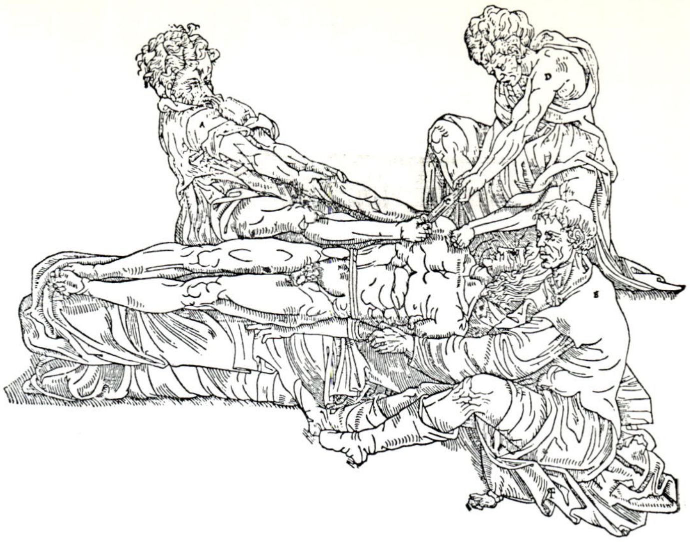

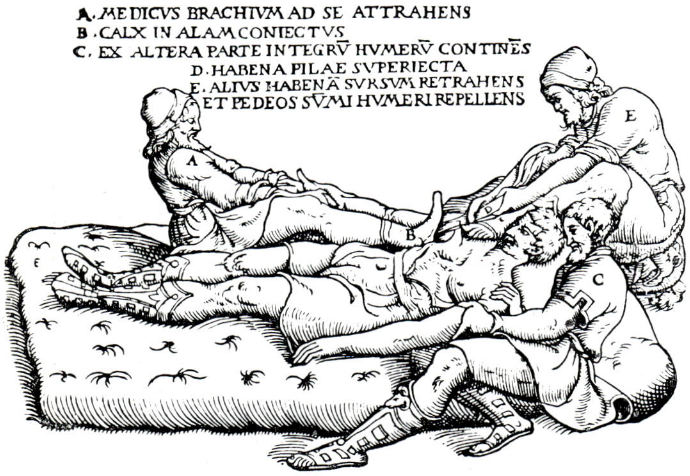

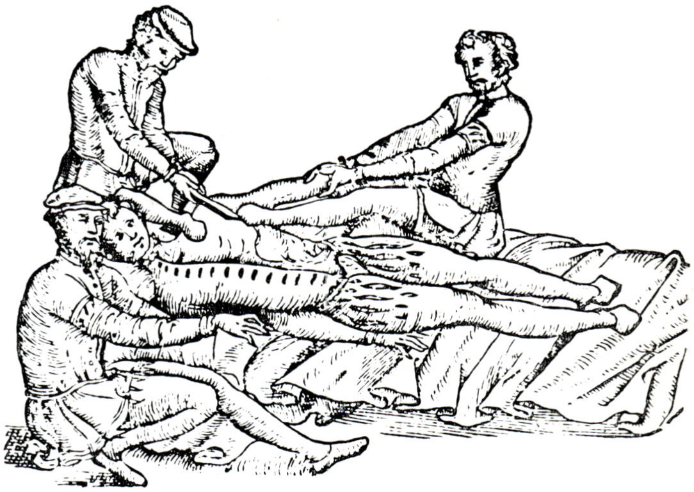

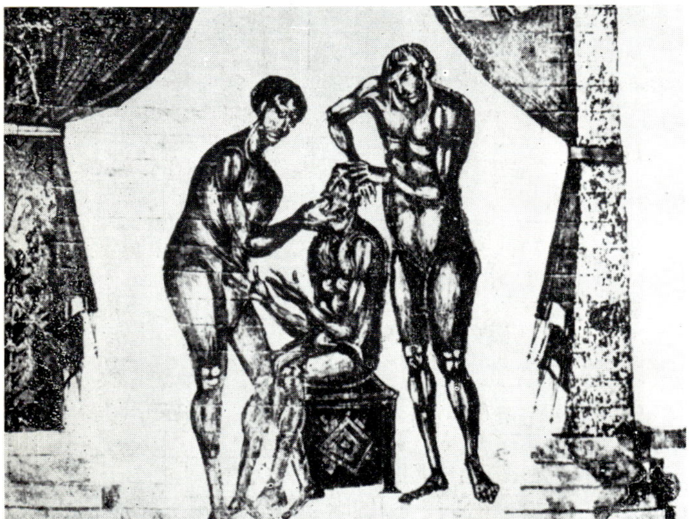

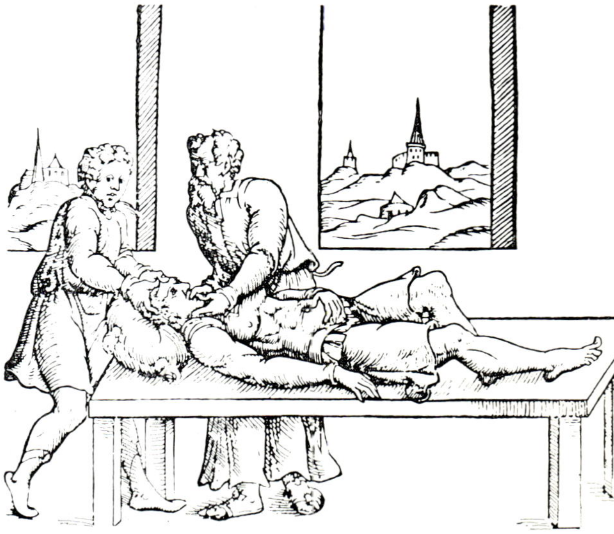

Plate XXVIII The two top rows show the history of an illustration of a shoulder dislocation, whose origin actually dates back to the Byzantine illustration in Peri arthron *(plate 1), and can be traced here from the watercolor copy ascribed to Primaticcio, to the print from Vidus Vidius's* Chirurgia è Graeco in latinum conversa, *Paris, 1544, and then to the two related textbooks from the second half of the 16th century. The bottom row illustrates the treatment of a dislocated jaw, drawn free-hand from a model, possibly only following the directions in the text. The second-row left illustration and the third-row right illustration derive from the Froben part of the Galen edition, Basel, 1562.*

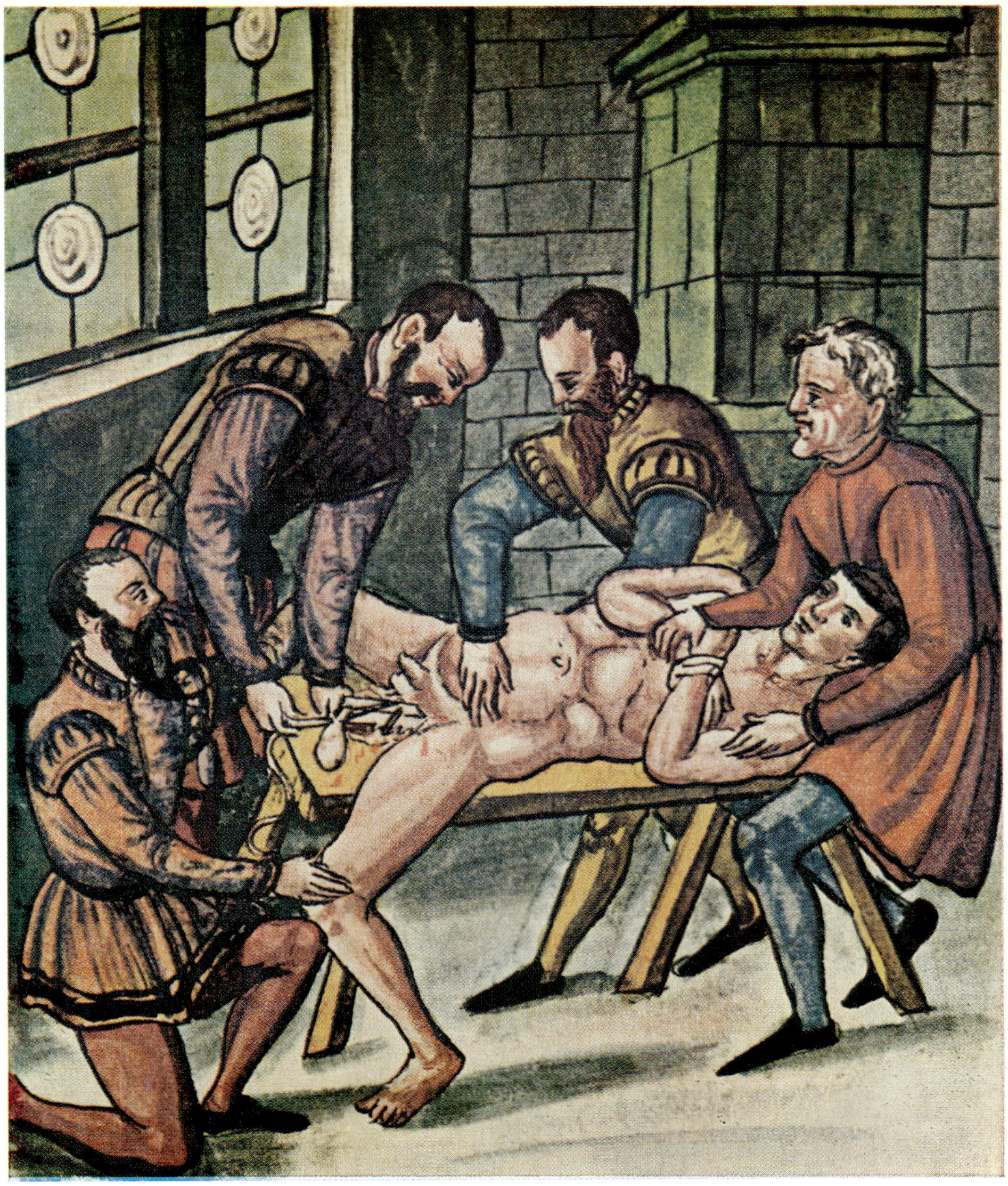

Plate XXIX Caspar Stromayr, Practica copiosa. *Manuscript with watercolor dated 1559, Lindau, Lake Constance. This scene is from a series of 7 illustrations depicting the procedure of an operation which the author himself criticizes. Enlarged 7 : 6, Staatsbibliothek, Lindau.*

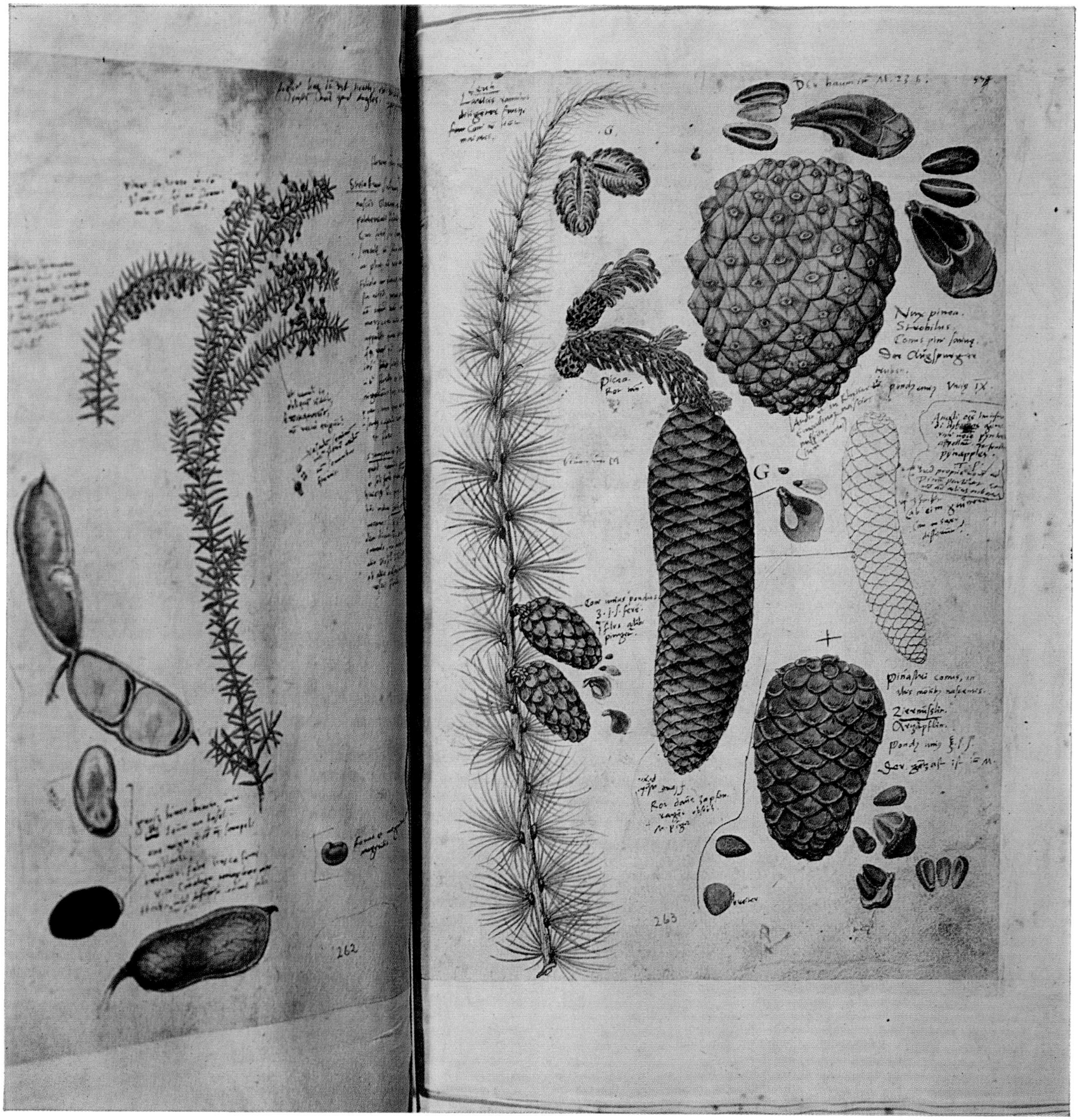

Plate XXX From Conrad Gessner's manuscript in the Trew Collection of the Universitäte-Bibliothek Erlangen. The plate on the right shows larch, spruce and fir, which have been traditional sources of effective pharmaceutics. 'Laricis ramulus,' the larch sprig (left picture), served as the model for a woodcut which appeared in the herbal of Matthioli Camerarius (see p. 160), fol. 25, 1586.

faithful drawings of individual specimens, he wanted them to depict the characteristic features of a particular kind of plant (fig. 287). Occasionally he was inclined to overreach himself and induce the draftsman to draw something which he could not possible have seen, but for the most part the illustrations represent an incomparable synthesis between didactic intention and botanical accuracy. The fact that the pictures are also very attractive artistic works speaks for a harmonious collaboration between author and illustrators, which finds its finest expression in the artists' portraits at the end of the work.

The excellent job done by the Basel printer makes FUCHS'S work comparable to VESALIUS'S *Fabrica*. It must be more than mere chance that two such superb books were produced in the same city, within approximately one year of each other.[34]

FUCHS'S book was quite successful. There soon followed editions in quarto, and some in even smaller sizes; and there were also pirated editions produced by the digest specialist EGENOLFF. The illustrations themselves were copied in German, French, Dutch, and English editions, as well as in one Spanish edition published in Antwerp in 1557. And, like the illustrations for the *Fabrica*, their influence can be traced to the present day.

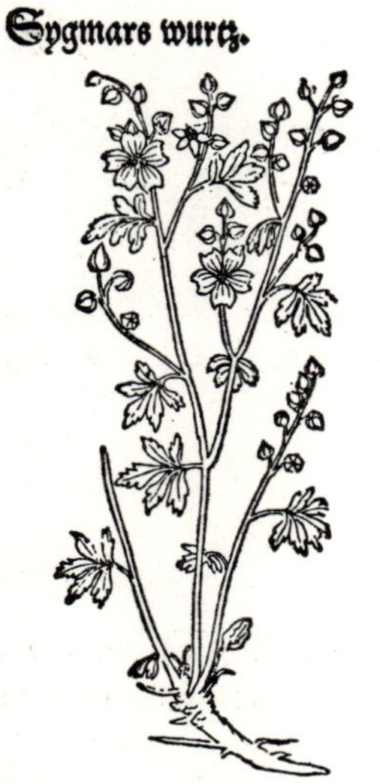

Fig. 288 Drawing of the mallow, from Bock, 1546. (Compare with figs. 286-287 and 289-290.)

FUCHS had planned an enlarged second edition; but, although many of the illustrations for this edition were transposed onto woodblocks,[35] the book itself never appeared. The woodblocks themselves are preserved in the Botanical Institute at the University of Tübingen (plate XXXIa).[36] The lines for the form-cutter to follow are drawn on the wood in black ink. If this was done by the same master who had already transposed the original drawings on the woodblocks for the first edition, then it is the work of HEINRICH FÜLLMAURER.

The third major 16th-century botanical author was the theologian HIERONYMUS BOCK, who was a vicar in Hornbach, near Zweibrücken. His *New Kreüter Buch* was first published without illustrations in 1539 by WENDEL RIHEL in Strasbourg. The second edition of 1546 was finally furnished with approximately 530 woodcuts drawn by DAVID KANDEL.[37] Although still very young, the artist executed his contract with a flourish, picking up ideas from WEIDITZ and FÜLLMAURER and even from the old *Hortus* illustrations of REWICH (see p. 47).

BOCK was also acquainted with CONRAD GESSNER,[38] a connection which leads us into the second half of the century. This eminent Zürich historian had collected the material for a large *Historia plantarum*, and upon his death he left over 1500 illustrations which had in part already been transposed onto the woodblock or even engraved. Among them there were several excellent watercolors which he had

[34] Historia stirpium, 1542; Fabrica, June 1543.

[35] For some of the illustrations, the woodblocks had actually been engraved and trial prints taken; in these cases, only the prints have been preserved (see RYTZ, *loc. cit.*, pp. 60 ff.).

[36] In 1898 there were 185 plates at the University Library at Tübingen.

[37] THIEME-BECKER *19*, 1926, pp. 514-15. In it further literature is specified up to and including the year 1923.

[38] A recent study which goes beyond NISSEN is that of ZOLLER, HEINRICH: Konrad Gessner als Botaniker, in: Gesnerus *22*, 1965, pp. 216-27.

painted himself.[39] In 1586, the Nuremberg physician Joachim Camerarius the Younger, who then owned Gessner's picture material, used it to illustrate a Matthioli edition published by Sigmund Feyerabend in Frankfurt. This *Kreutterbuch Dess Hochgelehrten und weitberühmten Herrn D. Petri Andreae Matthioli* demonstrates that the decline in quality which we have noted in other late 16th-century medical books affected pharmaco-botanical books as well: the material was spread thin, the illustrations were less carefully handled, and the book as a whole was less well designed and printed. Another group of illustrations similar to Gessner's was put together in Italy: Ulysse Aldrovandi of Bologna, the great teacher of two generations of physicians, had collected almost ten thousand botanical illustrations (Nissen), which like the Gessner papers have been preserved in all their stages of printing from the watercolor to the engraved printing block, but he did not publish them.[40]

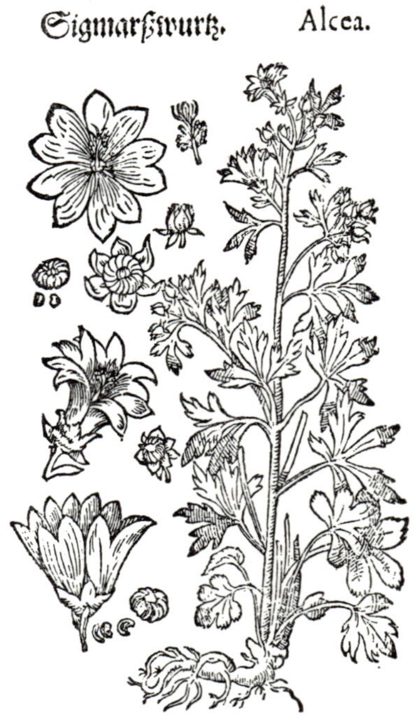

Fig. 289 Drawing of the mallow, from Camerarius, Kreutterbuch, *Frankfurt am Main, 1586.*

In the last decades of the 16th century, the initiative in the publication of original botanical texts shifted to Antwerp, where the publisher Christoph Plantin engaged three botanists who, with Camerarius, were the greatest living scholars in this field: Rembert Dodoens, Charles de L'Écluse and Matthias de L'Obel (Dodonaeus, Clusius, and Lobelius). Plantin modeled his illustrations on those of Fuchs. Finally, around 1590, two remarkably extensive works appeared which exemplify the long development that had taken place from the Mainz *Hortus* (1484) to a pharmaco-botanical encyclopedia with over two thousand illustrations: the *Neuw Kreüterbuch* of Tabernaemontanus (Jacob Theodor from Bergzabern), published in Frankfurt am Main by Nicolaus Basse in 1588-91; and an *Historia generalis plantarum,* containing 2751 woodcuts, published in Lyon by Roville in 1586-87. The reason it was possible to include so great a number of woodcuts in the *Historia generalis plantarum* is that the individual illustrations were quite small, less than five inches in height. Toward the close of the century, after the publication of these two encyclopedic works, copperplate engraving began to replace woodcuts in pharmaco-botanical works as well as in other kinds of medical books. By 1600, the victory of the copperplate was virtually complete.

Fig. 290 Drawing of the mallow, from Charles de L'Écluse, Rariorum plantarum historia, *Antwerp, 1601.*

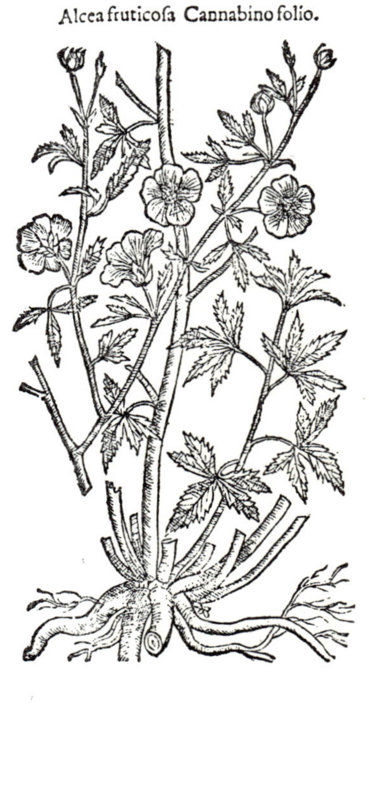

"Compound" situs illustrations

In the first half of the 16th century, a previously unknown publisher had had a new and completely original idea: he had the human abdominal viscera represented in a pseudo-three-dimensional form. The various stages of the situs were printed on separate small sheets; then the sheets were glued in the appropriate spot on a page containing a full-figure illustration, in such a way that the sheets could be

[39] After passing through different hands, the Gessner papers, together with the library of the Nuremberg physician Chr. J. Trew, were finally acquired by the University Library of Erlangen.

[40] The drawings and watercolors are in the University Library at Bologna, the woodblocks in the Orto Botanico.

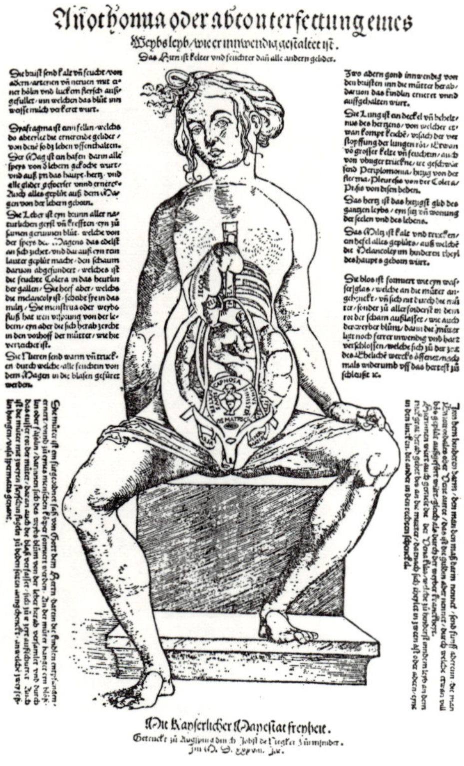

Fig. 291 'Eve.' A separate sheet published by Jobst de Necker, Augsburg, 1538. The sheet has nine flaps which can be folded back to reveal dissections of four different situses.

lifted and turned back like flaps to reveal the successive stages of an anatomical dissection.

Like the venesection tables and skeleton figures that we discussed in an earlier chapter (see p. 42), these situs figures were usually published as separate sheets, not bound into a book; thus only a small number of them have survived. On many of these, some of the flaps are missing and are probably lost forever. Nonetheless, there are enough of these separate sheets still extant so that we can trace the development of this kind of illustration from its beginning in the 16th century down to recent times.[41]

The earliest known examples were published in Augsburg and Strasbourg in the year 1538; other examples from Venice, Paris, and Nuremberg followed in 1539. VESALIUS also included in both the *Fabrica* and the *Epitome* a sheet of "cutouts"

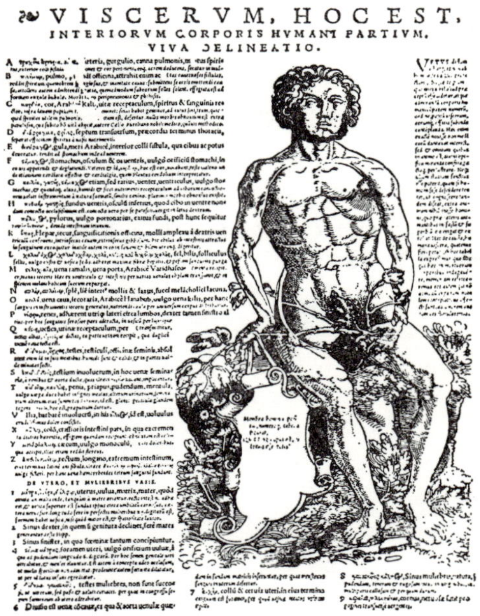

Fig. 293 Early pamphlet probably of southern German origin, 1538/39?, to which a corresponding female figure exists. Its date and place of origin are obviously related to tabulae VI or their direct copies (most specifically the sixth plate), Michigan Medical Center Library. The folding plate has four attached sheets.

Fig. 292 A "compound" situs sheet published in England about 1645, showing male and female figures in a bath chamber.

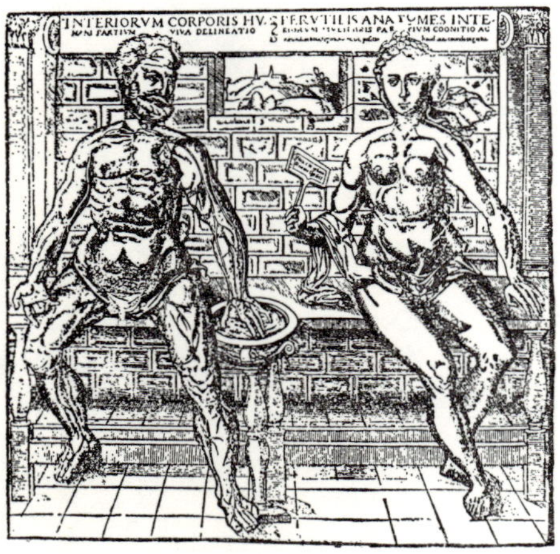

that could be taken out and made up into a compound illustration by the reader himself.[42] It is hardly surprising that the readers rarely did this, for VESALIUS'S text was so clear and complete that a study aid of this kind was not required.

The best-preserved 16th-century specimen of this type of illustration belongs to

41 CHOULANT-FRANK (footnote 1 on p. 54), pp. 156-67. CRUMMER, LEROY: Early anatomical fugitive sheets, in: Annals Med. Hist. *5*, 1923, pp. 189-209, and also: Further information on these early anatomical sheets, in: Annals Med. Hist *7*, 1925, pp. 1-2. WELLS, L. H.: A remarkable pair of anatomical fugitive sheets . . . in: Bull. Hist. Med., Baltimore, *38*, 1964, pp. 470-76. This work contains what is currently the most complete catalog and a literary reference.

42 Fabrica, 1543 edition, pp. 313-14; 1555 edition pp. 505-06. The Epitome is without pagination ("figurae ad tabulam aptandam paratae, illi agglutinandam"). According to the extensive directions for use, the various detail figures are to be cut out and glued together; they do not fit exactly, though.

the treasures of the Albertina in Vienna[43]: an "Eve" whose artistic execution is of excellent quality. It is dated 1538 and bears the inscription "Mit Kayserlicher Mayestat freyheit Gedruckt zu Augspurg durch JOBST DE NEGKER Fuormschnider." The precious and fragile sheet has no fewer than nine overlay flaps, covering four different situses (fig. 291).

Most of the 16th-century sheets are essentially pre-Vesalian in conception. The older sheets are in the tradition of the five-figure series of "squatting figures" (see p. 10): all the figures are drawn in a sitting position, with the legs spread apart. Originally there were probably a pair of figures involved – a male "Adam" doubtless accompanied the female "Eve." There is also a variation showing a pair of naked figures in a bath chamber: one such sheet was produced in London about 1545 (fig. 292), and another in Paris in 1585. We encounter quite complicated compound situs illustrations in the 17th and 18th centuries (REMMELIN, 1613; PICCOLOMINI FANTONI, 1745), and in the 19th century such illustrations experienced a resurgence of popularity. From the beginning up to the present day, however, this category of didactic illustration has always been on the borderline between popular lay literature and medical literature proper: *"Nosce te ipsum"* ("Know thyself") is inscribed on the small tablet held by Eve in the bath-chamber scene reproduced here (fig. 292).

[43] GEISBERG, MAX: Der deutsche Einblatt-Holzschnitt, Munich 1930, Cat. No. 1438. It is strange that this sheet has remained unnoticed by specialists in medical history.

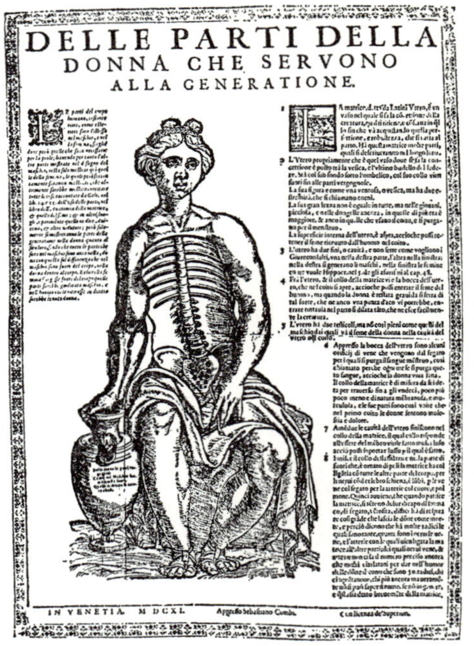

Fig. 294 A compound situs illustration from a 1611 Venetian pamphlet. The overlay flaps have all been lost; the final stage of dissection – which of course was printed on the bottom sheet – is all that remains.

16th-Century Title Pages

Several hundred years ago, anyone who wished to acquaint himself with newly published books had to travel to the Frankfurt or Leipzig booksellers' fair, where publishers displayed their forthcoming attractions to prospective buyers.[1] At that time, the title page of the book often served as a combination of advertisement and advance announcement. The title page, which was in many cases engraved and printed before the rest of the book was ready for production, had to offer the prospective buyer as much information as possible about the contents of the book; these decorative sheets, displayed on boards, adorned the entrances to the bookshops. It was in this way that a special category of graphic art developed: the embellished title page. In the beginning, woodcuts were used for these title pages; but by the end of the 16th century, copperplate engravings or etchings had almost entirely replaced the woodcut.

Title-page art has always played a special role in the history of medical illustration; because of its eyecatching nature, its importance has at times even been overestimated. The highpoint of title-page art was reached in the Baroque period, but in the 16th century the foundations were already laid for the developments that were to take place in the following century.

Title pages are of interest in our present study only to the extent that they are directly related to medical illustration; taken as a whole,[2] of course they should be treated as part of the history of printing.[3] For our purposes, we shall single out a few examples that are interesting because of their medical content and that can serve to represent the developments that took place in the course of the 16th century.

Fig. 295 Title page for Nicolò Leoniceno et al., Aureum opus, *Venice (De Garadis), 1516.*

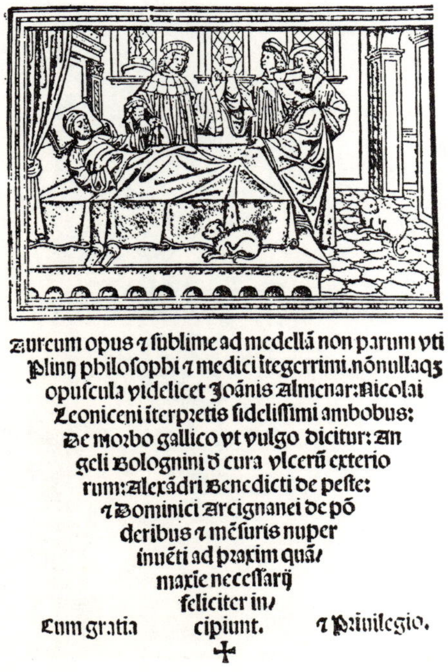

Aureum opus & sublime ad medellã non paruni vti
Pliniȝ philosophi & medici itegerrimi.nõnullaqȝ
opuscula videlicet Joãnis Almenar:Nicolai
Leoniceni iterpretis fidelissimi ambobus:
De morbo gallico vt vulgo dicitur:An
geli Bolognini d cura vlcerũ exterio
rum:Alexãdri Benedicti de peste:
& Dominici Arcignanei de põ
deribus & mẽsuris nuper
inuẽti ad praxim quã/
maxie necessarij
feliciter in/
Cum gratia cipiunt. & Priuilegio.

Figure 295 reproduces one of the earliest examples of 16th-century medical title pages, a title page from a medical anthology that was printed in Venice in 1516. (Venetian printers had produced another superbly illustrated work during the incunabula period, a quarter of a century earlier: JOHANNES DE KETHAM'S *Fasciculus medicinae* of 1491.) This anthology was compiled by various authors, of whom NICOLÒ LEONICENO (1428-1524) is the best known today. The top half of the title page shows a sickbed scene; the entire bottom half is devoted to the name of the book and the names of the authors. Had this book been printed during the incunabula period, there would doubtless have been a hand-painted miniature instead of

[1] GOLDFRIEDRICH, JOHANN: Geschichte des deutschen Buchhandels vom Westfälischen Frieden bis zum Beginn der klassischen Literaturperiode (1648-1740), Leipzig, Verlag des Börsenvereins, 1908.

[2] Title-page designs have been said to fall into three categories: (1) functional – containing type only, and no ornament; (2) decorative – containing decoration for its own sake, unrelated to the content of the book, and (3) illustrative – containing artwork that is related to the content. See SONDHEIM, MORITZ: Das Titelblatt, address to the Frankfurter Bibliophilen Gesellschaft, Frankfurt am Main, 1927; and HERMANN GLOCKNER, Logos *10*, 1922, pp. 58 ff.

[3] Unfortunately, a full-length study of title-page design has not yet been undertaken. Histories of book printing and book illustration usually mention title pages only in passing. The most extensively illustrated catalogue of medical title-page graphic art has been compiled by ALCIDE GAROSI: Inter artium et medicinae doctores, Florence, Olschki, 1963; this study deals with the material at the Biblioteca Comunale di Siena.

the woodcut, and there would probably have been a frame around the whole page. The absence of a frame is rather unusual; other title pages from the same period do generally have frames, as does the BERENGARIO title page of 1521 (fig. 296). On this page, the title itself is set in an architectural framework resembling an altarpiece; below the title is a picture of an anatomical scene that is represented as though it were a predella. The scene is in the medieval tradition; the anatomist is shown sitting at the foot of the corpse and lecturing; in the 1523 edition, the anatomist is actually identified by name in a label ("CARPUS"). As we have already remarked, graphic art in the early 16th century was still in a period of transition between the Middle Ages and the modern era. This small anatomical scene takes a medieval theme and partly translates it into modern terms – the treatment of the pictured space, for instance, is fairly realistic – without entirely departing from the older tradition.

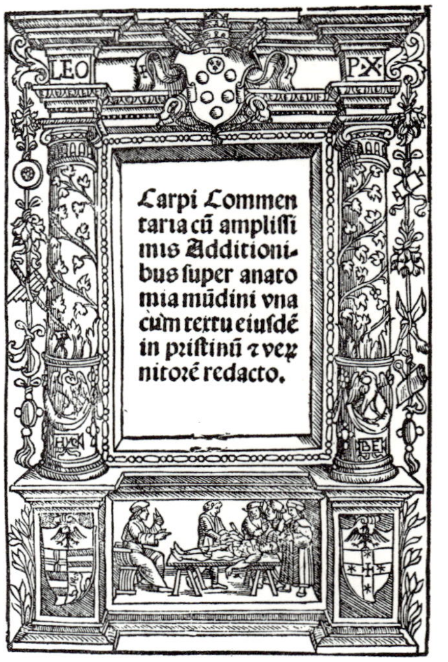

Fig. 296 Title page for Berengario da Carpi, Commentaria super anatomiam Mundini, *Bologna (De Benedictis), 1521.*

The three elements that are to be found in the BERENGARIO title page – framework, text, and picture – are also found in the title page of an edition of (H)ALI ABBAS that was printed in Lyon in 1523 (fig. 297). Here the title-page text is already somewhat diminished in size and importance, and the pictures have become more numerous and more elaborate. A fourth element also appears on this title page: the two shield-bearing figures that support the text and present it to the reader. Despite the relatively poor artistic quality of this sheet, it is a significant example for our study, for all four of these elements will appear again and again in the title-page art of the coming century.

All of the title-page pictures that we have discussed so far can be described as "modern" at least in the sense that they attempt to convey the illusion of real space to the observer. Only in the triangular pictures showing the shield-bearers does the artist fail to draw the various scenic elements in realistic proportion; the figures here seem to be dwarfed by the giant plants in the background. We notice, however, that the purely medical content of the title-page art has grown less in each successive example. While in the incunabula the medical scene was often the most prominent feature of the title page, in somewhat later works the place of prominence was given to other graphic devices: the publisher's colophon (figs. 137, 315-318), an allegorical scene, a coat of arms (fig. 299), or even the author's portrait (fig. 301). It often happened that a title-page woodcut that had originally been made for a specific medical book was reused in entirely different books. For instance, the page depicting the dispute between two Parisian anatomists, which served so aptly as title page for GALEN'S *De anatomicis administrationibus,* served the same function somewhat less aptly for GALEN'S *Methodus medendi* (fig. 298). This title page, which may be the work of JOLLAT,[4] succeeds in combining a number of title-page elements into a unified composition that is held together by an elaborate architectural framework. In many respects this design is avant-garde for

Fig. 297 Title page for (H)Ali Abbas, Liber totius medicine, *Lyon (J. Myt), 1523.*

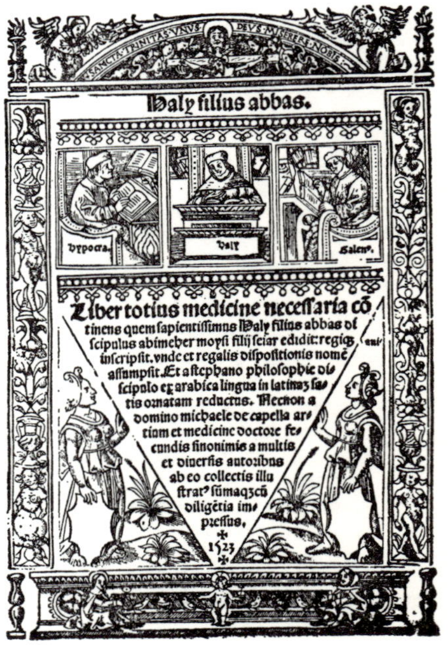

4 See BERNARD, AUGUSTE, *loc. cit.* (footnote 14, p. 88).

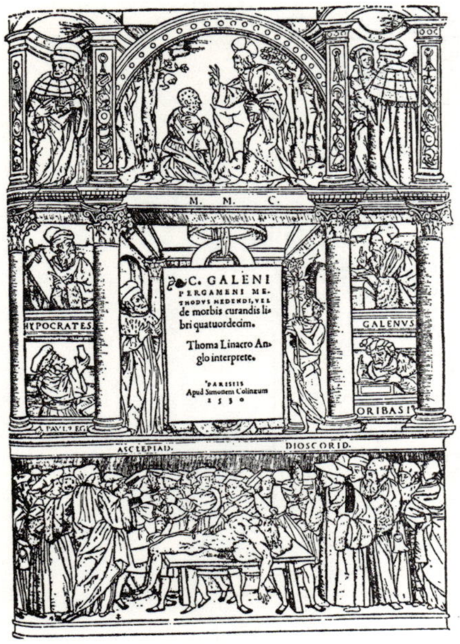

Fig. 298 Title page for Galen, Methodus medendi, *ed. Th. Linacre, Paris (S. de Colines), 1530.*

Fig. 299 Title page for Thomas Geminus, Compendiosa totius anatomie delineatio, *London (J. Herford), 1545.*

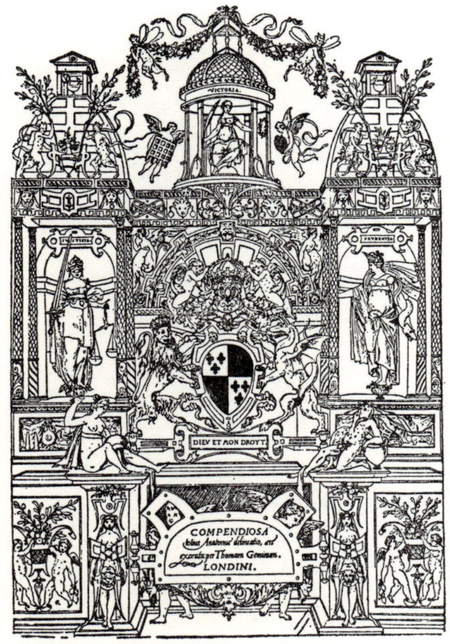

the year 1530: the surrealistic architecture of the central picture, the title-shield fancifully suspended from an enormous hook, and the shocking scene in the bottom picture are all Manneristic in conception, and even more or less Baroque. On the other hand, the artist is also indebted to the medieval tradition: the three scenes in the top row, with their Christian motifs, are strongly reminiscent of the small religious scenes depicted so often in 13th- and 14-century miniatures.

We shall not attempt a precise definition of "Baroque" at this point, but will use the term in its usual current sense, to refer both to a period in art history and to the style that is characteristic of that period. For WÖLFFIN it signifies the "decline of the Renaissance," cultural neglect and caprice, tension which has become form, the sum of opposites: systole and diastole simultaneously. It is the "presence of all diversity," as GOETHE once said. Material becomes spiritualized and spirit becomes materialized,[5] often in a way that seems tasteless or even macabre to us today. Many Baroque tendencies are already present in the illustrations for VESALIUS'S *Fabrica* – skeletons seem to be performing a *danse macabre*,[6] anatomical preparations hang from gallows like gruesome dolls, severed muscles swing from the hands, a diaphragm is affixed to a wall, and viscera issue from antique torsos.

In Paris at the mid-century, however, Mannerism still predominates. The anatomical art in ESTIENNE'S *De dissectione* is a little closer to Renissance "classicism," and one step further away from Baroque surrealism, than the Venetian art of the *Fabrica.* English graphic art at the mid-century is also still in the Mannerist phase, as the title page for THOMAS GEMINUS'S *Compendiosa* demonstrates (fig. 299). In fact, the architectural framework on this title page is a little disconcerting to the eye because of its virtually complete renunciation of three-dimensonal depth. The occasional sudden references to three-dimensional space may strike the observer as either humorous or disturbing: for instance, the male and female figures on the pilasters projecting from the front wall, or the figures of Justitia and Prudentia balanced on flower bowls inside pavilions, or the angel and the devil cavorting in empty space at the top of the framework on either side of the little pavilion containing the figure of Victory. This title page, by the way, as we mentioned earlier, is considered to be the first copperplate engraving to be used as the title page of a book.

The high esteem in which the famous title page of VESALIUS'S *Fabrica* (fig. 184) is held today should not mislead us into thinking either that it was particularly original or that it was particularly influential on later works of its own century. On the contrary, this type of title-page design was derived directly from the tradition of the medieval miniature. Such designs were employed only infrequently in the

5 BARTH, HANS: Die Zeitalter des Barocks und die Philosophie von Leibniz, in: Die Kunstformen des Barockzeitalters. Fourteen lectures, edited by RUDOLF STAMM (Sammlung Dalp 82), Bern, Franke, 1956.

6 ACKERKNECHT, ERWIN H.: Medical Art as a Psychological Safety-Valve. Bull. Medical Library Assoc., Milwaukee *43*, 1955, pp. 456-71.

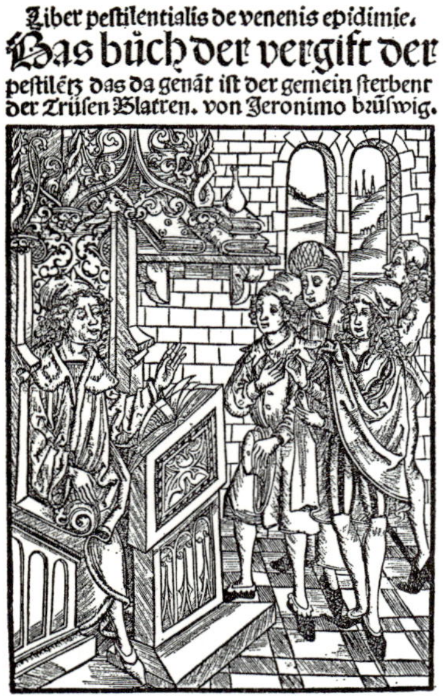

Fig. 300

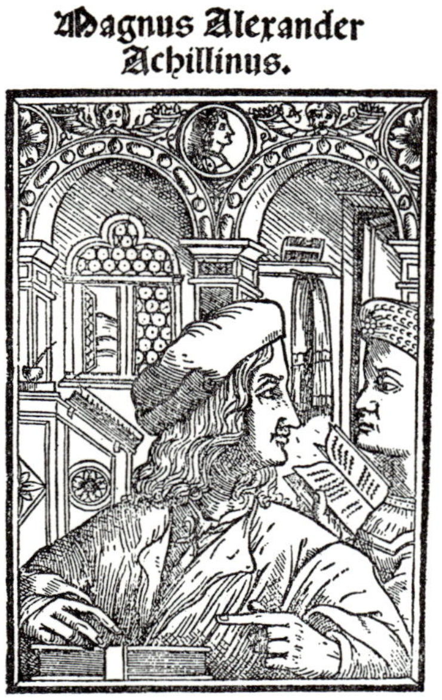

Fig. 301

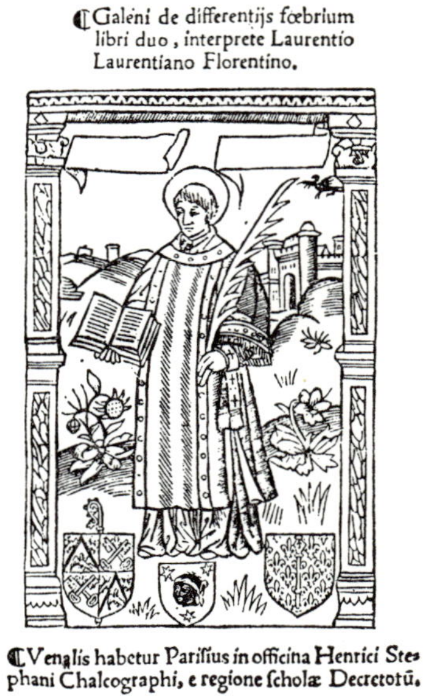

Fig. 302

Fig. 300 Title page for Brunschwig, Liber pestilentialis de venenis epidemie, *Strasbourg (Hans Grüninger), 1500. The woodcut had already been used in 1497 for the second title page of the* Buch der Cirurgia.

Fig. 301 Antiporta (title portrait) for A. Achillini, De humani corporis anatomia, *Venice, 1521.*

Fig. 302 Title page for Galen, De differentijs foebrium libri II, *published by Laurentius Laurentianus, Paris (Henri Estienne), 1512.*

16th century; VESALIUS'S title page itself does not seem to have exerted a direct influence on any later 16th-century title-page art, except perhaps for the frontispiece to the *De re anatomica* of REALDO COLOMBO, 1559, which was also produced in Venice (fig. 304).

Other 16th-century title pages that contain a single large picture fall into other categories. For instance, the title page for ALESSANDRO ACHILLINI'S *De humani corporis anatomia* (fig. 301) is an example of portrait art, in this case expanded into a dialogue scene by means of the second figure that has been added at the right. Another title page that might be said to be in the same genre as portrait art – although of course it is not portraiture – is the bizarre sheet that a second-rate Bruges printer produced for a 1569 edition of VESALIUS'S *Epitome* (fig. 305), which incorporates the macabre double figure by VALVERDE that was discussed on page 110.

Other title-page scenes usually are surrounded by decorative frames and often contain narrative elements. The title page for the *Sermonum liber scientiae medicinae (VIII)* of NICOLO FALCUCCI, for instance, shows the author in the surroundings of his study; he is clothed – quite correctly – in the Florentine dress of a century earlier, which of course was familiar from illuminated manuscripts.[7] The whole title page is bordered by an architectural framework that is more modern in style than the picture showing the author and that contains portraits of six famous physicians of antiquity, drawn to resemble sculptured reliefs: Aesculapius is enthroned Christ-like in the pediment, and the other five are shown in a row across the base. In accordance with the motto, "The more one shows, the better

[7] For example, the hospital scene in Ms. Gaddianus 24, in the Biblioteca Laurenziana, fol. 247.

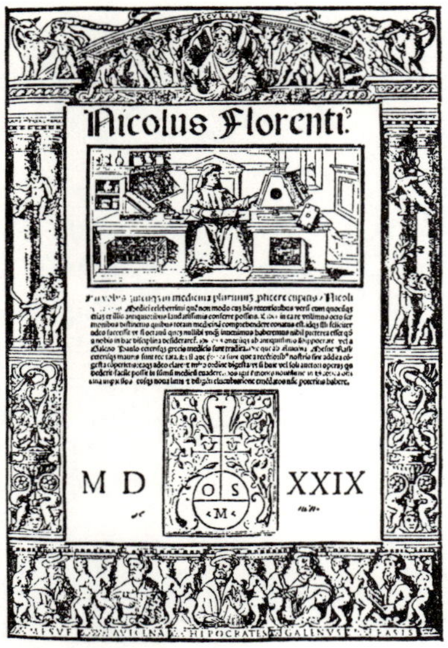

Fig. 303

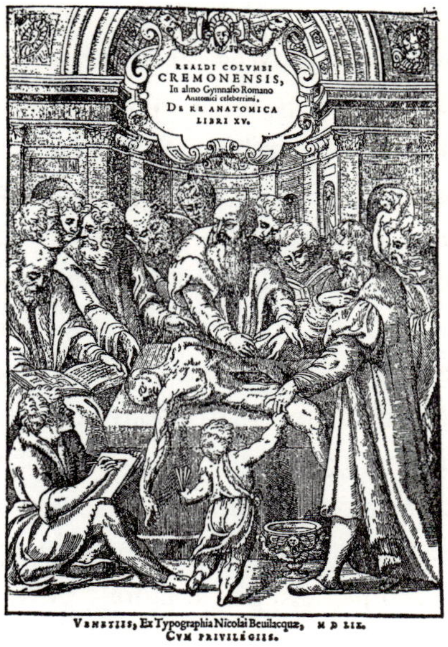

Fig. 304

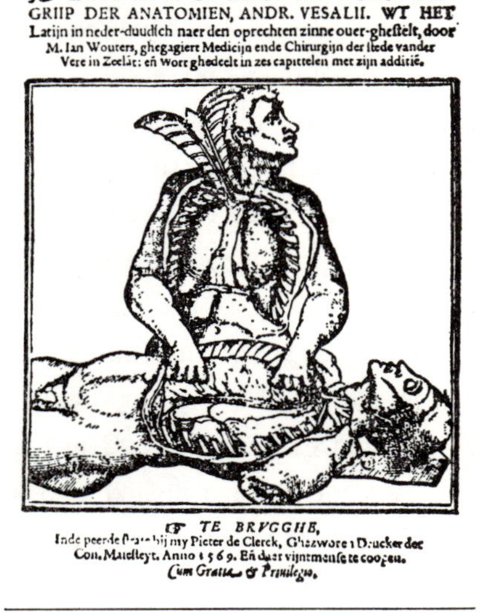

Fig. 305

Fig. 303 Title page for Nicolo Falcucci (Nicolus Florentinus), Sermonum liber scientiae medicinae, *Florence (off. Scotica), 1529.*

Fig. 304 Title page for Realdo Colombo, De re anatomica libri XV, *Venice, 1559. The design for this woodcut has been attributed to Paolo Veronese.*

Fig. 305 Title page for a Dutch edition of Vesalius's Epitome, *published by Jan Wouters, Bruges, 1569. The woodcut is a copy of a copperplate engraving from Valverde (fig. 202), which was in turn a combined copy of two figures from Vesalius (see p. 110).*

the chance of pleasing someone," the publishing house of SCOTUS also included its famous colophon.

A different type of 16th-century title page is the one whose design is dominated by a shield bearing the title of the book. The origin of this design can be traced back to examples such as the one reproduced in figure 295, where the text was so long that it demanded a graphic arrangement. A few years later (see figure 297), the originally unbordered text has been enclosed in a triangle, and two supporting figures have been added on the sides. It was not long before the triangle became a shield, and the two flanking figures began either to carry the shield or to point to the text inscribed on it. From Adam and Eve through Apollo and Aesculapius, Cosmos and Damian to Hippocrates and Galen, from skeletons to ecorchés, the kinds of flanking pairs utilized by illustrators of medical books were imaginatively diverse. Often when the title-shield device is combined with an architectural framework, the flanking figures appear as sculptures that are inserted into the architectural design: we can see this beginning to happen in the 1530 title page that is reproduced in figure 298, although the process is not complete until the last half of the century (see figures 307-312).

At this point in time, another variation on the title-shield motif makes its first appearance: instead of being shown as a sculptured plaque, the shield is sometimes transformed into a banner or a wall-hanging bearing the title of the book (fig. 307). Toward the end of the century, the wall-hanging in turn is transformed into a theatrical curtain, and the pointing figures are now shown as actors on a stage. (The idea of depicting a stage setting on the title page may have been derived from the illustrations that showed anatomical demonstrations taking place in a theater-like setting.)

In most late 16th-century title pages, however, the architectural theme remains dominant and does not give way to a theatrical scene. Whereas in the earlier title pages the human and mythological figures that are pictured in the architectural framework are relatively small, and the architectural setting itself relatively vast and complicated, the title pages of the latter part of the century emphasize the figures and reduce the architectural frame to a mere portico or a background for a statuary grouping. Both the figures and the setting tend to become more and more surrealistic as the century progress. The artist of the VALVERDE edition of 1586[8] (fig. 311) exercised his sense of humor in the figures that top his framework – a monkey and a pig (legitimate figures in anatomical illustration) pulling at the flayed skin of a satyr – and in the two flanking figures, the lower parts of whose bodies seem to have melted into architectural supports. When compared with the title page of the Rome edition of 1560 (see figure 230), the Baroque tendencies in the 1586 title page become apparent. The 1560 page, although more crowded with detail, shows a more tranquil scene: the architecture and the shield frame are flatter, and the monkey and the pig on the cornice are merely propped in heraldic positions against the bones on either side of the skull. The individual elements here are Baroque – the skeletons and the loose bones and skulls – but the design as a whole does not have the furious energy and macabre surrealism of the 1586 design.

A stylistically consistent development of the VALVERDE title page of 1586 can be found in another JUNTA title page, the one prepared for a 1611 edition of VIDIUS (fig. 312). Here, Death sits in the entablature with an apple and an hourglass in his hands; the two flanking figures have now become a man and a woman who are standing free in front of the pilasters, but who are represented as grisly anatomical preparations; and a pair of skeletons sit in front of the architecture in poses that became familiar in medical illustration after VESALIUS. Everything has become theatrical, a Baroque drama. This title-page framework can be compared with the somewhat similar framework used several decades earlier by the Basel etcher ABEL STIMMER for his portrait of FELIX PLATTER (fig. 245); STIMMER'S framework is typically Mannerist in conception and design.

The Italian Baroque influence did not reach northern France and the Netherlands until fairly late; up until the close of the 16th century, the title-page designs produced in Paris and Antwerp were frequently of an almost classical severity (figs. 308-310.)

One more type of title-page art remains to be mentioned briefly, the type that consists of a series of scenes arranged to form a rectangular frame around the title. This type, which was quite popular in the 16th century, was especially

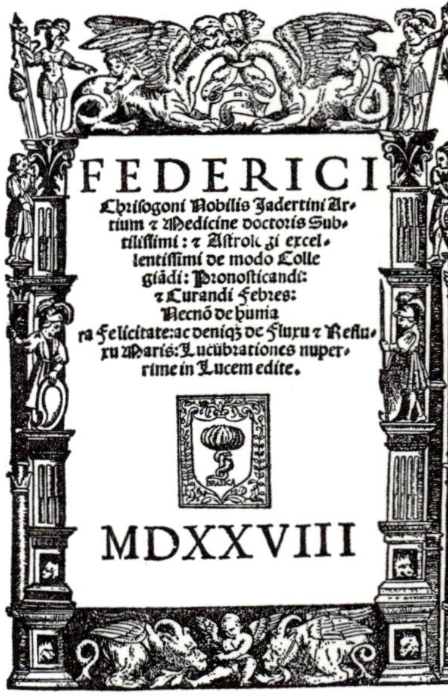
FEDERICI
Chrisogoni Nobilis Jadertini Artium & Medicine doctoris Subtilissimi: & Astrolo gi excellentissimi de modo Collegiādi: Pronosticandi: & Curandi Febres: Necnō de humana Felicitate: ac deniq3 de Fluxu & Refluxu Maris: Lucubrationes nuperrime in Lucem edite.
MDXXVIII

Fig. 306 Title page for F. Chrisogonus, De modo collegiandi, prognosticandi et curandi febres, *Venice (Joh. Ant. de Sabio), 1528.*

[8] WOLF-HEIDEGGER, GERHARD and ANNA MARIA CETTO: Die anatomische Sektion in bildlicher Darstellung, Basel, Karger, 1697. In No. 135/136, CETTO discusses the origins of the VALVERDE title-page engraving. However, she missed the fact that the plate for the Rome edition of 1560 was reworked and used again in the Venice edition of 1589 (CETTO No. 137).

Figures 307 to 312 Six title pages for 16th-century medical books, each designed with two flanking figures presenting the title.

Fig. 307 B. Pietragrassa, Politica medica, *Pavia, 1551.*

Fig. 308 G. Valverde, Anatomie oft levende beelden, *Antwerp (Plantin), 1568.*

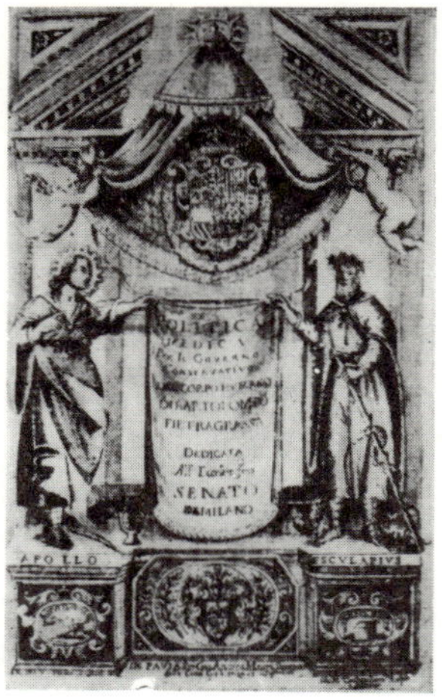

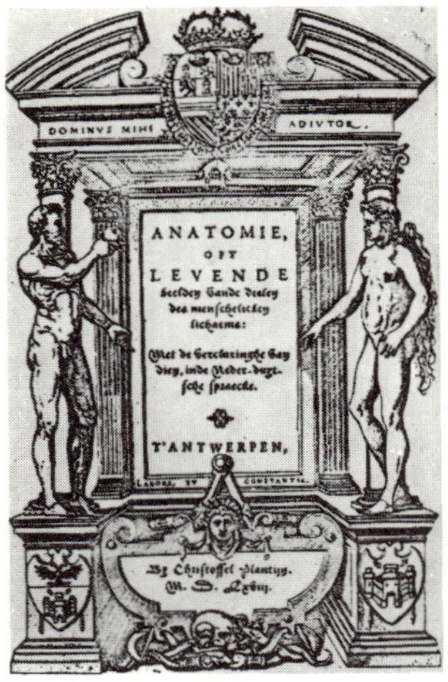

Fig. 309 P. Pena and M. de Lobel, Nova stirpium adversaria, *Antwerp (Plantin), 1576.*

Fig. 310 J. Guillemeau, Tables anatomiques, *Paris, 1586.*

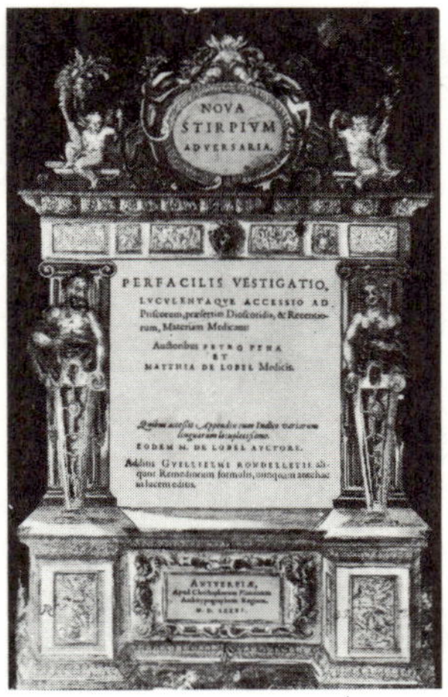

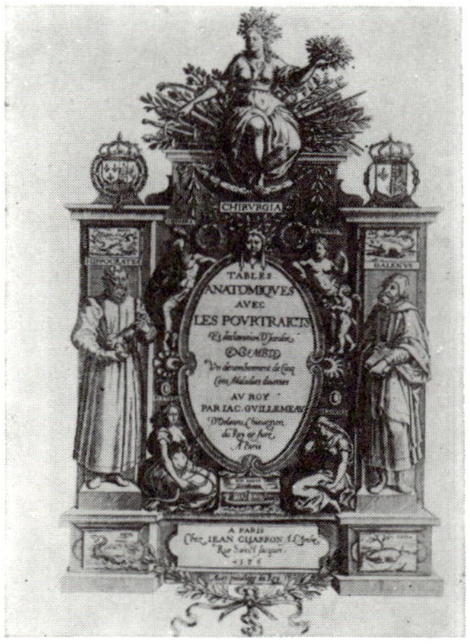

Fig. 311 G. Valverde, La anatomia del corpo umano, *Venice (Junta), 1586.*

Fig. 312 V. Vidius, De anatome corporis humani libri VII, *Venice (Junta), 1611.*

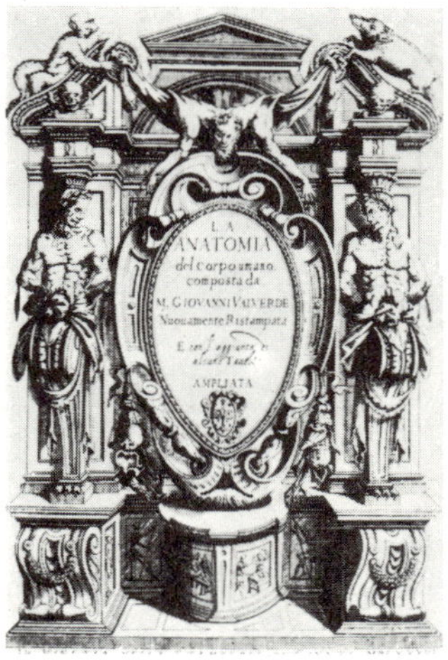

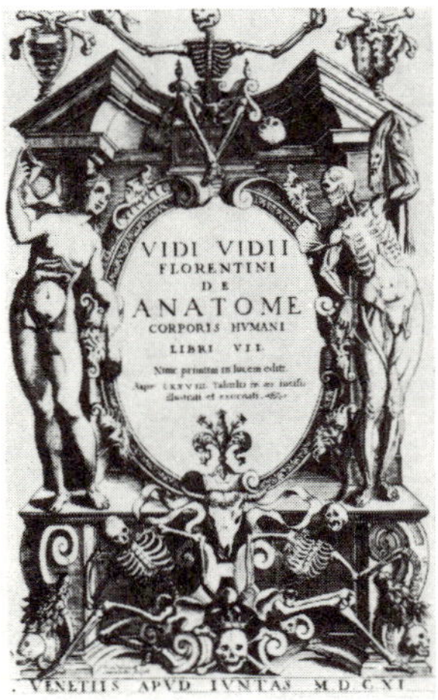

suitable for telling a story in pictures. For example, the pictures that frame the title of a medical anthology by ALESSANDRO BENEDETTI show scenes from the life of Aesculapius (fig. 313). German bookmakers developed a similar kind of frame; but the individual scenes in the German designs, instead of being narrative, tended to be decorative or symbolic (figs. 128, 314) – as if the German artists had imposed a regular rectangular design on the kinds of purely decorative or symbolic scenes that Italian artists had employed in fanciful architectural frameworks.

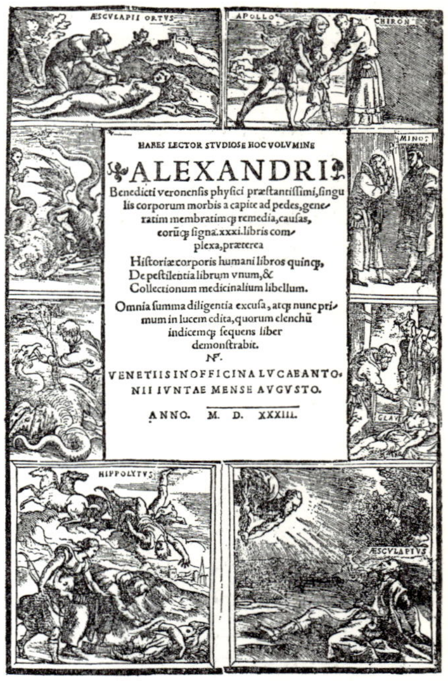

Fig. 313

Figures 313 and 314 Italian and German title pages with scenes arranged to form a rectangular frame around the title. Venice, 1533, and Strasbourg, 1529.

Fig. 314

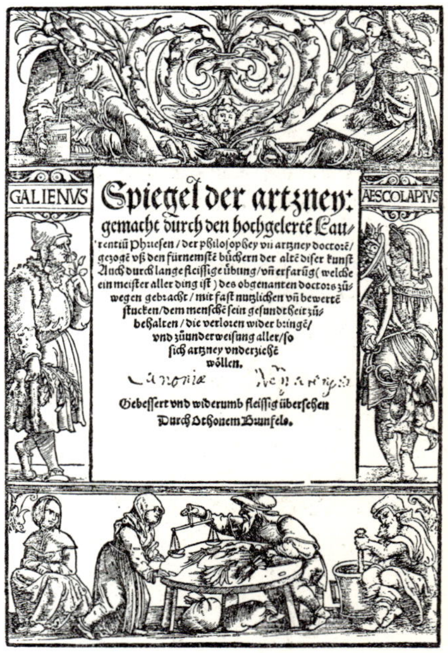

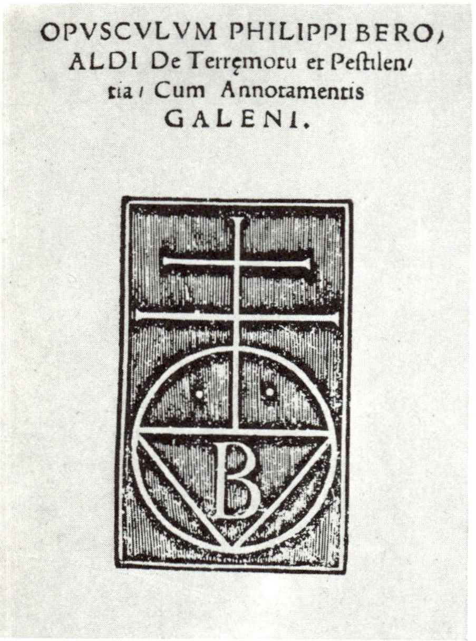

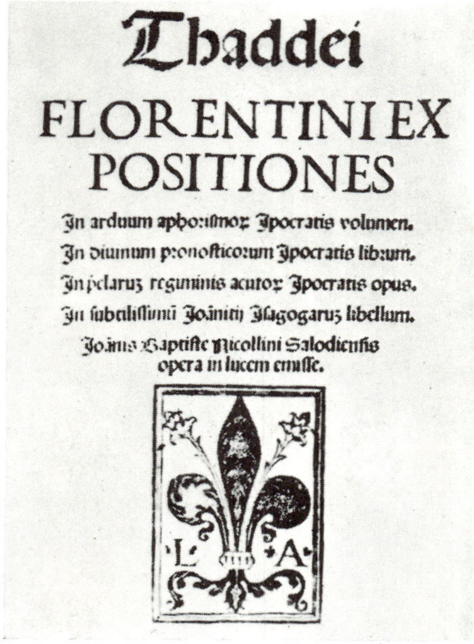

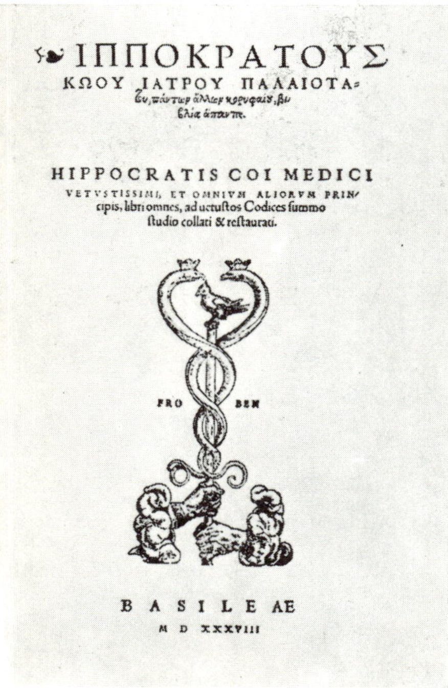

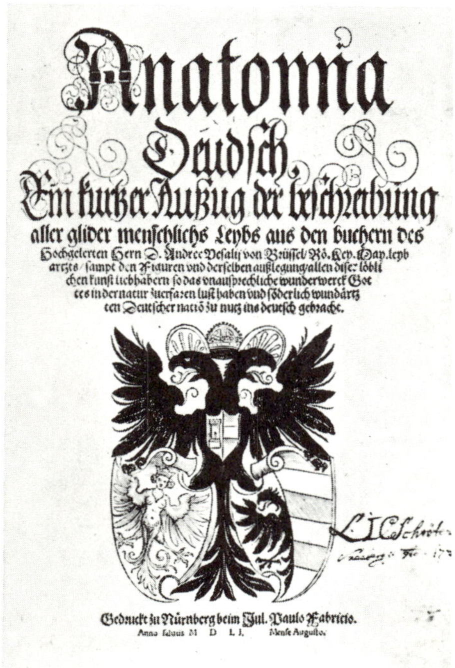

Figures 315 to 318 Four title pages on which the publisher's colophon is the dominant element; dating from 1505, 1527, 1538 and 1551.

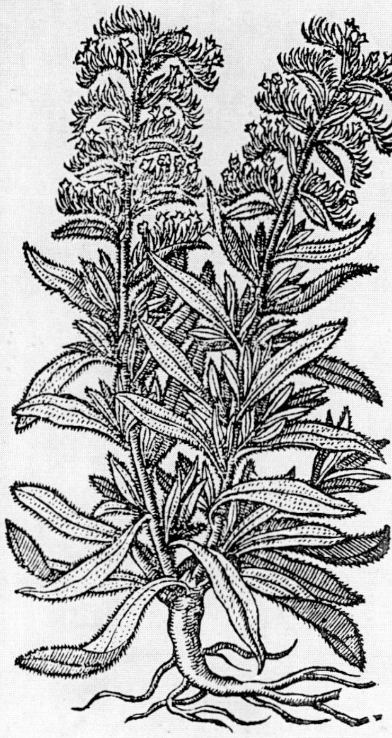

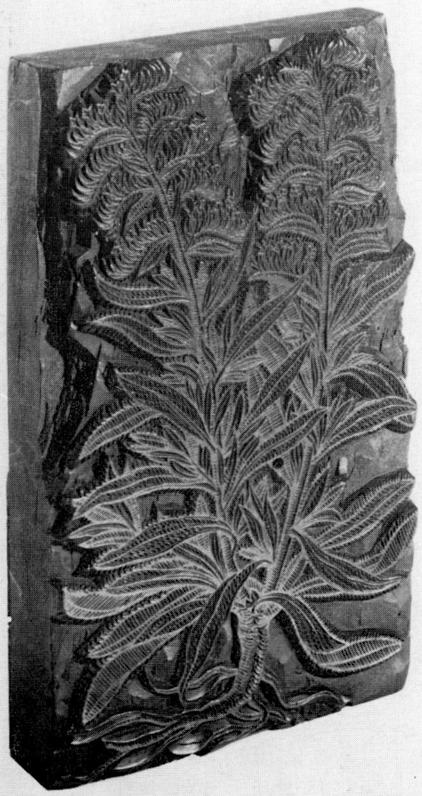

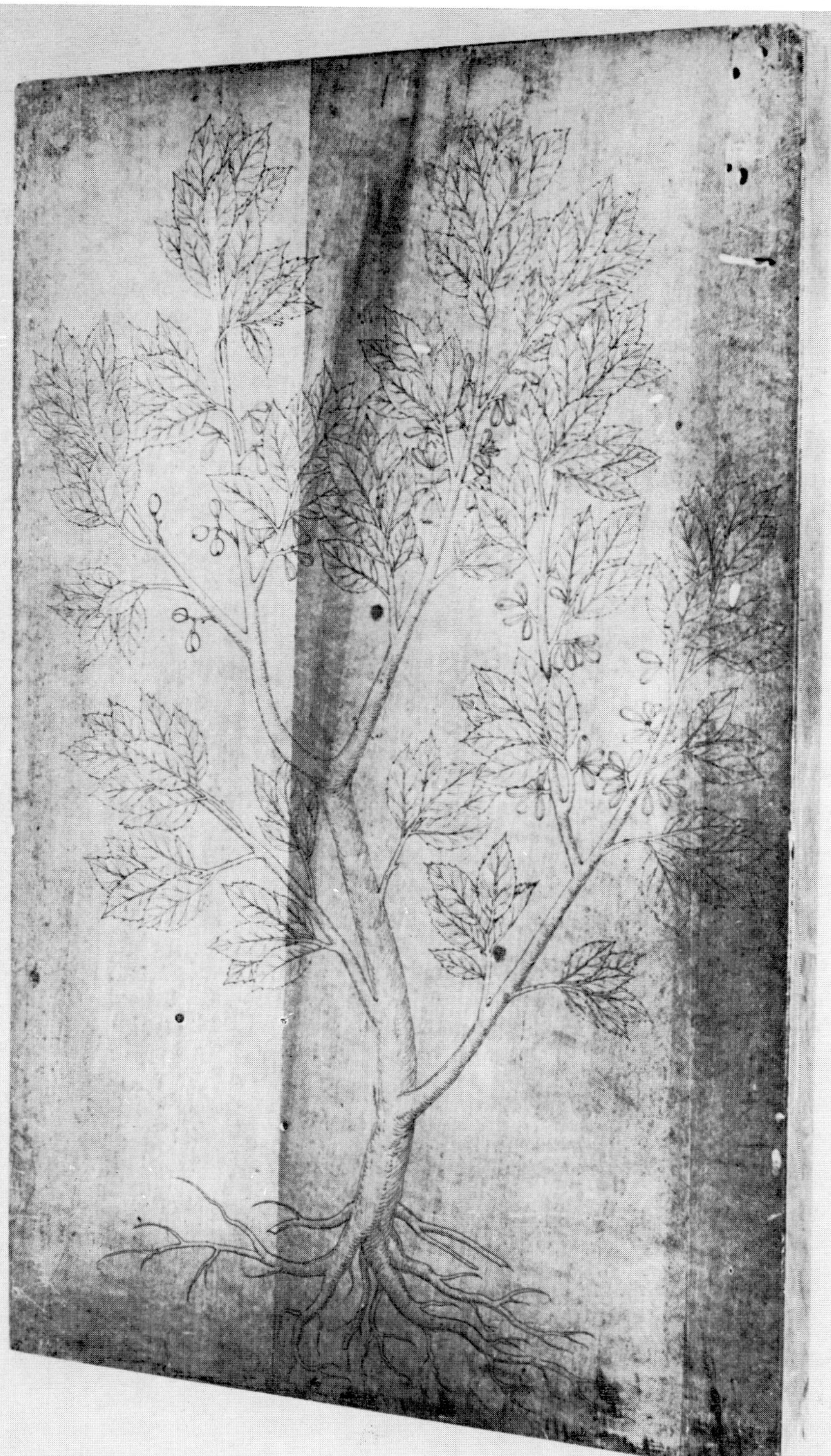

Plate XXXIa Above: A woodblock with a design for the unfinished illustration of a second edition of Fuchs's Historia stirpium. *With kind permission of the Botanisches Institut, Tübingen.*

Plate XXXI b and c Bottom left: a woodblock employed for the illustration of Matthias de Lobel's Plantarum seu stirpium Historia, *Antwerp (Plantin), 1576. Top left: The illustration printed from this woodblock. With kind permission of the Plantin-Moretus Museum, Antwerp.*

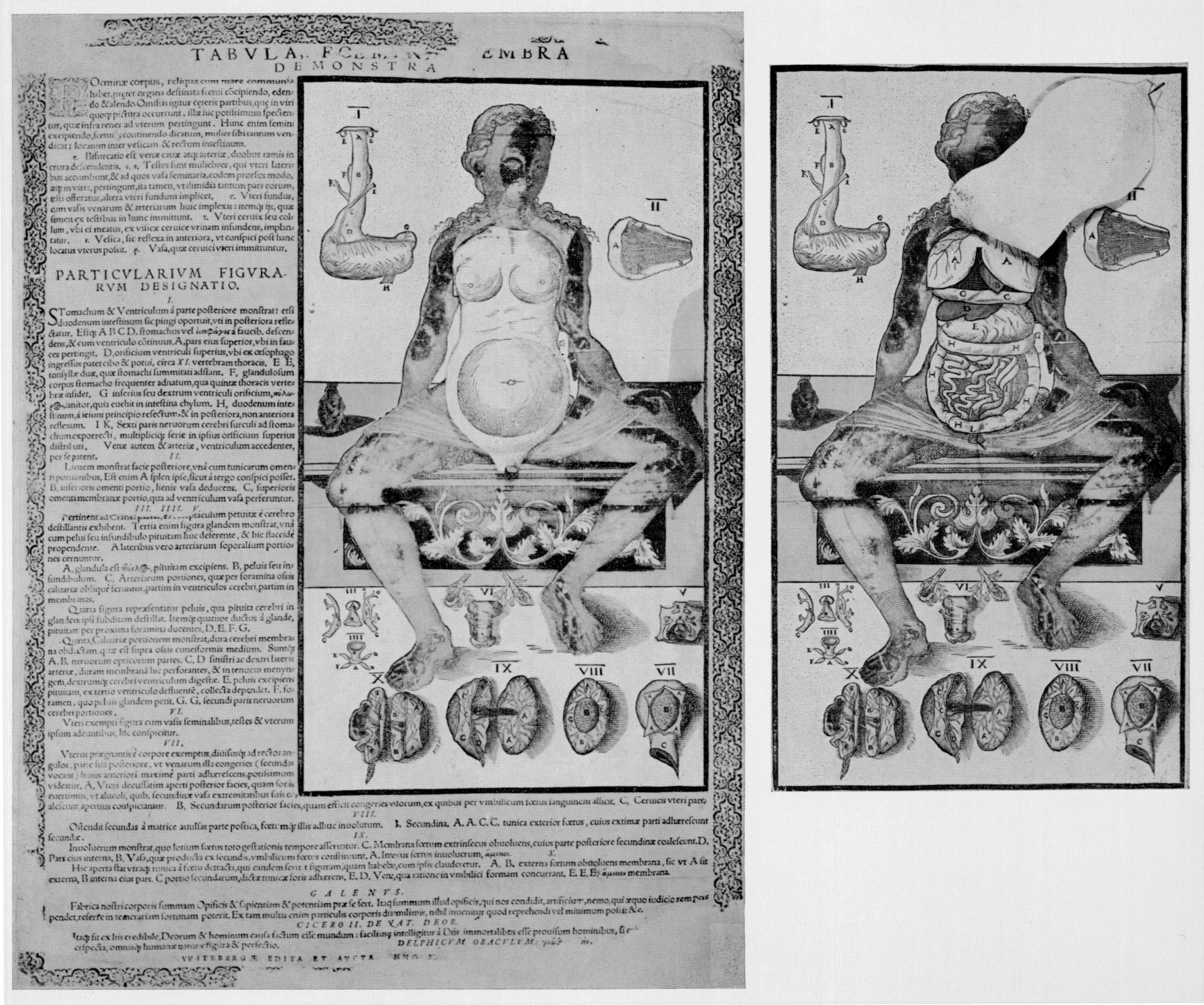

Plate XXXII German anatomical loose sheets with female viscera, Wittenberg (Simon Groneberg), 1589. With the exception of the two background figures, the design is virtually identical to the woodcut by Heinrich Vogtherr, Strasbourg, 1539. Our right hand illustration shows the viscera which are revealed upon folding back the anterior abdominal wall. With kind permission of the Print Department of the Germanisches Nationalmuseum, Nuremberg (H.B. 21847).

INDEX
AND
LIST OF SOURCES

Index

List of Sources

The following list gives the locations of manuscripts referred to in the text. After the name of the manuscript are the page numbers in the text where the manuscript is mentioned (the numbers given in parentheses are the plate numbers and figure numbers of illustrations reproduced from the manuscript).
The author and the publisher thank the libraries named for permission to reproduce the illustrations.

Basel, Stadt- und Universitätsbibliothek
Ms. D. II, 11 12 (II; 39)
Berlin, Deutsche Staatsbibliothek
Codex Hamilton 407 46
Bologna, Biblioteca Universitaria
Ms. 3632 29 (XII)
Brussels, Bibliothèque Royale
Ms. 3714 20 (V)
Cambridge, Trinity College
Ms. 1044 (0.1.20) 34
Chantilly, Musée Condé
Ms. 334 (ex 569) 41 (38)
Erlangen, Universitätsbibliothek
Ms. 2386/II 160 (XXX)
Florence, Biblioteca Laurenziana
Cod. Plut. LXXIII, 16 21
Cod. Plut. LXXIII, 41 16 (34)
Cod. Plut. LXXIV, 7 14, 15, 21, 22, 39, 143 (I, XXVIII, 16)
Ms. Gaddianus 24 166
Istanbul, Yeni Cami Bibliothek
Ms. 924 (52)
Leyden, Universiteitsbibliotheek
Ms. Voss. lat. 3 33, 53, 143 (XV)
Leipzig, Universitätsbibliothek
Ms. 1192 28 (XI)
Lindau, Stadtbibliothek
Stromayr ms. (XXIX)
London, British Museum
Ms. Egerton 2020 (XVIII a)
Ms. Harley 1585 32 (32)
Ms. Or. 2784 (XIX)
Ms. Sloane 1975 32 (III, XIII, XIV; 47)
Ms. Sloane 1977 33, 34 (XVI)
Prints & Engravings, Ms. 197.d.2 142
Milan, Biblioteca Trivulziana
Codex 836 (4)
Monte Cassino, Biblioteca Cassinensis
Codex 97 47
Munich, Bayerische Staatsbibliothek
Cod. lat. 161 (45)
Cod. lat. 13002 11 (5, 31)
Cod. lat. 13042 (40)
Cod. lat. 14300 (30)
Cod. lat. 17403 11
Nuremberg, Germanisches Nationalmuseum
H.B. 21847 (XXXII)
–, Stadtbibliothek
St. Med. 11 (XXIII b)
Oxford, Bodleian Library
Cod. Ashmolean 391 28
Cod. Ashmolean 399 12, 13 (43)
Cod. Ashmolean 789 (XI)
Ms. Rawlinson C 328 19, 20, 32 (VI)
Paris, Bibliothèque Nationale 15 (XXVIII)
Ms. français 2030 (37 a, b)
Ms. français 19994 43
Ms. lat. 7138 43
Ms. lat. 11229 (IX a, XI)
–, Bibliothèque Mazarine
Cod. 3599 42 (42)
Pisa, Biblioteca Universitaria
Cod. Roncioni 99 34, 59 (6, 7–9, 10, 14)
Rome, Biblioteca Casanatense
Ms. 1382 (A.II, 15) 19, 32, 33 (XV)
Stockholm, Kungliga Biblioteket
Ms. X 118 42 (XVII)
Tübingen, Universitätsbibliothek
Cod. arab. 91 (XVIII a)
M.d. 2 (VIII)
Vienna, Österreichische Nationalbibliothek
Juliana Anicia Codex (Cod. graec. I) 21, 45 (VI; 17, 18)
Cod. lat. 93 33, 143 (VII, XV)
Cod. S. n. 2641 (XVIII b)
Windsor Castle, The Royal Library
Leonardo sketchbook 67–79 (XX, XXI; 90–115)
Wolfenbüttel, Herzog-August-Bibliothek
Ms. 18, 2 28 (X)